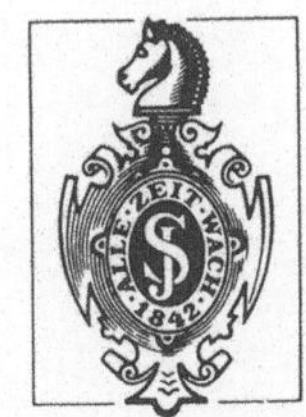
ALLEZEIT·NACH
S
·1842·

E. Gramer   A. Kampik (Hrsg.)

Pharmakotherapie am Auge

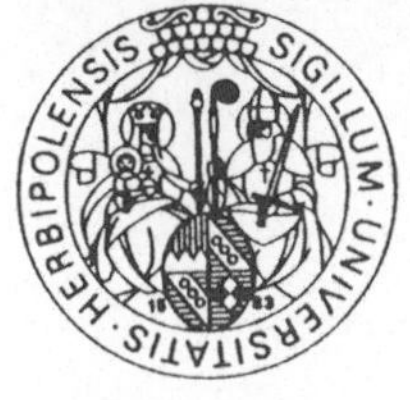

Internationales Symposium
der Universitätsaugenklinik Würzburg
10. November 1990

Mit 79 Abbildungen und 45 Tabellen

Springer-Verlag

Berlin Heidelberg New York
London Paris Tokyo
Hong Kong Barcelona
Budapest

Prof. Dr. med. Dr. jur. Eugen Gramer
Prof. Dr. med. Anselm Kampik
Universitätsaugenklinik, Josef-Schneider-Straße 11
W-8700 Würzburg, BRD

Die Deutsche Bibliothek – CIP-Einheitsaufnahme

Pharmakotherapie am Auge / E. Gramer, A. Kampik (Hrsg.)
Berlin; Heidelberg; New York; London; Paris; Tokyo; Hong Kong;
Barcelona; Budapest: Springer, 1992
ISBN-13: 978-3-540-55496-7   e-ISBN-13: 978-3-642-77532-1
DOI: 10.1007/ 978-3-642-77532-1

Die Wiedergabe von Gebrauchsnamen, Handelsnamen, Warenbezeichnungen usw. in diesem Werk berechtigt auch ohne besondere Kennzeichnung nicht zu der Annahme, daß solche Namen im Sinne der Warenzeichen- und Markenschutz-Gesetzgebung als frei zu betrachten wären und daher von jedermann benutzt werden dürfen.

Produkthaftung: Für Angaben über Dosierungsanweisungen und Applikationsformen kann vom Verlag keine Gewähr übernommen werden. Derartige Angaben müssen vom jeweiligen Anwender im Einzelfall anhand anderer Literaturstellen auf ihre Richtigkeit überprüft werden.

Satz: Mitterweger Werksatz GmbH, Plankstadt

25/3145-5 4 3 2 1 0 – Gedruckt auf säurefreiem Papier

Grußwort der Deutschen Ophthalmologischen Gesellschaft

H. E. Völcker

Zunächst danke ich Ihnen, lieber Herr Kampik, lieber Herr Gramer, für die Einladung zu dem von Ihnen initiierten und organisierten Internationalen Symposium der Universitätsaugenklinik Würzburg.

Es ist mir eine Ehre und Freude, Ihnen und allen Teilnehmern, insbesondere den Referenten, speziell denen aus Japan und den USA sowie aus den benachbarten europäischen Ländern Portugal, den Niederlanden, die Grüße der Deutschen Ophthalmologischen Gesellschaft in meiner Eigenschaft als Sekretär zu überbringen.

Internationalität und Weltoffenheit sind mehr denn je die Forderungen an eine moderne Universität, die den wissenschaftlichen Herausforderungen gerecht werden will.

Diese erfüllen Sie, Herr Kampik und Herr Gramer, in vorbildlicher Weise. Es ist Ihnen gelungen, weltweit anerkannte und bekannte Referenten zu gewinnen, die die komplexen Probleme der Therapie des Glaukoms und des trockenen Auges sowie die Probleme der antibiotischen wie antiproliferativen Therapie erörtern und diskutieren werden. Ich halte es für besonders verdienstvoll, daß Sie dieses Symposium therapeutischen Fragestellungen widmen, stellt doch die Therapie die Krönung aller unserer augenärztlichen Bemühungen dar.

Im Namen der Deutschen Ophthalmologischen Gesellschaft wünsche ich Ihnen und uns allen einen erfolgreichen Verlauf dieses wissenschaftlichen Symposiums mit zahlreichen Anregungen für unsere weiteren wissenschaftlichen und praktischen Tätigkeiten.

Da ich selbst in Würzburg studiert habe, kann ich voller Überzeugung sagen, daß auch das einmalige Ambiente dieser schönen Stadt Gelegenheit geben wird zu freundschaftlichen Begegnungen und der verdienten Entspannung.

Korrespondenzadresse
Professor Dr. med. H. E. Völcker
Direktor der Universitätsaugenklinik Heidelberg
Im Neuenheimer Feld 400, D-6900 Heidelberg

Vorwort

Die medikamentöse Therapie am Auge ist ein tägliches Problem in Praxis und Klinik. Mit diesem Symposium sollen einige Bereiche der Pharmakotherapie am Auge beleuchtet werden:

– Glaukom
– Trockenes Auge
– Antibiotikatherapie
– Antiproliferative Therapie bei proliferativen Vitreoretinopathien

Bei der Therapie des Glaukoms soll erörtert werden, inwieweit morphologische, diagnostische und klinische Aspekte die medikamentöse Therapie rationell beeinflußt und weiterentwickelt haben.

Für die Behandlung des trockenen Auges sollen diagnostische Möglichkeiten und neuere Therapiekonzepte dargestellt werden.

Schließlich werden aktuelle Probleme der Infektionsprophylaxe und Antibiotikatherapie in unterschiedlichen klinischen Situationen dargestellt.

Als Ausblick auf derzeitige Forschungsaspekte und therapeutische Möglichkeiten soll der jetzige Stand der intraokularen Applikation von Medikamenten sowie die Möglichkeit der Beeinflussung von proliferativen Vitreoretinopathien durch Medikamente beleuchtet werden.

Für die Darstellung dieser Probleme ist es uns gelungen, für das Internationale Symposium der Universitätsaugenklinik Würzburg „Pharmakotherapie am Auge" Experten unterschiedlicher Länder zu gewinnen. Der Fa. Alcon-Thilo, Pharma· GmbH, Freiburg, danken wir für die organisatorische und finanzielle Unterstützung dieses Symposiums und des Rahmenprogrammes.

Durch diese großzügige Unterstützung steht auch eine Simultanübersetzung zur Verfügung, um über Sprachbarrieren hinweg
eine Diskussion zu ermöglichen.

Der Rahmen des Symposiums auf der Festung Marienberg in
Würzburg wird sicherlich geeignet sein, die wissenschaftlichen
Inhalte auch im persönlichen Gespräch weiter diskutieren zu
können.

Würzburg, im November 1990   *E. Gramer*
                                                    A. Kampik

Inhaltsverzeichnis

Cornea

Autorenverzeichnis

Adachi, M., M.D.
Department of Ophthalmology, School of Medicine,
University of Tokyo, 7-3-1 Hongo, Bunkyo-ku, Tokyo 113,
Japan

Assil, K., M.D.
University of California, UCSD Eye Center, Department of
Ophthalmology, 9500 Gilman Drive, La Jolla, San Diego,
California 92093-0618, USA

Bacon, D. R., M.D.
Devers Eye Institute/Good Samaritan Hospital and Medical
Center, 1040 N.W. 22nd Ave. N 320, Portland, Oregon 97210,
USA

Baerveldt, G., M.D.
University of Southern California, School of Medicine,
Department of Ophthalmology, Glaucoma Services, Estelle
Doheny Eye Institute, 1355 San Pablo Street, Ste. 406E,
Los Angeles. CA 90033/USA

Baker, A. S., M.D.
Dana Center for Preventive Ophthalmology, Wilmer Institute,
Baltimore, MD 21265, USA

Bialasiewicz, A. A., Priv.-Doz. Dr. med.
Universitätsaugenklinik Münster, Domagkstraße 15,
D-4400 Münster

Cunha, L., M.D.
Departamento de Oftalmologia, Hospital Gracia de Orta,
Pragal-Almada, P-1600 Lisboa, Portugal

Diestelhorst, M., Dr. med.
Universitätsaugenklinik Köln, Joseph-Stelzmann-Str. 9,
D-5000 Köln 41

Freeman, W. R., M.D., Associate Professor
University of California, UCSD Eye Center, Department of
Ophthalmology, 9500 Gilman Drive, La Jolla, San Diego,
California 92093-0618, USA

Funk, R. H. W., Professor Dr. med.
Anatomisches Institut der Universität Erlangen–Nürnberg,
Krankenhausstr. 9, D-8520 Erlangen

Gariano, R., M.D., Ph.D.
University of California, UCSD Eye Center, Department of
Ophthalmology, 9500 Gilman Drive, La Jolla, San Diego,
California 92093-0618, USA

Gramer, E., Professor Dr. med. Dr. jur.
Universitätsaugenklinik Würzburg, Josef-Schneider-Str. 11,
D-8700 Würzburg

Heidenkummer, H.-P., Dr. med.
Universitätsaugenklinik Würzburg, Josef-Schneider-Str. 11,
D-8700 Würzburg

Heuer, D. K., M.D.
University of Southern California, School of Medicine,
Department of Ophthalmology, Glaucoma Services, Estelle
Doheny Eye Institute, 1355 San Pablo Street, Ste. 406E,
Los Angeles. CA 90033/USA

Hibberd, P. L., M.D. Ph.D.
Dana Center for Preventive Ophthalmology, Wilmer Institute,
Baltimore, MD 21265, USA

Hill, R. A., M.D.
University of California Irvine, Medical Plaza, Department of
Ophthalmology, Irvine, CA 92717/USA

Inoue, T., M.D.
Department of Ophthalmology, Gifu University School
of Medicine, Tsukasa – Machi 40, Gifu, 500 Japan

Iwata, K., M.D., Professor and Chairman
Department of Ophthalmology, Niigata University,
School of Medicine, 1 Asahimachi, Niigata-Shi, 951 Japan

Kampik, A., Professor Dr. med.
Direktor der Universitätsaugenklinik Würzburg,
Josef-Schneider-Str. 11, D-8700 Würzburg

Kenyon, K. R., M.D., FACS, Professor
Cornea Consultant, 100 Charles River Plaza, Boston,
MA 02114/USA

Kitazawa, Y., M.D., Professor and Chairman
Department of Ophthalmology, Gifu University School
of Medicine, Tsukasa – Machi 40, Gifu, 500 Japan

Klaassen-Broekema, N., M.D.
University Hospital Utrecht, Department of Ophthalmology,
P.O. Box 85500, NL-3508 GA Utrecht, Niederlande

Klauß, V., Professor Dr. med.
Universitätsaugenklinik München, Mathildenstr. 8,
D-8000 München 2

Knaut-Speath, M.
Universitätsaugenklinik Würzburg, Josef Schneider-Str. 11,
D-8700 Würzburg

Koseki, N., M.D.
Department of Ophthalmology, School of Medicine,
University of Tokyo, 7-3-1 Hongo, Bunkyo-ku, Tokyo 113,
Japan

Krieglstein, G. K., Professor Dr. med.
Direktor der Universitätsaugenklinik Köln,
Joseph-Stelzmann-Straße 9, D-5000 Köln 41

Lee, M., Ph. D.
University of Southern California, School of Medicine,
Department of Ophthalmology, Glaucoma Services, Estelle
Doheny Eye Institute, 1355 San Pablo Street, Ste. 406E,
Los Angeles. CA 90033/USA

Listhaus A., M.D.
University of California, UCSD Eye Center, Department of
Ophthalmology, 9500 Gilman Drive, La Jolla, San Diego,
California 92093-0618, USA

Lütjen-Drecoll, E., Professor Dr. med.
Vorstand des Anatomischen Institutes, Lehrstuhl II,
Universität Erlangen–Nürnberg, Krankenhausstr. 9,
D-8520 Erlangen

Maier, H.
Universitätsaugenklinik Würzburg, Josef-Schneider-Straße 11,
D-8700 Würzburg

Marquardt, R., Professor Dr. med.
Direktor der Universitätsaugenklinik Ulm, Prittwitzstr. 43,
D-7900 Ulm

Martone, J. F., M.D.
University of Southern California, School of Medicine,
Department of Ophthalmology, Glaucoma Services, Estelle
Doheny Eye Institute, 1355 San Pablo Street, Ste. 406E,
Los Angeles. CA 90033/USA

Minckler, D. S., M.D., Professor and Director
University of Southern California, School of Medicine,
Department of Ophthalmology, Glaucoma Services, Estelle
Doheny Eye Institute, 1355 San Pablo Street, Ste. 406E,
Los Angeles. CA 90033/USA

Munguia, D.
University of California, UCSD Eye Center, Department of
Ophthalmology, 9500 Gilman Drive, La Jolla, San Diego,
California 92093-0618, USA

Schein, O. D., M.D.
Dana Center for Preventive Ophthalmology, Wilmer Institute,
Baltimore, MD 21265, USA

Schneiderman, T., M.D.
University of California, UCSD Eye Center, Department of
Ophthalmology, 9500 Gilman Drive, La Jolla, San Diego,
California 92093-0618, USA

Siebert, M., Dr. med.
Universitätsaugenklinik, Würzburg, Josef-Schneider-Straße 11,
D-8700 Würzburg

Shiose, Y., M.D., Professor, Director
Division of Ophthalmology, Aichi Prefectural Center of
Health Care, 3-2-1 San-no-maru, Naka-ku, Nagoya, Japan

Shirato, S., M.D., Assistant Professor
Department of Ophthalmology, School of Medicine,
University of Tokyo, 7-3-1 Hongo, Bunkyo-ku, Tokyo 113,
Japan

Soudijn, W., Ph.D., Professor of Medical Chemistry
Gorlaeus Laboratories, Leiden University, P.O. Box 9502,
N-2300 RA Leiden, Niederlande

Starck, T., M.D.
Dana Center for Preventive Ophthalmology, Wilmer Institute,
Baltimore, MD 21265, USA

Sugiyama, K., M.D.
Department of Ophthalmology, Gifu University School
of Medicine, Tsukasa – Machi 40, Gifu, 500 Japan

Svendsen, P., B.S.
University of California, UCSD Eye Center, Department of
Ophthalmology, 9500 Gilman Drive, La Jolla, San Diego,
California 92093-0618, USA

Taniguchi, T., M.D.
Department of Ophthalmology, Gifu University School
of Medicine, Tsukasa – Machi 40, Gifu, 500 Japan

van Bijsterveld, O. P., M.D., Ph.D.
Department of Ophthalmology, University Eye Hospital
Utrecht, P.O. Box 85500, NL-3508 G.A.-Utrecht, Niederlande

van Buskirk, E. M., M.D., Professor and Chairman
Devers Eye Institute/Good Samaritan Hospital and Medical
Center, 1040 N.W. 22nd Ave, N 320, Portland, Oregon 97210,
USA

Völcker, H. E., Professor Dr. med.
Direktor der Universitätsaugenklinik Heidelberg,
Im Neuenheimer Feld 400, D-6900 Heidelberg

Wiedemann, P., Professor Dr. med.
Universitätsaugenklinik Köln, Josef-Stelzmannstr. 9,
D-5000 Köln 41

Wiley, C. A., M.D., Ph.D.
University of California, UCSD Eye Center, Department of
Ophthalmology, 9500 Gilman Drive, La Jolla, San Diego,
California 92093-0618, USA

Yamagami, J., M.D.
Department of Ophthalmology, School of Medicine,
University of Tokyo, 7-3-1 Hongo, Bunkyo-ku, Tokyo 113,
Japan

Glaukom

Low-Tension Glaucoma – Prevalence and Background Factors

Y. Shiose

Introduction

Low-tension glaucoma (LTG) is defined as the condition consisted of characteristic glaucomatous disc and visual field defects, an open angle and intraocular pressure (IOP) within the statistically normal range.

Reappraisal of earlier epidemiologic studies (Hollows and Graham, 1966; Leibowitz et al., 1980; Armaly, 1980; Bengtsson, 1981) has recently highlighted that LTG is not an unusual condition as it has been thought, but prevails commonly as primary open angle glaucoma (POAG) (Leske, 1983; Sommer, 1989; Sponsel, 1989). Shiose et al. (1981) conducted a mass screening of glaucoma by way of tonometry and assessment of fundus photographs on subjects who underwent automated multiphasic health testing services and found that a prevalence of LTG was almost equal to that of POAG in the population. This becomes a matter of grave concern, since it raised a fundamental question as to the causal relationship between IOP and glaucomatous change in the disc and visual field.

During 1988 and 89, we conducted a population-based, multicenter study of glaucoma survey with the technique employed in the previous study (Shiose et al., 1981). This project was prosecuted with collaboration of glaucoma experts in seven districts across Japan under the auspices of Japan Ophthalmologist's Association (Shiose, 1990a; Shiose et al., 1990).

In this text epidemiologic aspects of LTG in Japan will be presented and secondly, possible genesis and background factors will also be discussed.

Epidemiology of LTG

Study Design

Defined Population. This screening project is intended to investigate the prevalence of various types of glaucoma in seven districts across Japan from lattitude of 33° to 44° north (Hokkaido, Iwate, Yamanashi, Aichi, Gifu, Hyogo and Kumamoto). During two-year period from 1988 through 1989, we could examine a total of 8,126 persons among the target population of 16,078 residents above 40 years (participation rate; 50.54%).

Gramer/Kampık (Hrsg.) Pharmakotherapie am Auge
© Springer-Verlag Berlin Heidelberg 1992

About 50% of nonparticipants was also investigated by way of random sampling (785 persons) to compare the background (age and professional constitution, subjective symptoms and family history of glaucoma), there was no statistical difference between these factors between participants and nonparticipants.

Method for Screening. An overall control center located at Nagoya standardizes methodology and planning for all districts. The center was wholly responsible for establishing diagnostic criteria and detailed screening procedures.

The screening used in the survey consisted of two stages; namely the first stage included a questionnaire, autorefractometry, visual acuity testing, slit-lamp examination, gonioscopy, tonometry, and fundus photography. Automatic visual field test was conducted as the second stage, only for those with suspected glaucoma either by tonometry (Goldmann's pressure $\geqq 21$ mmHg) or by disc assessment of fundus photographs. The most characteristic feature in this screening is the assessment of fundus pictures taken by non-mydriatic camera. The use of non-mydriatic camera greatly facilitated fundus photography to shorten time and avoided possible hazzard caused by mydriatics. This camera enabled to take amazingly beautiful pictures even in the elderly, unless otherwise the eye with hazy media or extremely miotic pupil.

All of the pictures taken at each district were immediately delivered to the center at Nagoya, and assessed exclusively by the author. Assessment of the fundus photograph was carried out on an enlarged screen image by a standardized manner. Major features noted were both disc signs; abnormality in pallor and cupping of the disc, and retinal signs, i.e. retinal nerve fiber layer defect (RNFLD) and splinter hemorrhage at the disc margin. Disc assessment was performed in such a way that the upper and lower sectors of the rim were specifically inspected applying the "Quantitative Disc Pattern" based on disc topography (Shiose, 1979; Shiose, 1981). All eyes with pathologic changes in the disc were drawn on the chart specifying possible locations of visual field loss and sent back to each district by tele-fax.

Visual field test was conducted on Humphrey's automatic perimeter, using Armaly's central 30° three zone strategy. The method used for the assessment of field defect is designed to determine whether or not the location of the field defect corresponds with that predicted by disc evaluation. These defects were categorized as paracentral scotoma, nasal step, arcuate scotoma including Bjerrum scotoma, and nasal depression. Observations in agreement with the disc findings were regarded as glaucomatous. Nonspecific type of defect or unconvincing results were reexamined employing some other testing strategies.

Diagnostic Criteria. Table 1 outlines the basic criteria for an automated diagnosis processed on a computer. This appeared to be most reliable and efficient method of standardizing diagnosis. After the completion of the

Table 1. Criteria for automated diagnosis. POAG primary open-angle glaucoma; LTG low-tension glaucoma; PACG primary angle-closure glaucoma; SG secondary glaucoma; OH ocular hypertension

Diagnosis	IOP[a]	Disc	Field	Angle[b]	Slit-lamp[c]
POAG	+	+±	+	−	−
LTG	−	+±	+	−	−
PAOG	+	+−	+−	+	−
SG	+	+−	+−	+−	+
OH	+	−	−	−	+

[a] IOP(+): applanation pressure $\geq$ 21 mmHg.
[b] Angle(+): Becker-Shaffer's Grade 0–1.
[c] Slit-lamp(+): inflammatory sign, rubeosis, trauma etc.

screening, a summarized printout table for all eyes was made including automated and physician's diagnoses, with the data of IOP, disc, visual field, slit-lamp exams and the history of glaucoma treatment. In case that there was any inconsistensy between automated and physician's diagnoses, all findings were thoroughly rechecked to finalize diagnosis.

Prevalence of LTG

Prevalence at the Time of Screening. Figure 1 shows the prevalence of glaucoma and ocular hypertension (OH) screened on 8,126 persons over 40 years. There is extremely high prevalence of LTG and very low prevalence of OH compared with Western populations (7–10%) (Hollows and Graham, 1966; Leibowitz et al., 1980).

Prevalence by age in different types of glaucoma and OH is shown in Fig. 2. Noteworthy is a sharp increase of LTG with age, while OH tends to decrease with age as opposed to the finding in Westerners.

Corrected Estimate with the Follow-up Study. Among 119 cases of LTG diagnosed at 1988 Survey, 94 patients were able to follow for one year. The result indicated that 73 patients (77.7%) were confirmed to be LTG, and 11 cases (11.7%) changed diagnosis of POAG. Five cases (5.3%) showed

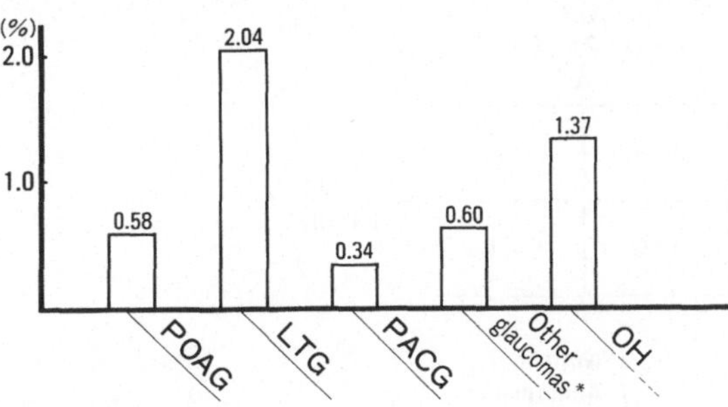

Fig. 1. Prevalence of glaucoma and ocular hypertension at the time of screening. Total: 8,126 persons over 40 years. *Secondary glaucoma, capsular glaucoma, congenital glaucoma, developmental glaucoma, absolute glaucoma etc.

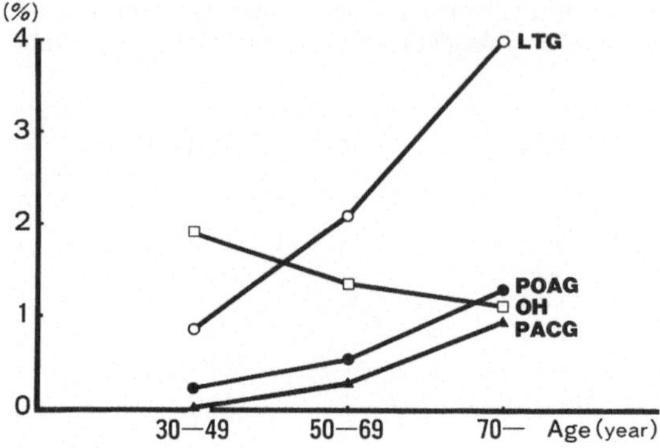

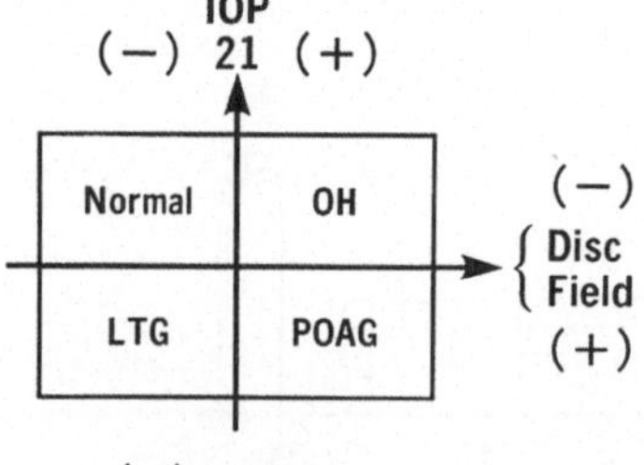

Fig. 2. Prevalence of glaucoma and ocular hypertension by age at the time of screening. Total: 8,924 persons over 30 years

some inflammatory sign to be categorized as secondary glaucoma, and the rest of cases (5.3%) were not considered from glaucomatous origin. On the basis of these findings estimated prevalence of LTG in final diagnosis would be 1.58%. Though original data revealed POAG/LTG ratio to be 1/3, it would finally be settled around 1/2 among Japanese population.

Background Factors that Cause High Prevalence of LTG

Figure 3 outlines diagnostic criteria of open-angle glaucoma and associated conditions. A vertical line indicates the cut-off level of IOP (21 mmHg) that separates Normal from OH, and LTG from POAG. When one is dealing with the population with relatively low IOP, like Japanese, cut-off of 21 mmHg is too high and the line should be moved toward right. Similarly, the horizontal line indicates both disc and visual field abnormalities that separates Normal from LTG, and OH from POAG. Therefore, in case that sufficiently sensitive methods are employed for the assessment of disc and visual field as in this study, the line should be shifted upwardly which, in turn, results prevalences of LTG and POAG higher. Shifts of the two lines as indicated, prevalence of LTG becomes very high on one hand, that of OH becomes much less on the other.

Fig. 3. Diagnostic concept of open angle glaucoma and associated conditions

Figure 4 illustrates a frequency distribution of IOP measured on all subjects who underwent the first year's Survey (1988). The rate of occurrence in visual field defect was plotted on each range of IOP. There is a beautiful relationship between IOP and field defect at the range above 15 mmHg, and this becomes especially remarkable above 20 mmHg. The most important observation, however, is a presence of visual field defect of approx. 1.2% of corresponding population below 15 mmHg, even at the lowest end of the pressure.

Though the relative risk to develop visual field loss would be 5 to 10 times higher in the pressure level above 21 mmHg than the level below, there is only 2% of the total population above 21 mmHg. Accordingly, estimated number of LTG patients becomes much higher than that of POAG.

Possible Genesis and Background of LTG

Low tension glaucoma is not a single clinical entity, but appears to be consisted of diseases with different mechanisms. Almost constant rate in occurrence of visual field defect below 15 mmHg strongly suggests that there is some other factor than IOP is playing an important role for the generation of LTG (see Fig. 4). Figure 5 is a hypothetical schema showing the underlying mechanism of LTG based on the result presented in Fig. 4. Pathogenically, LTG can be classified in Groups 1 and 2 (Levene, 1980). Group 1 LTG is categorized in POAG with low normative pressure and therefore, a pressure reduction may effectively stop further progression of visual field defect. It is most likely that the pressure range of Group 1 LTG would be from 15 to 21 mmHg as shown in the figure.

Group 2 LTG, on the other hand, is thought to be pressure-indifferent, and possibly be caused by vascular insufficiency associated with aging. Eyes with maximum IOP below 15 mmHg should be fallen in this category, however, it is quite probable that the same mechanism is being operated at any level of pressure as shown in the schema. This implies that a pressure-indifferent mechanism cannot be ruled out even in high-tension side above 21 mmHg as well as low-tension side.

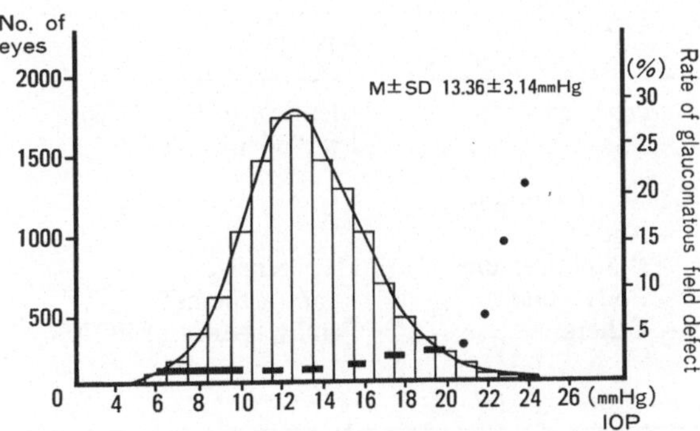

Fig. 4. Rate in occurrence of visual field defect at each range of IOP measured on 12,952 eyes

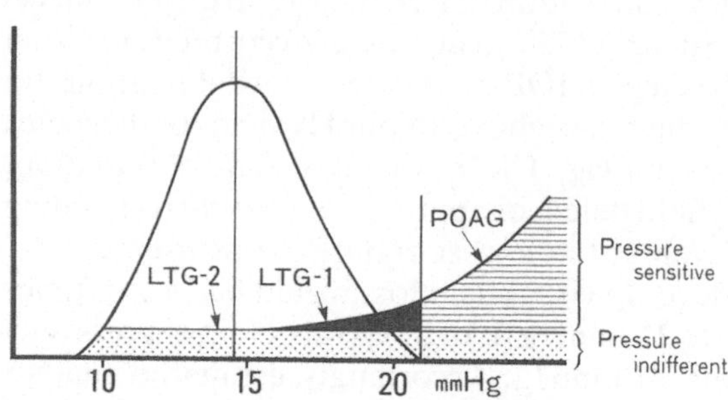

Fig. 5. The schema illustrating possible pathogenic mechanisms consisted of pressure-sensitive and pressure-indifferent components. A pressure-sensitive component becomes proportionately greater with the increase in IOP above 15 mmHg, while pressure-indifferent component seems constantly existing throughout all levels of IOP

Table 2 summarizes possible systemic conditions of Groups 1 and 2 LTG. Group 1 is more likely to be old, systemically hypotensive with asthenic in statue, since these conditions are shown to have physiologically low IOP (Shiose, 1984; Shiose and Kawase, 1986; Shiose, 1990b). Group 2 LTG is not a well defined entity that includes various factors causing optic disc damage. Systemic blood pressure is not always hypotensive, but occasionally is rather hypertensive. Many studies have indicated that there is a positive correlation between systolic blood pressure and IOP (Bengtsson, 1972; Bulpitt et al., 1975; Klein and Klein, 1981; Leske and Podger, 1983; Shiose, 1984; Shiose and Kawase, 1986). Systemic blood pressure in LTG is shown to be significantly lower than that in OH (Goldberg et al., 1981; Shiose et al., 1984), but higher than that in age-matched normals (Shiose et al., 1984). Since a majority of LTG is categorized in Group 2 (Levene, 1980), clinical features of LTG as a whole may represent characteristics of Group 2 LTG. Angiosclerosis is assumed to diminish the filtering rate of aqueous even under the influence of systolic hypertension (Shiose and Kawase, 1986), resultant IOP may stay proportionately low.

From topical point of view, visual field defect in low-tension and high-tension glaucoma is shown to be different; i.e. the former reveals

Table 2. Possible difference in general aspects between LTG-1 (Group 1) and LTG-2 (Group 2)

	LTG-1	LTG-2
Pathogenesis:	Identical to POAG with low "normative IOP"	Vascular insufficiency at the optic nerve head
Systemic condition:		
– Age	–	Over middle age
– Blood pressure	Hypotensive	Occasionally hypertensive
– Body build	Lean (asthenic)	–
– Others	Family history of POAG	Hemodynamic crisis Cardiovascular diseases Respiratory diseases

Table 3. Possible difference in local findings between LTG-1 and LTG-2

	LTG-1	LTG-2
IOP:	15 ~ 21 mmHg	< 21 mmHg
Ocular fundus:		
– Disc cupping	Generalized	Localized
– RNFLD	Diffuse	Localized
– Disc hemorrhage	Absent	Present
Visual field	Bjerrum scotoma with diffuse loss	Steep-sided scotoma close to the fixation

steep-sided scotoma close to the fixation, while the latter shows more diffuse defect (Hitchings and Anderton, 1983; Caprioli and Spaeth, 1984; Flammer, 1985; Drance et al., 1987). The results tended to point that increased pressure may affect visual function diffusely, whereas localized defect may be less influenced by IOP (Flammer, 1985; Drance et al., 1987).

Earlier, Shiose (1979) has shown that there are two modes in progression of glaucomatous cupping; i.e. unidirectional encroachment (localized type) and expansive enlargement (generalized type). It is of great interest to note that localized cupping is typically seen in LTG accompanying sharply localized RNFLD with frequent occurrence of disc hemorrhage (Shiose, 1983), while generalized cupping is predominantly seen in high-tension glaucoma (Pederson and Anderson, 1980; Shiose et al., 1987). It would appear that there is an essential difference in local findings between typical high-tension and low-tension glaucoma. In view of the fact that LTG with extremely low pressure possibly represent Group 2 condition, whereas Group 1 LTG is thought to belong the category of POAG, it is tempting to speculate that characteristic found in high-tension and low-tension glaucoma may be applied to Groups 1 and 2 LTG, respectively (Table 3).

Concluding Remarks

It was shown that prevalence of LTG is unexpectedly high, especially in the elderly population. This result may indirectly suggest that the main cause of LTG is most likely to relate the common process of aging; i.e. arteriosclerosis. Chronic or intermittent type of anterior ischemic optic neuropathy due to angiosclerosis would possibly be a main mechanism of pressure-indifferent component of LTG. Though pressure-indifferent mechanism is typically seen in "low-tension" side, the same mechanism is involved in "high-tension" side as well. Complicated is the fact that in most glaucoma cases with intermediary pressure level, both pressure-sensitive and pressure-indifferent components are indistinguishably mixed to reveal complicated clinical features.

The current definition of LTG adopting a given pressure level is clearly artificial and the practice has come under much criticism, but there exists no alternatives so far. Recognition of local and systemic features peculier to Groups 1 and 2 LTG may possibly give some clue for the management of these conditions.

Acknowledgments. The author is greatly indebted to following collaborators of the glaucoma survey; Y. Kitazawa MD, S. Tsukahara MD, T. Akamatsu MD, K. Mizokami MD, R. Futa MD, H. Katsushima MD, H. Kosaki MD. He also wishes to thank Banyu, Santen Pharmaceutical Cos. Chibret International, Humphrey SKB and Canon Cos. for their contribution to the study.

References

Armaly MF, Krueger DE, Maunder L et al (1980) Biostastical analysis of the collaborative glaucoma study. I. Summary report of the risk factors for glaucomatous visual field defects. Arch Ophthalmol 98: 2163–2171

Bengtsson B (1972) Some factors affecting the distribution of intraocular pressure in a population. Acta Ophthalmol 50: 33–46

Bengtsson B (1981) The prevalence of glaucoma. Br J. Ophthalmol 65: 46–49

Bulpitt CJ, Hodes C, Everitt MG (1975) Intraocular blood pressure and systemic blood pressure in the elderly. Br J. Ophthalmol 59: 717–720

Caprioli J, Spaeth GL (1984) Comparison of visual field defects in the low tension glaucomas with those in the high tension glaucomas. Am J. Ophthalmol 97: 730–737

Drance SM, Douglas GR, Airaksinen PJ (1987) Diffuse visual field loss in chronic open-angle and low-tension glaucoma. Am J. Ophthalmol 104: 577–580

Flammer J (1985) Psychophysics in glaucoma. A modified concept of the disease. In: Greve EL, Leydhecker W, Raitta C (eds) The Second European Symposium. W. Junk, The Hague, pp 11–15

Goldberg I, Hollows FC, Kass MA et al (1981) Systemic factors in patients with low-tension glaucoma. Br J. Ophthalmol 65: 56–62

Hitchings RA, Anderton SA (1983) A comparative study of visual field defects seen in patients with low-tension glaucoma and chronic simple glaucoma. Br J Ophthalmol 67: 818–821.

Hollows FC, Graham PA (1966) Intraocular pressure, glaucoma and glaucoma suspects in a defined population. Br J. Ophthalmol 50: 570–586

Klein BE, Klein K (1981) Intraocular pressure and cardiovascular risk variables. Arch Ophthalmol 99: 837–839

Leibowitz HM, Krueger DE, Maunder LR et al (1980) The Framingham Eye Study Monograph. Surv Ophthalmol (suppl) 24: 355–610

Leske MC (1983) The epidemiology of oen-angle glaucoma: A Review. Am J Epidemiol 118: 166–191

Leske MC, Podger MJ (1983) Intraocular pressure: cardiovascular risk variables and visual field defects. Am J Epidemiol 118: 280–287

Levene RZ (1980) Low-tension glaucoma. A critical review and new material. Surv Ophthalmol 24: 621–664

Pederson JE, Anderson DR (1980) The mode of progressive disc cupping in ocular hypertension and glaucoma. Am J Ophthalmol 98: 490–495

Shiose Y (1979) "Quantitative disc pattern" as a new parameter for glaucoma screening. Glaucoma 1: 41–49

Shiose Y (1983) Prevalence and clinical aspects of low-tension glaucoma. In: Henkind P (ed) Acta XXIV International Congress of Ophthalmology. Lippincott, Philadelphia, pp 587–591

Shiose Y (1984) The aging effect on intraocular pressure in an apparently normal population. Arch Ophthalmol 102: 883–887
Shiose Y (1990a) Method for glaucoma screening in a multicenter, collaborative study in Japan. Chibret International J Ophthalmol 7: 42–49
Shiose Y (1990b) Intraocular pressure: New perspectives. Surv Ophthalmol 34: 413–435
Shiose Y, Kawase Y (1986) A new approach to stratified normal intraocular pressure in a general population. Am J Ophthalmol 101: 714–721
Shiose Y, Komuro K, Ito T et al (1981) New system for mass screening of glaucoma, as part of automated multiphasic health testing services. Jpn J Ophthalmol 25: 160–177
Shiose Y, Ito T, Komuro K et al (1984) Prevalence and background of ocular hypertension and low-tension glaucoma. Acta Soc Ophthalmol Jpn 88: 806–813
Shiose Y, Ito T, Amano M et al (1987) Relationship between mode of disc cupping and clinical features in primary open-angle and low-tension glaucoma. Glaucoma 9: 150–162
Shiose Y, Kitazawa, Y, Tsukahara S et al (1990) A collaborative glaucoma survey in Japan – Result of 1988. Jpn Clin Ophthalmol 44: 653–659
Sommer A (1989) Intraocular pressure and glaucoma. Am J Ophthalmol 107: 186–188
Sponsel WE (1989) Tonometry in question: Can visual screening tests play a more decisive role in glaucoma diagnosis and management? Surv Ophthalmol (Suppl) 33: 291–300

Corresponding Address

Professor Y. Shiose, M.D.
Director of the Division of Ophthalmology, Aichi Prefectural Center of Health Care,
3-2-1 San-no-maru, Naka-ku, Nagoya, Japan

Is Low-Tension Glaucoma a Real Glaucoma?

Histopathological Studies and Their Therapeutic Significance

K. Iwata

Recent epidemiological and follow-up studies of glaucoma in Japan revealed that the frequency of low-tension glaucoma (LTG) was twice as high as that of primary open angle glaucoma (POAG). The therapy for LTG, however, has not yet been established because of the ignorance about the mechanism of optic nerve damage. For better understanding of the mechanism of optic nerve damage in LTG, we need histopathological studies at every stage. As far as we know, there are no reports on the histopathology of LTG in the literatur.

Recently we had the opportunity to perform histopathological studies on an advanced LTG eye in a 76 year-old man. His bilateral senile cataracts had been operated on some year previously, and marked glaucomatous cupping had been found in both eyes. The IOP ranged from 13 to 18 mmHg, and LTG was suspected but not treated. Nine years after the cataract-surgery his right eye was enucleated because of developing malignant choroidal melanoma. The visual field of the left eye showed further deterioration 4 years after the right eye enucleation. The findings indicated typical progressive LTG in both eyes.

Histopathological examination revealed that the tumor excised from the right eye was epithelioid malignant melanoma. The intraocular pressure (IOP) had ranged from 12 to 16 mmHg in the right eye and from 14 to 18 mmHg left eye. The patient had no history of elevation of IOP, shock, or migraine, and systemic blood pressure was 130/75 mmHg. No abnormal laboratory findings were noted. The optic nerve head was cut vertically and microscopically studied. Remarkable cupping and backward bowing of lamina cribrosa (LC) was noticeable (Fig. 1). In the normal eye the laminal layers usually display a horizontal parallel arrangement; however, in this patient the laminal layers were partially compressed and disarranged and had lost the original regular multilayered structure. In the upper middle part of the optic disc, the channel structure was crushed, and among the crushed channels shrunken axons and connective tissue proliferation were observed. These findings are characteristic of glaucoma, not simple atrophy. As Hogan and Zimmerman (1962) stated in their textbook *Ophthalmic Pathology*, in simple optic atrophy LC does not reveal the compression and posterior bowing that are typical of glaucoma. Therefore, the above findings indicate glaucomatous change of LC in this patient. It should be noted that these

Gramer/Kampık (Hrsg) Pharmakotherapıe am Auge
© Sprınger-Verlag Berlın Heıdelberg 1992

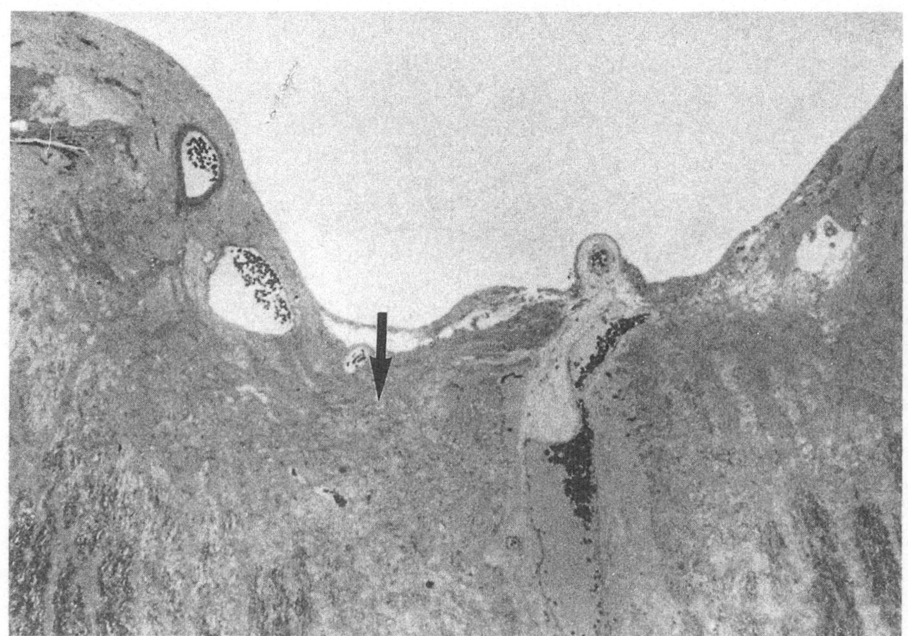

Fig. 1. Remarkable cupping and backward bowing of LC. Laminal layers are compressed and disarranged. *Arrow* indicates crushed laminal layers

changes had developed under normal IOP. Our findings concerning the mechanism of optic nerve fiber damage were very impressive and suggestive. Due to the progressive backward expansion of LC the axons passing through LC were overstretched, and at the termination of Bruch's membrane they were strongly angulated (Fig. 2). As a result, axoplasmic flow stagnated and induced swelling of axons. The sensory retina was forced away from the disc margin by this swelling. The axonal swelling partly resulted in degeneration. The same axonal swelling and degeneration were found everywhere at the channel edge of LC (Fig. 3).

The histopathological findings suggest that due to its weakness glaucomatous LC cannot sustain even normal IOP, and as a result develops backward bowing and invades the axons mechanically.

Attention should be drawn to the vascular change, because in LTG the main cause of optic nerve damage is generally believed to be ischemia (Begg, Drance, Sweeney, 1971). As far as our microscopic examination went, we did not find any abnormal structure of capillaries. Even in the area of axonal mass degeneration, the capillary distribution seemed to be relatively rich and showed no abnormality (Fig. 4). In the area of marked axonal swelling, no vascular abnormality was found. In the atrophied portion of LC vascularity seemed to be normal and again no abnormality of capillaries was found. If optic nerve damage were induced by ischemia, the capillaries in the optic disc would have to show clearer abnormality. That is not the case. Therefore, the

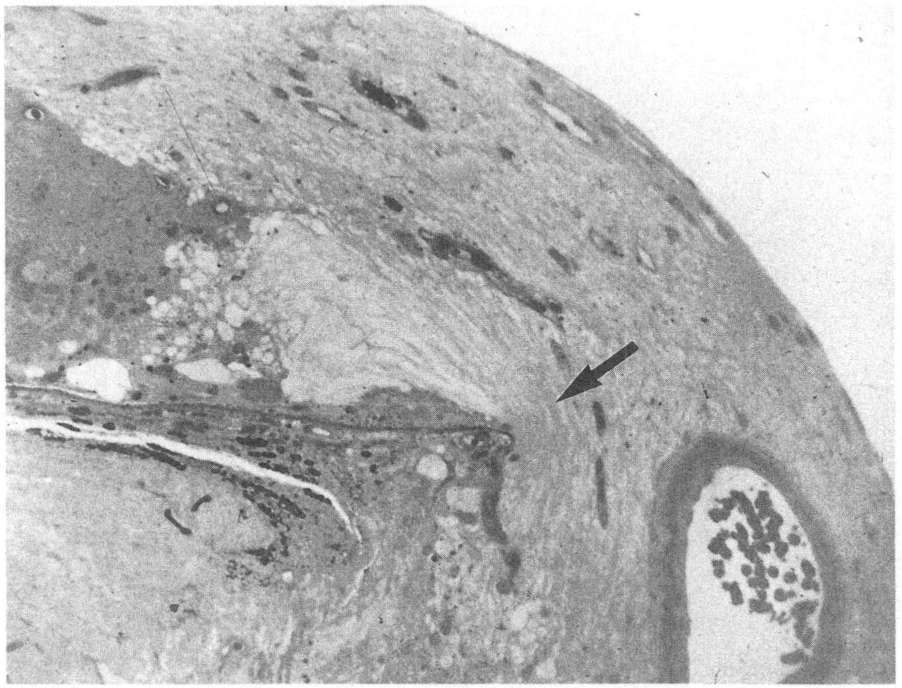

Fig. 2. At the termination of Bruch's membrane (*arrow*) axons were strongly angulated and the resulting stagnation of axoplasmic flow induced marked swelling and degeneration of axons

absence of vascular abnormality may suggest that in this case of LTG the damage to axons was not induced by vascular pathology.

The above-mentioned histopathological findings may be common to all cases of LTG, because Albert et al. (1972), and Brownstein et al. (1980) reported the same findings in one and two cases, respectively, without paying any regard to LTG. From all of the findings it can be concluded that to prevent the progression of optic nerve damage in LTG, LC has to retain its original form and position despite the IOP.

In our long follow-up study of ten cases of bilateral LTG, the average IOP was 16 mmHg and one eye of each patient was trabeculectomized with 5-FU administration. After the surgery IOP was reduced to 10 mmHg, and in 90% of cases no further progression of visual field defects was observed during three years. Stereo image analysis (Imagenet TOPCON) revealed only slight recovery of cupping. Therefore, IOP of 10 mmHg is indispensable to maintain the visual field unchanged. The other eyes of each patient was followed up as a control, and β-blocker and pilocarpine drops were given every day. The IOP was 15–17 mmHg over a period of 3 years, and surprisingly all 10 partner eyes showed progressive visual field defect even with the medication. This means that 10 mmHg IOP is safe and 16 mmHg IOP is harmful. Even IOP between

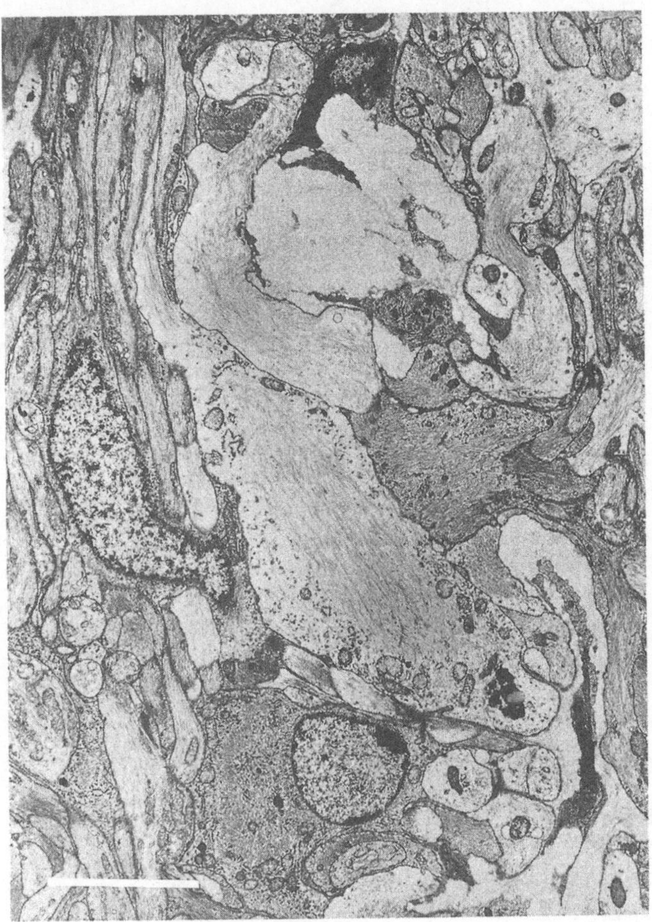

Fig. 3. Axonal swelling and degeneration were found everywhere at the channel edge of LC. *Bar* = 5 μm

11 and 15 mmHg is potentially dangerous. Usually IOP of 10 mmHg can be obtained only by trabeculectomy in combination with subconjunctival administration of 5-FU. According to our experience, administration of pilocarpine, β-blocker, and epinephrine in the form of eye drops reduces the IOP of LTG eyes by only 2–2.5 mmHg on average. Laser trabeculoplasty is also largely ineffective.

Therefore, when we administer such medication we must recognize the fact that most LTG patients will show further progressive visual field damage. The lower the IOP, the better the prognosis for the visual field.

I previously reported another histopathological finding indicating the necessity of very early therapy before the disarrangement of laminal channels (Iwata, 1989). In experimental glaucoma in monkey, typical glaucomatous

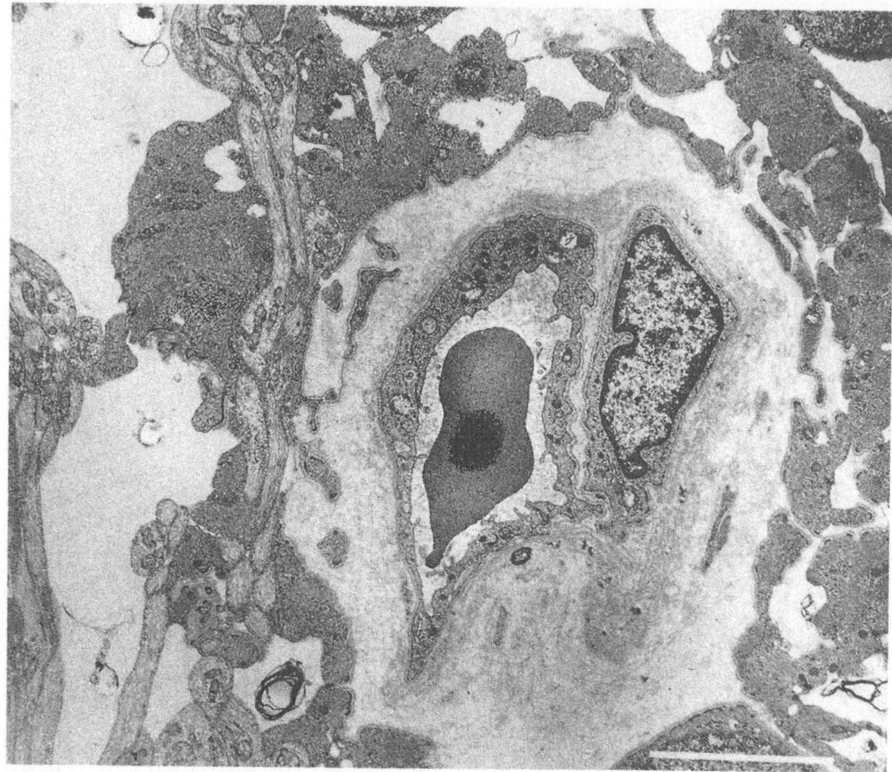

Fig. 4. Even in the area of axonal mass degeneration the capillary microstructure was normal. *Bar* = 5 μm

cupping was induced, as shown in Fig. 5. The IOP of this experimental glaucoma then reduced to 12 mmHg spontaneously. No further change of the optic disc was then found. Two months later the monkey was killed and examined. It is noticeable that in spite of 2 months of normal IOP of 12 mmHg, the compression of axons by the laminal beam was not released, and as a result the remarkable swelling of axons caused by stagnation of axoplasmic flow remained unchanged (Fig. 5). Such abnormal axons may become sensitive to slight changes in IOP. This means that already disarranged LC channels cannot recover and that axons are damaged even after IOP reduction in advanced glaucoma. Therefore, to maintain the optic nerve fiber continuously intact we should prevent the disarrangement of LC channels in the early stage.

In summary, we ophthalmologists should pay attention to the increase in the number of LTG patients. The histopathological findings indicate that the optic nerve damage is mainly attributable to mechanical compression, strangulation, and overstretching of nerve fibers by the disarrangement and backward bowing of LC. The LC cannot sustain itself against normal IOP

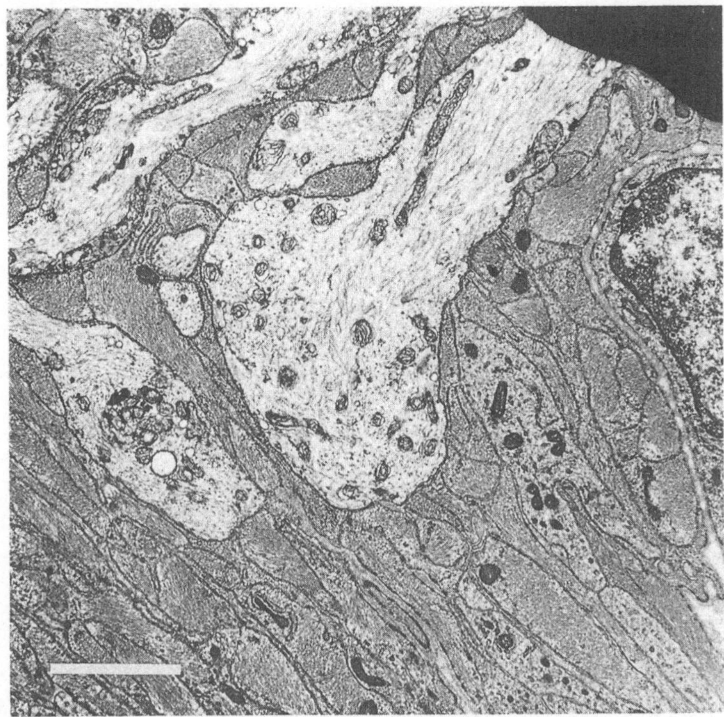

Fig. 5. In experimental glaucoma of monkey, even after 2 months of IOP reduction to 12 mmHg the axoplasmic stagnation was not released

because of progressive weakness of laminal beams. Today, what we can do to arrest the progression of visual field damage in LTG is to reduce the IOP as much as possible. Empirically IOP of 10 mmHg is ideal. To obtain such low IOP, we have to perform trabeculectomy and administer 5-FU. The usual eye-drop combination of pilocarpine, β-blocker, and epinephrine reduces IOP only by 2–2.5 mmHg, insufficient to arrest the progressive damage of LTG. The development of eye drops containing agents such as acetazolamide and prostaglandins can be expected. Acceleration of uveoscleral flow by prostaglandins may be especially promising, and further investigation is needed.

References

Albert DM, Gaasterland DE, Zimmerman LE et al (1972) Bilateral metastatic choroidal melanoma, nevi, and cavernous degeneration, involvement of the optic nerve head. Arch Ophthalmol 87: 39–47

Begg IS, Drance SM, Sweeny VP (1971) Ischemic optic neuropathy in chronic simple glaucoma. Br J Ophthalmol 55: 73–90

Brownstein S, Font RL, Zimmerman LE, Murphy SB (1980) Nonglaucomatous cavernous degeneration of the optic nerve. Arch Ophthalmol 98: 354–358
Hayreh SS (1975) Anterior ischemic optic neuropathy. Springer, Berlin Heidelberg New York, pp 74–88
Hogan MR, Zimmerman LE (1962) Ophthalmic pathology, an atlas and textbook. Saunders, Philadelphia, p. 626
Iwata K (1989) Mechanism of optic nerve damage in glaucoma.
Ophthalmological Mook No. 40, Kanehara Medical Book Publisher, Tokyo, pp 81–89

Corresponding Address

Professor K. Iwata, M.D.
Chairman, Dapartment of Ophthalmology, Niigata University, School of Medicine, 1 Asahimachi, Niigata-Shi, 951 Japan

Intraocular Pressure Treatment in Low-Tension Glaucoma?

Asymmetric Visual Field Defects and Their Relation to Unequal Outflow Facility in Low-Tension Glaucoma – A Clinical Study

L. Cunha and E. Gramer

Abstract

Forty-six eyes of 23 patients with low-tension glaucoma (LTG) were examined by means of automated perimetry (Prog. 31, Octopus 201) and Leydhecker's tonography test.

In an intraindividual comparison 40 eyes of 20 patients with LTG and asymmetric visual field (difference between total loss of right and left eye higher than 200 dB) were examined. In 85% of the patients the eye with more advanced visual field damage also had the worse tonography test values.

Regarding the sensitivity of the tonography test in the diagnosis of LTG, 60.9% of patients with LTG received the tonography test diagnosis "nonpathologic".

The mean visual field loss of eyes with tonography test diagnosis "nonpathologic" and "pathologic" were compared. Eyes with the diagnosis "pathologic" had a significantly higher mean visual field loss than eyes with the diagnosis "nonpathologic".

The therapeutic consequence of these results is the first-line use of drugs (pilocarpine and adrenaline derivates) which improve the outflow facility. If progression of visual field damage occurs or if the patient cannot tolerate these drugs, a topical betablocker may be indicated. If this is not sufficient and if the known systemic risk factors are corrected as much as possible, filtering surgery may be called for.

Elevated intraocular pressure is widely accepted as the main risk factor in primary open angle glaucoma. In low-tension glaucoma (LTG) which by definition features intraocular pressure (IOP) within the normal range, many authors [1–19] have postulated other risk factors, most of them related to vascular insufficiency of the optic nerve head.

An important question is now: Are there IOP-related damaging factors in LTG?

Some arguments implicate IOP in the pathogenesis. In LTG the most frequent intraocular pressure is 19 mmHg [20], higher than the most frequent IOP in normals (16 mmHg; Fig. 1) [21, 22]; there is, in LTG a shift to higher IOP levels within the normal range. A second argument is the higher diurnal

Gramer/Kampik (Hrsg.) Pharmakotherapie am Auge
© Springer-Verlag Berlin Heidelberg 1992

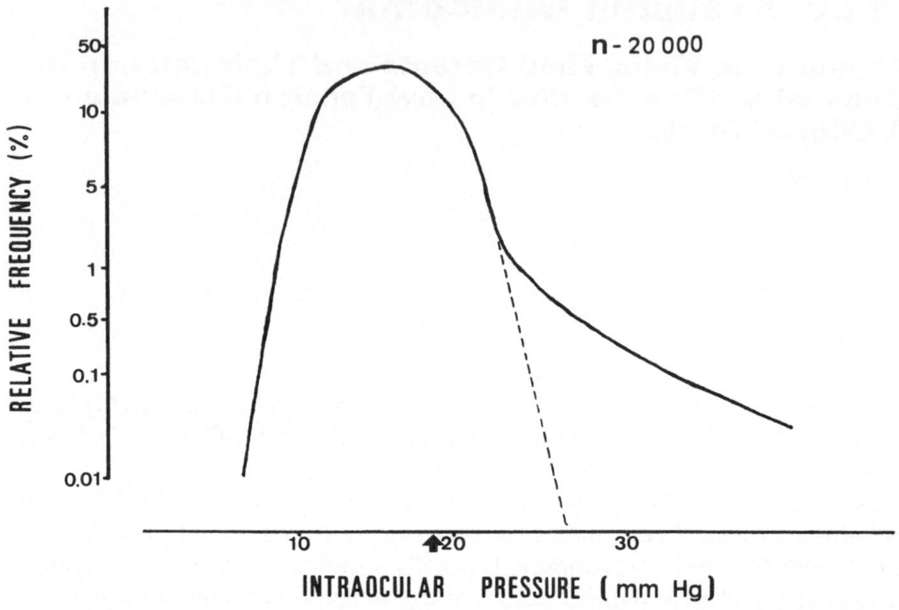

Fig. 1. IOP distribution in 20 000 normal eyes. (From [32])

variation of IOP in LTG (8.0 mmHg) than in normals (3.7 mmHg; Table 1). This higher variation may have a harmful influence [20].

Two studies relating asymmetries in IOP and visual field defects between the right and left eyes of patients with LTG (intraindividual study design) have recently been performed [23, 24]. These studies clearly show that when IOP is asymmetric in LTG, the visual field damage appears greater on the side with higher mean IOP.

In LTG – in our definition glaucoma with IOP of 21 mmHg or less – we did not expect clear differences in IOP between the right and the left eye. So we

Table 1. Diurnal tension variation in eyes with primary open angle glaucoma (POAG), ocular hypertension (OH), low tension glaucoma (LTG) and normals. (From [20])

		Eyes (n)	Δ IOP $\pm$ SD
POAG	Kitazawa (1979)	73	13.3 $\pm$ 0.83
	Katavisto (1964)	329	11.3 $\pm$ 4.2
	Gramer (1982)	22	11.75 $\pm$ 4.27
OH	Kitazawa (1979)	71	8.4 $\pm$ 0.3
LTG	Gramer (1982)	21	8.09 $\pm$ 2.42
Normals	Kitazawa (1979)	42	6.4 $\pm$ 0.2
	Drance (1960)	404	3.7 $\pm$ 1.8
	Katavisto (1964)	100	3.17 $\pm$ 1.2

looked, using an intraindividual study design, for differences in the tonography test values (C3–7, P3/C3–7) in eyes with asymmetric visual fields.

We were interested in answering the questions:

1. Has the eye with the more advanced visual field defect the worse tonography test values?
2. How often does the tonography test yield the diagnosis "pathologic" in LTG?
3. Do the eyes with the tonography test diagnosis "pathologic" display a significantly greater mean total loss than the eyes with the diagnosis "nonpathologic"?

Material and Methods

Forty-six eyes of 23 patients with LTG diagnosed at the University Eye Clinic in Würzburg were included in this study. All these patients had, in both eyes, IOP lower than 21 mmHg (measured using isolated Goldmann tonometry and diurnal tensional curves), glaucomatous visual field damage, glaucomatous optic disc changes, and open chamber angle. Patients were either on no medication or symmetric medication. No patient had used topical or systemic corticosteroids (this excluded former steroid glaucoma). No systemic beta-blockers were being used at the time of the examination (this excluded the lowering effect of these drugs). All patients underwent neurological examination, including computed tomography, to exclude neurological disease. At the time of the examination the patients' mean age was 58 ± 10 years (range 30 – 78 years).

All patients underwent visual field assessment and tonographic evaluation in the same week. The visual fields were evaluated by threshold automated perimetry (Prog. 31, Octopus 201). The visual field defects are quantified by the sum of the loss of sensitivity (in dB) in 69 of the 73 points of this program (excluding four points in the area of the blind spot). This value is referred to as total loss (TL) and is quantified by program Delta. Visual field asymmetry is defined as a difference in total loss between right and left eye of more than 200 dB (Fig. 2).

The threshold strategy was used because it possesses a higher sensitivity and specificity in the detection and quantification of visual field defects than Goldmann perimetry and the automated suprathreshold strategies [25–31].

The tonography test described by Leydhecker in 1958 was used [32]. Its concept is different from the original method in that it does not claim to measure a physiological parameter and its results are expressed as dimensionless numbers [33]. It consists of 7 min tonography with an electronic impression tonometer. The so-called coefficient of outflow facility was calculated using the Fridenwald calibration of 1955, between the 3rd and the 7th min (C3–7). The ratio between the IOP in the 3rd min (P3) and the

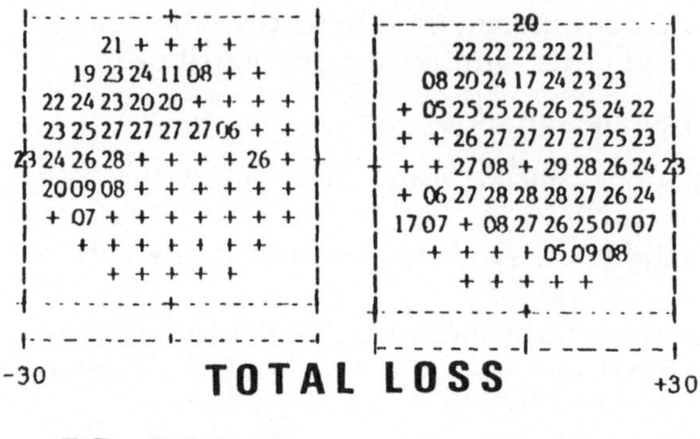

Fig. 2. Definition of asymmetric visual fields. Δ-total loss between right and left eye greater than 200 dB

coefficient of outflow facility (P3/C3–7) was also calculated (Fig. 3). The main advantage of this tonographic test over Grant tonography lies in the exclusion of the first 3 min, which show many variations in normal and glaucomatous eyes on repeated testing. These variations are probably due to changes in aqueous secretion and blood content of the choroid, which stabilizes during the first few minutes of testing.

Based on the results of his tonography test, Leydhecker [32] calculated, in healthy eyes, the mean results and the standard deviation. The values beyond the statistical m ± 2SD (mean value plus or minus two standard deviations) are called "probably pathologic" and the values beyond the statistical m ± 3SD are called "pathologic".

Using this methodology the limits of each group are:

Tonographic diagnosis	C3–7	P3/C3–7
– Nonpathologic	> 0.09	< 160
– Probably pathologic	0.06–0.08	161–213
– Pathologic	< 0.06	> 213

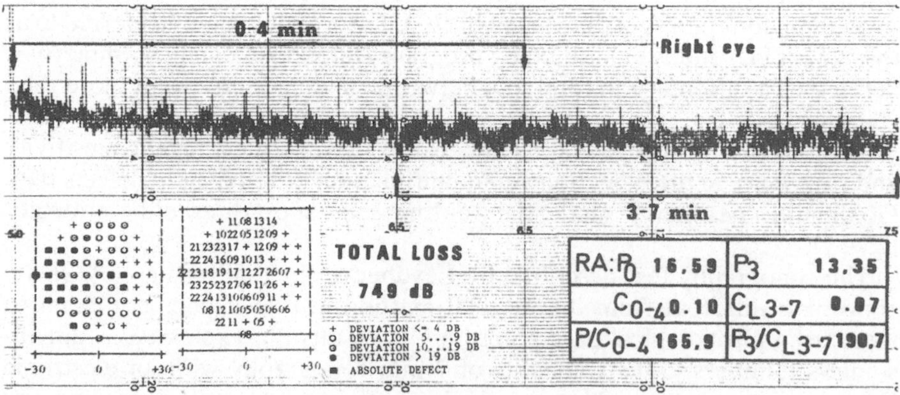

Fig. 3. Tonography test values and total loss in visual field (prog. 31/Delta) of the right eye of a patient with LTG

Tonography test values were compared intraindividually between right and left eyes presenting asymmetric visual field damage. Asymmetry was defined as a difference in total loss of more than 200 dB (Fig. 2). Intraindividual comparison was used to exclude the influence of systemic factors.

In addition we evaluated how often the tonography test diagnosis "pathologic" was assigned in LTG and looked for significant differences in visual field loss between groups of eyes with different tonography test diagnoses.

The Mann-Whitney U test was used for statistical evaluation

Results

Intraindividual comparison of tonography test values was performed in 20 patients with LTG and asymmetric visual field defects (difference in total loss of more than 200 dB). Seventeen (85%) of the patients had the worse tonography test values in the eye with higher visual field defects.

We found that 28 eyes (60.9%) were assigned the diagnosis "nonpathologic", 10 eyes (21.7%) "probably pathologic", and 8 eyes (17.4%) "pathologic". The visual field loss in the 28 eyes with the tonographic diagnosis of "nonpathologic" was 399.53 ± 226.26 dB, significantly different ($p < 0.05$) from that in the 8 eyes with the diagnosis "pathologic" (625.62 ± 246.11 dB) (Table 2).

Table 2. Tonography test diagnosis and m-total loss in visual field in 46 eyes with LTG

Eyes	Tonography Test Diagnosis	m-Total Loss ± 1 SD
28	"Non pathologic"	399.53 ± 226.26
10	"Probably pathologic"	565.20 ± 309.37
8	"Pathologic"	625.62 ± 246.11
46	Total	474.64 ± 262.56

Discussion

Ocular hypertension is widely accepted as an important damaging factor in primary open angle glaucoma (POAG) [34, 48, 49]. Nevertheless this damaging influence is difficult to prove, because the cardiovascular risk factors differ among individuals. It is well known that there are patients with POAG in whom the visual field deteriorates in treated eyes within IOP with the statistical normal range [34, 44–47].

Only by intraindividual comparison of IOP and visual field loss can the damaging impact of elevated IOP be shown. Cardiovascular risk factors affect both eyes similarly, and they are more or less excluded when we ask the question: Has the eye with the more severely damaged visual field the higher IOP?

In an earlier study [34] involving intraindividual comparison of 108 eyes in 54 patients with POAG we demonstrated that patients with four times greater visual field loss in one eye than the other had significantly higher maximum IOP in the eye with the more severe damage. This definition of visual field asymmetry guarantees that a clear asymmetry exists, but such a study design is not easy to use for LTG because such clear asymmetry in IOP can hardly be found in low-tension eyes.

In spite of this, two recent studies [23, 24] used this intraindividual study design to examine the relation between IOP and the amount of visual field defect. It is important to look at the definitions of asymmetry in visual field and IOP used by the authors of these studies. Cartwright and Anderson [23] defined IOP asymmetry as "an average asymmetry of IOP between the two eyes of at least 1 mm Hg. The IOP asymmetry had to be regularly present, with 90% of the asymmetric readings in the same direction on all clinical visits while not receiving treatment or while receiving symmetric treatment". The definition of visual field asymmetry was based on the reader decision, sometimes using a forced decision method so that one eye was necessarily designated worse. The authors found a corresponding asymmetry in visual field defects in 12 of 14 patients with asymmetric mean IOP.

In the other study, Crichton and al. [24] defined IOP asymmetry according to the difference between the mean pressures of the two eyes. Patients in whom IOP in any of the pairs of pressure readings was higher by more than 1 mmHg in the eye with the lower mean IOP were excluded. The definition of LTG in this study included IOP never greater than 23 mmHg.

The visual fields were judged to be clearly asymmetric if the more affected eye had more glaucomatous scotomata than the other; for instance, both hemifields involved in one eye and only one in the other. In the absence of such obvious asymmetry the defects were quantified "in automated perimetry by visual field indices, in Goldmann perimetry by planimetry. Fields are judged to be asymmetric when the more affected eye had scotomata three times greater than the fellow eye".

A mean IOP difference between the eyes greater than 2 mmHg was found in five patients, and all five showed a corresponding asymmetry of their visual field defects. A mean IOP difference of 1 mmHg or greater was found in 17 patients, 13 of whom showed a corresponding visual field asymmetry. A mean IOP difference of 0.5 mmHg occurred in 32 patients, and in 22 of whom corresponding visual field defect existed.

These studies clearly show that when IOP is asymmetric in LTG, the visual field defects appear to be greater on the side with higher mean IOP.

In LTG, defined by us as glaucoma with maximum IOP of 21 mmHg or less, we did not expect clear differences in IOP between the right and the left eye. So we looked for differences in the tonography test values (C3–7, P3/C3–7) between right and left eye in patients with asymmetric visual fields defects. We tested whether the eye with the more advanced visual field defects also had the worse tonography test values.

Whether these tonography test values are physiologic or not is irrelevant, because we merely wanted to ascertain whether there is asymmetry between these dimensionless values according to the asymmetry of visual field damage. The close relation we found – 85% of the patients with asymmetric visual field defects had the worse tonography test values in the eye with more advanced visual field defect – could be a further argument for IOP as a risk factor in LTG. However, this is only an indirect conclusion from the intraindividual differences in the dimensionless tonographic values.

Is the classification of tonography test results into "nonpathologic", "probably pathologic", and "pathologic" helpful in LTG? In the present study 28 (60.9%) of the 46 eyes studied were assigned the diagnosis "nonpathologic" and only 8 received the diagnosis "pathologic". Thus 60% of these cases of LTG would not have been detected by the tonography test alone. We can conclude that tonography test diagnosis within the limits of the definition used is not sensitive enough for the single LTG patient.

Evaluating not single patients but tonography test diagnosis groups, we found that eyes with the diagnosis "pathologic" had significantly greater mean visual field loss (625 dB) than eyes with the diagnosis "nonpathologic" (399 dB; $p < 0.05$). This may be a further argument for IOP-related risk factors in LTG.

Many different therapeutic approaches have been proposed for LTG. The first step in the management of LTG is directed at the systemic risk factors which can be at least partially eliminated – heart failure compensated with digitalis [35], ocular or systemic vasospasm diagnosed by Doppler blood flow measurements in the fingers and a cold test and treated with calcium antagonists [36–38].

Besides these systemic risk factors, the IOP-related factors that we have described in this study have to be treated. We believe it is logical to lower IOP in LTG, probably first using drugs that increase outflow facility (miotics and adrenaline derivatives). If the therapeutic effect of these drugs is insufficient and the progression of visual field defects occurs in spite of IOP under 15 mmHg, or their secondary adverse effects are not acceptable to the patients, a betablocker may be indicated. The patients treated with local betablockers, calcium antagonists or clonidine derivatives should be carefully monitored with respect to blood pressure and cardiovascular status, looking for important hypotensive or negative inotropic effects. Our earlier studies [19] showed that patients with LTG have low blood pressure and hypotensive crises more frequently than patients of the same age with POAG. This was the only difference between these two groups with respect to risk factors. If the visual field damage progresses in spite of all medical therapy, filtering surgery could be indicated [30–43].

Our visual field follow-up [44] comparing 45 eyes of 45 patients with LTG treated with IOP-lowering therapy (pentoxifylline and digitalis if indicated) and 232 eyes of 232 patients with POAG featuring IOP less than 21 mmHg treated with IOP lowering drugs, in the same observation time showed no difference in the frequency or amount of visual field deterioration [44, 45]. In other words, patients with LTG did not show a worse prognosis for the preservation of visual field, when treated, than patients with POAG. This is an argument which at least does not speak against IOP-lowering treatment in low-tension glaucoma.

References

1. Chumbley LC, Brubaker RF (1976) Low tension glaucoma. Am J Ophthalmol 81: 761–767
2. Drance SM (1972) Some factors in the production of low tension glaucoma. Br J Ophthalmol 56: 229–242
3. Drance SM, Sweeney VP, Morgan RW, Feldman F (1973) Studies of factors involved in the production of low-tension glaucoma. Arch Ophthalmol 89: 457–465
4. Geijssen HC et al (1985) Fluorescein fundus angiographic studies in various types of glaucoma. Invest Ophthalmol Vis Sci 26 (ARVO Suppl): 42
5. Goldberg I et al (1981) Systemic factors in patients with low-tension glaucoma. Br J Ophthalmol 65: 56–62
6. Hayreh SS (1987) Factors determining the glaucomatous optic nerve head damage. In: Krieglstein GK (ed) Glaucoma Up-Date III. Springer, Berlin Heidelberg New York Tokyo, pp 40–46
7. Hiatt RL, Deutsche AR, Ringer G (1971) Low-tension glaucoma. Ann Ophthalmol 3: 85–92
8. Hitchings RA, Spaeth GL (1977) Fluorescein angiography in chronic simple and low-tension glaucoma. Br J Ophthalmol 61: 126–132
9. Hoyng PFJ, Greve EL, Frederikse K et al (1985) Platelet aggregation and Glaucoma. Doc Ophthalmol 61: 167–173
10. Lambrou GN, Sindhunata P, Van Den Berg TJTP, Geijssen C, Vyborny P, Greve EL (1989) Ocular pulse measurements in low-tension glaucoma. In: Lambrou GN, Ocular blood flow in glaucoma. Greve EL (eds) Kugler and Ghedini Publications, Dordrecht, pp 115–120
11. Levine RZ (1980) Low-tension glaucoma: A critical review and new material. Surv Ophthalmol 24: 621–664
12. Perkins ES, Phelps CD (1984) The ocular pulse in low-tension glaucoma. Klin Monatsbl Augenheilk 184: 303–304
13. Perkins ES, Phelps CD (1982) Open angle glaucoma, ocular hypertension, low-tension glaucoma, and refraction. Arch Ophthalmol 100: 1464–1467
14. Phelps CD, Corbett JJ (1985) Migraine and low-tension glaucoma. Invest Ophthalmol Vis Sci 26: 1105–1108
15. Spaeth GL (1975) Fluorescein angiography: Its contribution towards understanding the mechanisms of visual loss in glaucoma. Trans Am Ophthalmol Soc 73: 491–553
16. Sugar HS (1979) Low tension glaucoma: A practical approach. Ann Ophthalmol 11: 1155–1171
17. Winder AF (1977) Circulating lipoprotein and blood glucose levels in association with low tension and chronic simple glaucoma. Br J Ophthalmol 61: 641–645
18. Gramer E, Leydhecker W (1985) Zur Pathogenese des Glaukoms ohne Hochdruck. Z Prakt Augenheilkd. 6: 329–333
19. Gramer E, Leydhecker W (1985) Glaukom ohne Hochdruck. Eine klinische Studie. Klin Monatsbl Augenheilkd. 186: 262–267
20. Gramer E, Mohamed J, Krieglstein GK (1982) Der Ort von Gesichtsfeldausfällen bei Glaucoma simplex, Glaukom ohne Hochdruck und ischämischer Neuropathie. Indikationen zur vasoaktiven Therapie. Medikamentöse Glaukomtherapie, JF Bergmann Verlag, München
21. Kahn HA, Leibowitz HM, Ganley JP et al (1977) The Framingham eye study. 1. Outline and major prevalence findings. Am J Epidemiol 106: 17–32

22. Leydhecker W, Akiyama, K, Neumann HG (1958) Der intraokulare Druck gesunder menschlicher Augen. Klin. Monatsbl. Augenheilkd 133: 622
23. Cartwright MJ, Anderson DR (1988) Correlation of asymmetric damage with asymmetric intraocular pressure in Normal Tension Glaucoma. (Low-Tension Glaucoma). Arch Ophthalmol 106: 898–900
24. Crichton A, Drance SM, Douglas GR, Schulzer M (1989) Unequal intraocular pressure and its relation to asymmetric visual field defects in Low-Tension Glaucoma. Ophthalmol 96: 1312–1314
25. Gramer E (1982) Der Informationsgehalt der computergesteuerten Perimetrie für die Diagnostik und Verlaufskontrolle von Augenkrankheiten. Würzburg, Habilitationsschrift
26. Gramer E, Pröll M, Krieglstein GK (1980) Die Reproduzierbarkeit zentraler Gesichtsfeldbefunde bei der kinetischen und der computergesteuerten statischen Perimetrie. Klin Monatsbl Augenheilk. 176: 374–383
27. Gramer E, Krieglstein GK (1983) The role of computerized perimetry in the management of optic nerve diseases. Chibret Int J Ophthalmol 1: 41
28. Gramer E, Leydhecker W (1984) Zum gegenwärtigen Stand der Perimeterentwicklung. Teil II. Z Prakt Augenheilk. 5: 221–236
29. Gramer E (1985) Gegenwärtiger Stand der Perimeterentwicklung. Teil III. Z Prakt Augenheilk. 6: 334–346
30. Gramer E (1985) Lesen von Gesichtsfeldbefunden bei der automatischen Perimetrie. Z Prakt Augenheilk. 6: 353–364
31. Krieglstein GK, Schrems W, Gramer E, Leydhecker W (1981) Detectability of early glaucomatous field defects. A controlled comparison of Goldmann versus Octopus perimetry. Doc Ophthalmol Proc Ser. 26: 19–24
32. Leydhecker W (1958) Tonography in the early diagnosis of glaucoma. Trans Ophthal Soc UK, 73: 553–564
33. Leydhecker W (1986) Are there reliable clinical methods to study aqueous humor dynamics? New Trends in Ophthalmology Vol I N° 1 129–136
34. Gramer E, Althaus G (1990) Bedeutung des erhöhten intraokularen Drucks für den glaukomatösen Gesichtsfeldschaden. Eine klinische Studie. Klin. Mbl. Augenheilk. 197, pp 218–224
35. Drance SM (1975) LTG and its management. In Symposium on Glaucoma, Trans. New Orleans Academy of Ophthalmology. pp 257–265
36. Flammer J, Guthauser U, Mahler F (1987) Do ocular vasospasms help cause Low Tension Glaucoma? Doc Ophthalmol Proc Ser 397–9
37. Gasser P (1989) Ocular vasospasm: A risk factor in the pathogenesis of Low-Tension Glaucoma. Int Ophthalmol 13: 281–290
38. Kitazawa Y, Shirai H, GO JF (1989) The effect of Ca^{2++}-antagonist on visual field in Low-Tension Glaucoma. Arch Clin Exp Ophthalmol 408–412
39. Schwartz LS, Perman KI, Whitten M (1984) Argon laser trabeculoplasty in progressive Low Tension Glaucoma. Ann Ophthalmol 16: 560–566
40. Thomas JV, Simmons RJ, Belcher III CD (1982) Argon laser trabeculoplasty in the presurgical glaucoma patient. Arch Ophthalmol 89: 187–197
41. Hitchings RA (1988) Low Tension Glaucoma – is treatment worthwhile? Eye 2 636–640
42. Abedin S, Simmons RJ, Grant M (1982) Progressive Low Tension Glaucoma. Ophthalmol 89: 1–6
43. De Jong N, Greve EL et al (1989) Results of filtering procedure in Low Tension Glaucoma. Int Ophthalmol 13-1/2: 131–139
44. Gramer E, Althaus G (1987) Risikofaktoren bei Niederdruckglaukom. Klinische Studie zur Quantifizierung der Gesichtsfeldverschlechterung bei Glaukom ohne Hochdruck und Glaucoma simplex mit reguliertem intraokularem Druck mit dem Programm Delta des Octopus-Perimeters 201. Z Prakt Augenheilkd 8: 388–399
45. Gramer E: Gesichtsfeldänderung bei der Langzeittherapie des Glaukoms. Langzeitverlaufskontrolle glaukomatöser Gesichtsfeldausfälle bei Glaucoma simplex mit

reguliertem intraokularem Druck und bei Glaukom ohne Hochdruck zur computer-perimetrischen Quantifizierung des augeninnendruckabhängigen Glaukomschadens. In: M Mertz (Hrsg) Neue Gesichtspunkte zur Entdeckung und Behandlung des Glaukoms, 19–41, W Zuckschwerd-Verlag München 1990
46. Gramer E, Althaus G (1992) Risk factors for deterioration of visual field defects in primary open angle glaucoma. Invest. Ophthalmol. Vis. Sci. Vol 33, No 4, p 1278
47. Gramer E, Althaus G (1992) Einfluß des systolischen Blutdruckes auf die Lage der Gesichtsfeldausfälle in oberer und unterer Gesichtsfeldhälfte bei Patienten mit Glaucoma chronicum simplex. Ophthalmologe (im Druck)
48. Gramer E (1992) Zur Beurteilung des Therapieeffektes bei Glaukom. In: G. K. Krieglstein (Hrsg), Glaukom. Verlag ad manum medici, München, S. 39–64
47. Gloor B (1990) Verlaufskontrolle beim Glaukom. Fortschr. Opthalmol 87 [Suppl], S. 163–171

Corresponding Address
Professor Eugen Gramer, MD, LLD
University Eye Hospital Würzburg, Josef Schneider-Straße 11, D-8700 Würzburg

Unterschiede in der Form der Papillen-
exkavation bei Glaucoma chronicum
simplex und Glaukom ohne Hochdruck –

Eine klinische Studie
mit dem Laser Tomographic Scanner

H. Maier, M. Siebert und E. Gramer

Zusammenfassung

Das konfokale Untersuchungsprinzip des Laser Tomographic Scanners (LTS) erlaubt neue Papillenparameter zu errechnen, die erstmals dazu verwendet werden, die Steilheit der Exkavationsränder zu quantifizieren.

153 Augen von 82 Patienten der Diagnosegruppen Gesund, okuläre Hypertension, Glaucoma chronicum simplex und Glaukom ohne Hochdruck werden mit dem Laser Tomographic Scanner (LTS) und dem Octopus Perimeter 201 untersucht.

Geprüft wurde, ob sich die Diagnosegruppen unterscheiden: 1. In der Tiefe der Papillenexkavation, 2. in der Form der Papillenexkavation und 3. in den Papillenparametern Exkavationsvolumen, Exkavationsfläche und Verhältnis Exkavationsfläche zu Papillengesamtfläche.

Der Vergleich erfolgte bei Augen mit Glaucoma chronicum simplex und Glaukom ohne Hochdruck bei gleichem Stadium des Gesichtsfeldausfalls.

1. Augen mit Glaukom ohne Hochdruck zeigten im Vergleich zu Augen mit Glaucoma chronicum simplex bei gleichem Stadium des Gesichtsfeldausfalls
   - eine kleinere maximale und mittlere Tiefe der Papillenexkavation in allen Stadien mit Ausnahme des Stadium 1.
   - signifikant steilere Exkavationsränder und einen flacheren Exkavationsboden im Stadium 1 und 2. In den fortgeschrittenen Stadien 3 bis 5 bestehen keine Unterschiede in der Steilheit der Exkavationsränder und der Form des Exkavationsbodens.
   - im Stadium 1 ein signifikant größeres Exkavationsvolumen und eine signifikant größere Exkavationsfläche.
   - im Stadium 1 bereits steile Exkavationsränder, während Augen mit Glaucoma chronicum simplex erst im Stadium 2 steile Exkavationsränder zeigen, das bedeutet: Ein Erkrankungsstadium später.
2. Gesunde Augen, Augen mit okulärer Hypertension und Augen mit Glaucoma chronicum simplex Stadium 1 zeigten keine signifkanten Unterschiede in der Steilheit der Exkavationsränder und der Form des Exkavationsbodens.
   Augen mit okulärer Hypertension zeigten gegenüber gesunden Augen ein signifikant größeres Exkavationsvolumen.

Gramer/Kampik (Hrsg.) Pharmakotherapie am Auge
© Springer-Verlag Berlin Heidelberg 1992

Zwischen Augen mit Glaucoma chronicum simplex und Glaukom ohne Hochdruck wurden von uns in früheren Studien Unterschiede in Lage und Tiefe der Gesichtsfeldausfälle, Unterschiede in der Größe der Papillenexkavation und Unterschiede in der Fläche der neuroretinalen Randzone bei gleichem Stadium des Gesichtsfeldausfalls gefunden. In der vorliegenden Arbeit wurden hinsichtlich der Morphologie der Papille mit Hilfe des konfokalen Untersuchungsprinzips nun auch Unterschiede in der Steilheit der Exkavationsränder belegt.

Diese Unterschiede in der Morphologie der Papille weisen auf Unterschiede in den Schädigungswegen und Risikofaktoren in den Anfangsstadien bei Glaucoma chronicum simplex und Glaukom ohne Hochdruck hin.

Die Therapie des Glaukoms ohne Hochdruck muß daher diese zusätzlichen Risikofaktoren berücksichtigen.

Einleitung

Unterschiede in der Lage und Tiefe der Gesichtsfeldausfälle [24, 26, 31–34, 36, 38, 39, 43, 46, 48] sowie Unterschiede in der Morphologie der Papille bei Glaucoma chronicum simplex und Glaukom ohne Hochdruck [9, 15, 28, 35, 45, 49, 50, 91] weisen auf Unterschiede in den Schädigungswegen bei Glaukom mit bzw. ohne Augeninnendruckerhöhung hin. Quantifizierende Untersuchungsmethoden der Gesichtsfeldausfälle und der Papille erlauben diese Fragestellungen nun quantitativ und unter Anwendung statistischer Methoden besser zu beantworten als dies bisher möglich war. So hat z.B. für die Perimetrie das Octopus Perimeter 201 mit dem Programm Delta, für die Papille z.B. der Laser Tomographic Scanner (LTS) und der Optic Nerve Head Analyzer (ONHA) zur verbesserten Quantifizierung des Glaukomschadens beigetragen.

Bei einer quantifizierenden Untersuchung mit dem Laser Tomographic Scanner (LTS) oder Heidelberger Retina-Tomographen (HRT) werden neue Meßdaten erhoben, die Rückschlüsse auf die Form der Papillenexkavation, die Steilheit der Exkavationsränder und die Form des Exkavationbodens bei Glaucoma chronicum simplex und Glaukom ohne Hochdruck zulassen. Neue, bisher nicht verfügbare Papillenparameter werden dazu errechnet und dargestellt.

Diese Papillenparameter sind:

1. effektive mittlere Tiefe (HE) der Papillenexkavation;
2. maximale Tiefe (HM) der Papillenexkavation;
3. drittes zentrales Moment der Tiefenwerte der Papille.

Fragestellung

Mit dieser Arbeit werden diese neuen Papillenparameter für folgende drei Fragestellungen im Vergleich von gesunden Augen, Augen von Patienten mit okulärer Hypertension, Glaucoma chronicum simplex und Glaukom ohne Hochdruck erstmals angewandt:

1. Tiefe der Papillenexkavation: Bestehen Unterschiede in der Tiefe der Papillenexkavation (definiert als a) maximale Tiefe (HM) und b) effektive mittlere Tiefe (HE) der Papillenexkavation) bei Augen mit Glaucoma chronicum simplex und Glaukom ohne Hochdruck?
2. Form der Papillenexkavation: a) Bestehen Unterschiede in der Form der Exkavation (definiert als Verhältnis zwischen effektiver mittlerer Tiefe (HE) zu maximaler Tiefe der Papillenexkavation oder definiert als drittes Zentralmoment der Tiefenwerte) bei gesunden Augen, Augen mit okulärer Hypertension, Glaucoma chronicum simplex und Glaukom ohne Hochdruck bei gleicher Größe des Gesichtsfeldausfalls?
   b) Tritt eine Änderung der Steilheit der Exkavationsränder beim Glaukom ohne Hochdruck bereits in früheren Stadien der Glaukomerkrankung auf als beim Glaucoma chronicum simplex?
3. Papillenparameter: Zeigen Augen mit Glaucoma chronicum simplex und Glaukom ohne Hochdruck bei gleichem Stadium des Gesichtsfeldausfalls Unterschiede in folgenden Papillenparametern des Laser Tomographic Scanners (LTS): a) Exkavationsvolumen, b) Exkavationsfläche und c) Verhältnis Exkavationsfläche zu Papillengesamtfläche?

Methodik

Patienten

153 Augen von 82 Patienten der Diagnosegruppen Gesund, okuläre Hypertension, Glaucoma chronicum simplex und Glaukom ohne Hochdruck wurden mit dem Laser Tomographic Scanner (Abb. 1) unter standardisierten Bedingungen an der Universitäts-Augenklinik Würzburg untersucht (Tabelle 1). 70 Augen von 37 Patienten waren gesund. 4 Augen von 2 Patienten zeigten erhöhte Druckwerte bei normalem Gesichtsfeldbefund und unauffälligem Papillenbefund (okuläre Hypertension). 61 Augen von 33 Patienten hatten ein Glaucoma chronicum simplex. Für die statistische Auswertung wurde nach dem Zufallsprinzip nur jeweils ein Auge eines Patienten ausgewählt. Danach waren 26 Augen mit Glaucoma chronicum simplex im Stadium 1 der Glaukomerkrankung, 3 Augen im Stadium 2 und 4 Augen in den fortgeschrittenen Stadien 3 bis 5. Bei 18 Augen von 10 Patienten lag ein Glaukom ohne Hochdruck vor. Unter den 10 in die Studie aufgenommenen Augen wiesen 6 Augen ein Stadium 1, 2 Augen ein Stadium 2 und 2 Augen fortgeschrittene Stadien der Glaukomerkrankung auf (vgl. Tabelle 1).

Bei den meisten Patienten lag eine Langzeitbeobachtung über mehrere Jahre in unserer Poliklinik mit Papillenfotographie und regelmäßigen Gesichtsfelduntersuchungen vor. In die vorliegende Studie wurden nur Patienten aufgenommen, die einen Visus von 0.8 oder besser hatten, und

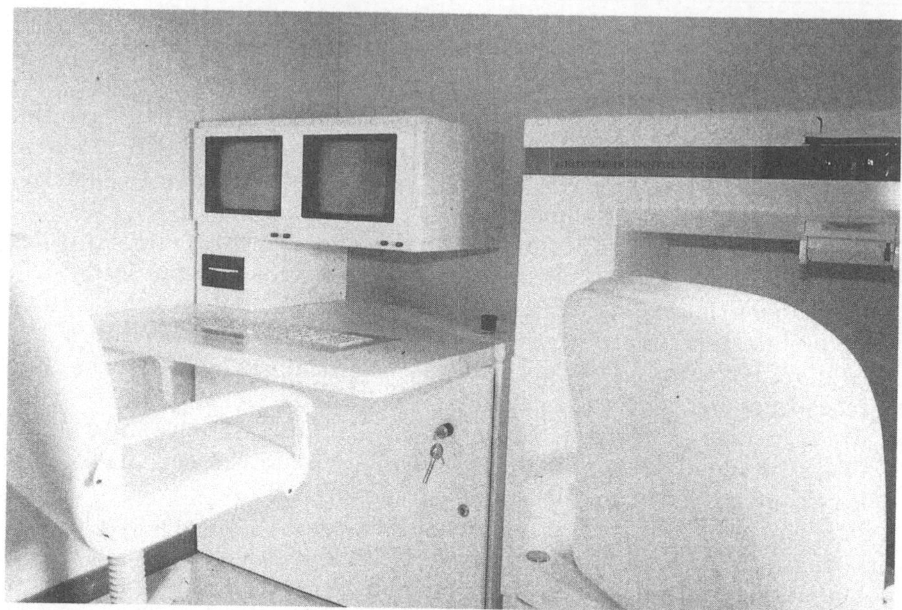

Abb. 1. Laser Tomographic Scanner (LTS) von Heidelberg Instruments. *Links:* Untersuchereinheit mit Rechner, Laufwerk für optische Speicherplatten (zur Archivierung der Untersuchungsergebnisse) und zwei Monitore zur Einstellung des Patientenauges und zur Bilddokumentation, sowie die Tastatur zur Steuerung aller Systemfunktionen. *Rechts:* Patienteneinheit mit Helium-Neon Laser und Scanner

deren Ametropie maximal ± 3 dpt betrug, um Refraktionsskotome auszuschließen und Unsicherheiten bei der Bestimmung objektiver Meßdaten möglichst gering zu halten, da sich der Vergrößerungsfaktor der Papille bei großer Ametropie stark ändert.

Ausschlußkriterien waren Augen mit Aphakie, hoher Myopie, fortgeschrittener Katarakt oder nicht glaukombedingten pathologischen Verände-

Tabelle 1. Diagnose und Anzahl der mit dem Laser Tomographic Scanner untersuchten und nach dem Zufallsprinzip ausgewählten und ausgewerteten Augen

Diagnose	Untersuchte Augen	Patienten = ausgewertete Augen	Glaukomstadien I	II	III bis V
Gesund	70	37			
Okuläre Hypertension	4	2			
Glaucoma chronicum simplex	61	33	26	3	4
Glaukom ohne Hochdruck	18	10	6	2	2
Insgesamt	153	82			

rungen, eine diabetische Retinopathie und der Zustand nach okulären Entzündungen oder Gefäßerkrankungen. Glaukompatienten nach systemischer oder lokaler Steriodtherapie (Steriodglaukom) oder systemischer β-Blocker Therapie (Senkung des Augeninnendrucks) wurden nicht in die Studie aufgenommen.

Patienten mit Glaucoma chronicum simplex zeigten computerperimetrisch quantifizierte Gesichtsfeldausfälle, eine glaukomatöse Papillenexkavation und maximale Augeninnendruckwerte ohne Medikation von mehr als 21 mmHg. Im Mittel betrug der maximale Augeninnendruck ohne Medikation in dieser Gruppe 31.2 ± 2.7 mmHg. Der Kammerwinkel war weit und offen.

Alle Patienten mit Glaukom ohne Hochdruck sind über viele Jahre langzeitbeobachtet, so daß eine Zuordnung dieser Diagnose, die ja eine Ausschlußdiagnose darstellt, mit hoher Sicherheit gegeben ist. Die Diagnose Glaukom ohne Hochdruck wurde dann gestellt, wenn eine glaukomatöse Papillenexkavation und ein glaukomatöser Gesichtsfeldausfall vorlag, wobei wiederholte Tagesdruckkurven ohne Medikation und frühere Messungen des Augeninnendrucks keine Werte größer als 21 mmHg ergeben haben. Der Augeninnendruck lag bei den Patienten mit Glaukom ohne Hochdruck im Mittel bei 18.7 ± 1.3 mmHg und damit an der oberen Grenze des Normbereiches. Die Patienten waren neurologisch untersucht inklusive einer kraniellen Computertomographie und einer Dopplersonographie der Arteria carotis interna, um eine andere Ursache der Gesichtsfeldausfälle auszuschließen. Das mittlere Alter der Patienten mit Glaucoma chronicum simplex lag bei 49,3 Jahren, das der Patienten mit Glaukom ohne Hochdruck bei 51,9 Jahren.

Patienten mit okulärer Hypertension zeigten bei mehrmaligen Kontrollen des Augeninnendrucks erhöhte Werte aber keine computerperimetrisch quantifizierbaren Gesichtsfeldausfälle. Das mittlere Alter der Patienten mit okulärer Hypertension betrug 41,3 Jahre. Der Augeninnendruck bei den Patienten mit okulärer Hypertension lag im Mittel bei 24.1 ± 2.2 mmHg.

Bei gesunden Augen war durch ophthalmoskopische und biomikroskopische Untersuchung einschließlich einer computergesteuerten Gesichtsfelduntersuchung eine Augenerkrankung ausgeschlossen worden. Der Augeninnendruck der Gesunden lag im Mittel bei 15.1 ± 1.7 mmHg. Der Augeninnendruck Gesunder lag damit niedriger als die durchschnittlichen Druckwerte der Patienten mit Niederdruckglaukom dieser Studie, der bei 18.7 ± 1.3 mmHg lag. Im Mittel waren die gesunden Probanden 30,4 Jahre alt.

Gesichtsfeldausfall

Bei allen Patienten lag eine Untersuchung des Gesichtsfeldes mit dem Programm 31 oder Programm G1 des Octopus Perimeters 201 vor. Die Außengrenzen waren mittels Goldmann-Perimeter bestimmt worden. Die Stadieneinteilung der Glaukomerkrankung erfolgte anhand des Gesichtsfeldausfalls [5, 26] – bei Untersuchung mit dem Programm 31 anhand des Total Loss (TL), errechnet mit dem Programm Delta [30], beim Programm Gl anhand des Mean Defects (MD). Die Mean Defect Werte wurden anhand der Umrechnungsgeraden [36] in Total Loss Werte umgerechnet, so daß eine Stadieneinteilung anhand der Total Loss Werte erfolgte.

Konfokales Untersuchungsprinzip des Laser Tomographic Scanners (LTS)

Mit dem Laser Tomographic Scanner (LTS) ist eine dreidimensionale Untersuchung des Augenhintergrundes auch ohne medikamentöse Mydriasis möglich. Der Laser Tomographic Scanner (LTS) besteht aus einer Untersuchereinheit und einer Patienteneinheit. Im Untersucherteil des Gerätes befinden sich der Rechner für die quantitative Auswertung der aufgenommenen Bilder, zwei Monitore für die Benutzerführung und die Bilddokumentation, ein Laufwerk für optische Speicherplatten mit einer Speicherkapazität von je 800 Megabite zur Archivierung der Untersuchungsergebnisse und eine Tastatur zur Steuerung aller Systemfunktionen (vgl. Abb. 1, linker Bildteil). Der Patiententeil enthält die Bildaufnahme-Einheit mit dem Helium-Neon Laser (vgl. Abb. 1. rechter Bildteil).

Nach Bestimmung der Distanz zwischen beiden Pupillen fixiert der Patient mit dem nicht untersuchten Auge einen Leuchtpunkt. Dieser läßt sich mittels Tastatur im Blickfeld des Patienten bewegen, wodurch die Blickrichtung des Patienten gesteuert wird. Eine Videokamera filmt währenddessen das kontralaterale Auge, an dem die Untersuchung der Papille durchgeführt werden soll. Das Bild der Pupille wird auf den linken Bildschirm der Untersuchereinheit übertragen. Durch Veränderung der Stirn- und Kinnstütze des Patienten und ein seitliches Verschieben der Lasereinheit mit Hilfe der Tastatur wird die Pupille des untersuchten Auges auf dem linken Monitor zentriert. Dadurch ist gewährleistet, daß der Laserstrahl die Pupille passieren kann und keine Lichtenergie verloren geht. Mit Hilfe des Fixationspunktes wird die Blickrichtung des Patienten so verändert, daß die zu untersuchende Struktur auf dem rechten Monitor der Untersuchereinheit erscheint.

Bei Untersuchung der Papille fertigt der LTS in einem Bereich (Tiefenbereich), der vom Untersucher festgelegt wird, ähnlich einem Computertomogramm während des Untersuchungsablaufs 32 transversale Schichtbilder (Transversalschnitte) des ausgewählten Objekts – in unserem Fall der Papille – an. Die einzelnen transversalen Schichtbilder erzeugt der LTS über das konfokale Aufnahmeprinzip [49, 50, 56, 60, 62, 69, 80, 100, 102, 104–106], (Abb. 2a, b):

Ein Laserstrahl (HeNe-Laser, $\lambda = 633$ nm) wird durch eine Scanneinrichtung und ein Mikroskopobjektiv zeilenweise über das zu untersuchende Objekt gelenkt. Das vom Objekt reflektierte Licht wird durch einen halbdurchlässigen Spiegel zurückgeleitet und über eine Linse auf den Detektor fokussiert. Vor dem Detektor befindet sich eine *konfokale Blende*, die das Licht ausblendet, das nicht aus der Fokalebene (Ebene des Brennpunktes des Laserlichts = Ebene eines Transversalschnittes) stammt (vgl. Abb. 2a, b).

Liegt das Objekt in der Fokalebene des Laserstrahls, so passiert das reflektierte Licht vollständig die konfokale Blende und wird auf dem Detektor abgebildet. Ein starkes Meßsignal ist die Folge (vgl. Abb. 2a).

Befindet sich das Objekt hinter der Fokalebene, so liegt der Brennpunkt des reflektierten Laserlichts vor der konfokalen Blende und nur ein Streulichtanteil erreicht den Detektor (vgl. Abb. 2b). Ein schwaches Meßsignal ist die Folge. Auf einem Transversalschnitt, der einem konfokalem Bild entspricht, erscheint also nur diejenige Struktur hell, die sich in der Fokalebene des Laserlichts befindet.

Der Laser Tomographic Scanner verschiebt die Fokalebene während eines Untersuchungsganges schrittweise über das zu untersuchende Objekt und nimmt bei jedem Schritt ein konfokales Bild auf. Bei der Untersuchung der

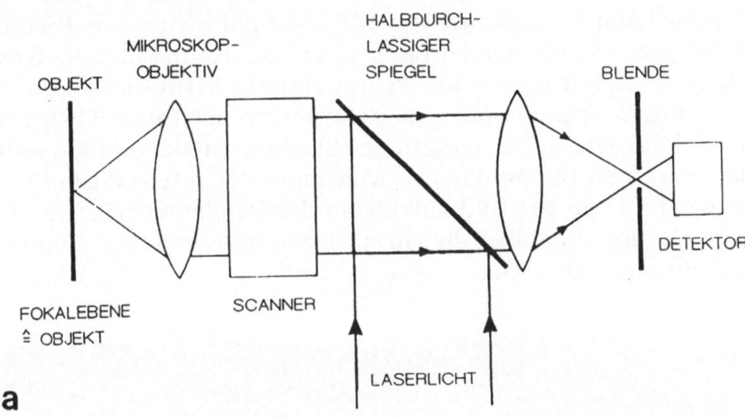

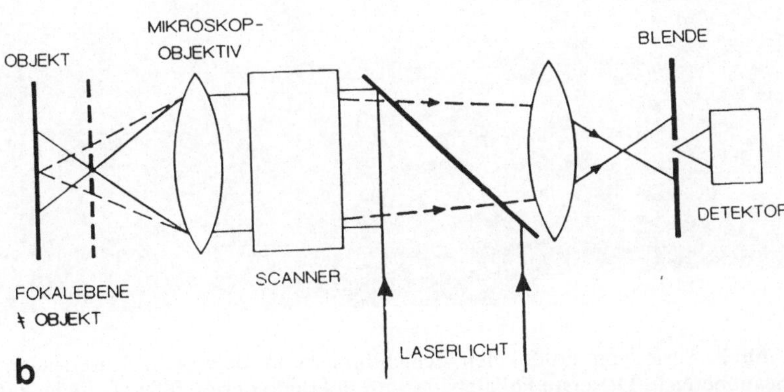

Abb. 2a, b. Das kofokale Untersuchungsprinzip des Laser Tomographic Scanners: **a** Strahlengang des Lasers, wenn sich das Objekt in der Fokalebene befindet; **b** Strahlengang des Lasers, wenn das Objekt hinter der Fokalebene liegt

Papille mit dem konfokalen Untersuchungsprinzip des LTS legt der Untersucher die erste Fokalebene etwa 100 µm oberhalb der Papillengefäße und die letzte Fokalebene etwa 100 µm unterhalb des Exkavationsbodens fest, um eine maximale Information über die dreidimensionale Struktur der Papille zu erhalten. In diesem Bereich, der je nach Exkavationstiefe 1 bis 2 mm beträgt, fertigt der LTS 32 Transversalschnitte an (Abb. 3). Das entspricht einem Abstand der einzelnen Schichtbilder von 30 bis 60µm. Die Aufnahme der 32 Schichtbilder dauert 5 Sekunden. Augenbewegungen des Patienten während dieser Zeitspanne gleicht der Laser Tomographic Scanner (LTS) durch einen Bildlageausgleich der 32 Transversalschnitte bei der Auswertung automatisch aus.

Da sich in der ersten und letzten Fokalebene keine reflektierende Struktur befindet, und das Licht, das aus einer anderen Ebene stammt, ausgeblendet wird, sind diese Bilder bis auf das Grundrauschen dunkel (vgl. Abb. 3 links oben und rechts unten). Dies ist ein Zeichen dafür, daß die gesamte Papillentiefe im Meßbereich enthalten ist. Während der Untersuchung werden beim Verschieben des Mikroskopobjektives in Richtung Exkavationsboden hintereinander die Gefäße, die Retina und die Exkavation hell (Abb. 4). Somit durchläuft das reflektierte Licht eines jeden Bildpunktes eine Intensitätskurve mit einem Ansteigen der Intensität bei Näherrücken der Fokalebene an die anatomische Struktur mit der größten Reflektivität für den einzelnen Bildpunkt. Das Maximum der Intensitätskurve definiert die räumliche Lage des Bildpunktes an der Papillenoberfläche, indem es eine Tiefeninformation über die am stärksten reflektierende anatomische Struktur gibt (vgl. Abb. 4).

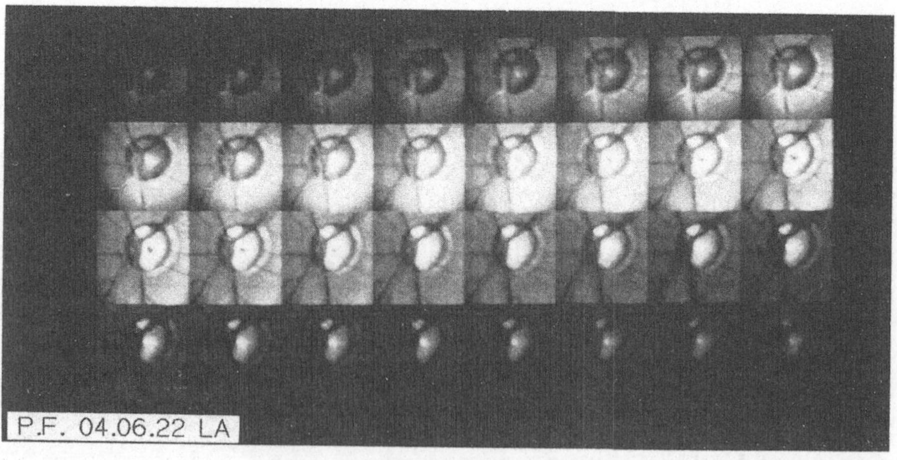

Abb. 3. Serie von konfokalen Schichtbildern in dem vom Untersucher festgelegten Scannbereich. Die erste Fokalebene wird oberhalb der Gefäße (*1. Reihe links*), die letzte unterhalb des Exkavationsbodens (4. Reihe rechts unten) gelegt, so daß der gesamte Tiefenbereich der Papillenexkavation erfaßt wird. Aus diesen 32 Schichtbildern wird die räumliche Struktur errechnet

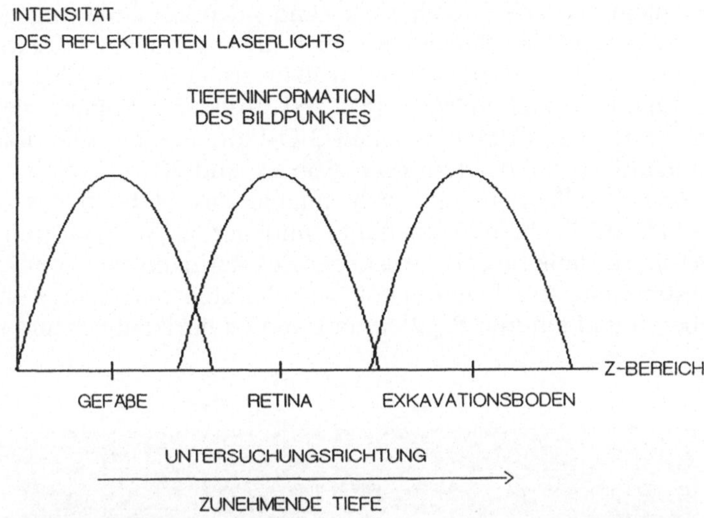

Abb. 4. Intensitätsverteilung des reflektierten Lichts eines Bildpunktes parallel zur optischen Achse während der Untersuchung mit dem Laser Tomographic Scanner. Beim Verschieben der Fokalebene in die Tiefe wird die Intensität des reflektierten Lichts umso größer, je näher die Fokalebene an die anatomische Struktur mit der größten Reflektivität rückt. Bei einer Untersuchung der Papille wird somit jeweils in der Gefäßebene und dem Exkavationsboden ein Intensitätsmaximum erreicht, das eine Tiefeninformation über die jeweilige anatomische Struktur liefert

Befunddarstellungen des Laser Tomographic Scanners

Die einzelnen Schichtbilder setzt der Computer des Laser Tomographic Scanners zu einem Ergebnisbild zusammen (Abb. 5a, oben), das einem Papillenfoto (Abb. 5a, mitte) mit großer Schärfentiefe entspricht. Das zum Papillenbefund gehörige Gesichtsfeld zeigt der Differenzausdruck des Octopus Perimeters 201 in Abb. 5a unten. Um dem Untersucher einen räumlichen Eindruck der Papille zu geben, ist es möglich, die Oberflächenstruktur der Papille, die aus 32 konfokalen Schichtbildern errechnet wird, im Winkel von + 30° bis − 30° auf dem Monitor unter unterschiedlichen Bildwinkeln darzustellen [49, 50].

Die einzelnen Intensitätsmaxima, die für den Computer eine Tiefeninformation der Bildpunkte in dem von uns gewählten 10° Bildausschnitt darstellen, setzt der Computer zu einer Zahlenmatrix zusammen. Durch Farbcodierung dieser Matrix (= Falschfarbendarstellung) erhält man auf dem Monitor ein sogenanntes Höhenbild (Abb. 5b, links unten), auf dem tieferliegende Strukturen heller dargestellt werden als höherliegende. Durch dieses Höhenbild können im Bereich einer Markierung (Cursor) Profilschnitte durch die Papille in der x- und y-Achse (Abb. 5b, rechts unten, links oben) gelegt werden. Dabei wird die räumliche Lage des Cursors auf der

Papillenoberfläche durch x-, y- und z-Koordinaten angegeben (Abb. 5b, rechts oben). Die Anpassung der bisher noch nicht refraktionskorrigierten Meßwerte an die effektiven Größenverhältnisse am Fundus ist durch die Littmann-Formel möglich [67, 68]. Aus der Summe der Profilschnitte errechnet der Computer einen 3-D-Plot, der die Oberfläche der Papille dreidimensional darstellt (vgl. Abb. 9c und 9f).

Der Papillenrand läßt sich anhand des Höhenbildes (meist an einer zirkulären leichten Aufhellung) und der x- und -y-Profilschnitte mittels Scrollertechnik (leichtes Ansteigen des Retinaniveaus vom Papillenrand aus) bestimmen. Aus Koordinaten von Punkten am rechten und linken, bzw. oberen und unteren Papillenrand werden horizontaler und vertikaler Papil-

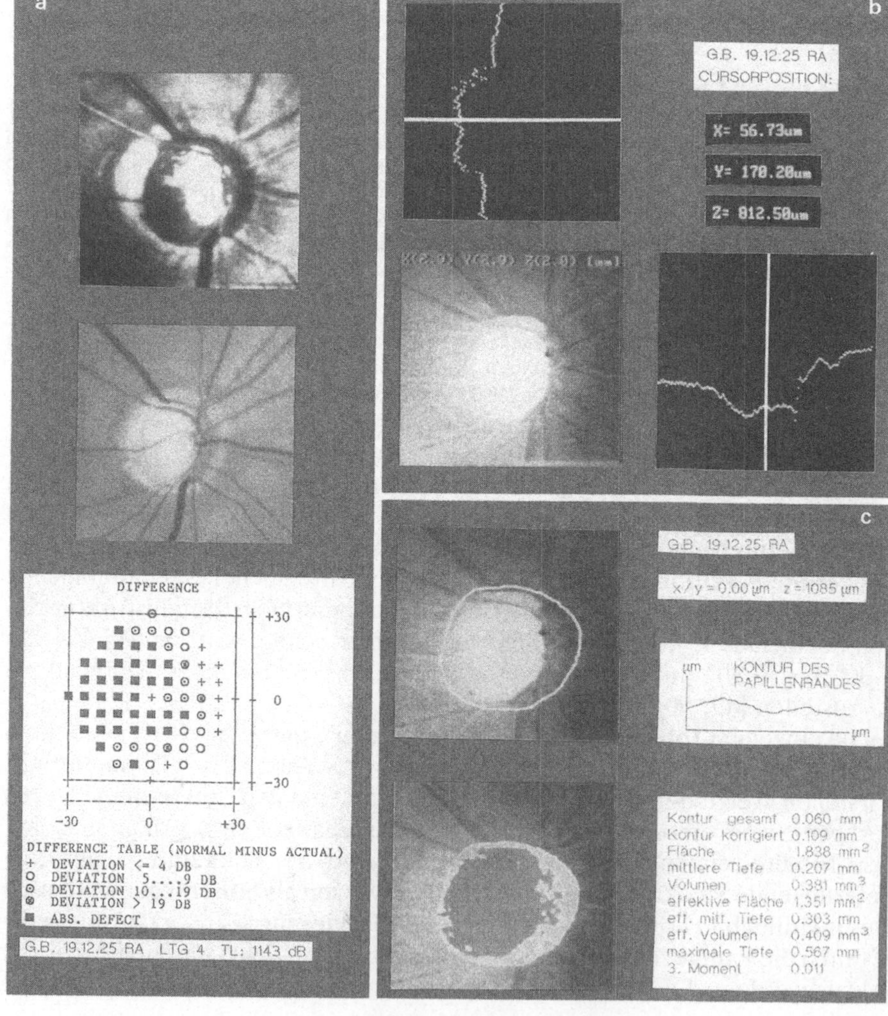

lendurchmesser bestimmt. Dabei wird die Lage der entsprechenden Bildpunkte jeweils mit dem Cursor festgelegt.

Papillenparameter des Laser Tomographic Scanners

Nach Festlegen des Papillenrandes, durch den Untersucher (Abb. 5c, links oben) berechnet der LTS die weiteren Papillenparameter wie z.B. Exkavationsvolumen, Papillengesamtfläche und Exkavationsfläche (effektive Fläche der Papille) und als Tiefenwerte die mittlere und maximale Tiefe der Papillenexkavation (Abb. 5c, rechts unten).

Die Gesamtfläche ergibt sich aus den Bildpunkten, die innerhalb der Konturlinie liegen, die alle Papillenrandpunkte enthält. Da diese Konturlinie dem Papillenrand folgt, weist sie Höhenunterschiede auf. Die Verbindungslinie aus den Höhenwerten am Papillenrand gibt die Referenzebene für die Berechnungen von Exkavationsvolumen und Exkavationsfläche an. Somit ist die Referenzebene, die zur Berechnung der Papillenparameter herangezogen wird, keine gerade Ebene, sondern eine in sich vielgestaltig gekrümmte Oberfläche, die dem Konturverlauf des Papillenrandes aufliegt [21]. Die Konturlinie des Papillenrandes im gesamten Umfang des Papillenrandes zeigt Abb. 5c, rechts oben. Die beiden Gipfel stellen den oberen bzw. unteren Papillenpol mit den Gefäßen dar. Die Exkavationsfläche, vom Computer unter der Bezeichnung effektive Fläche ausgedruckt (vgl. Abb. 5c, rechts unten), errechnet sich aus den Bildpunkten, die unterhalb der Referenz-

Abb. 5. a. Papille und Gesichtsfeldbefund des linken Auges einer 65jährigen Patientin mit Glaukom ohne Hochdruck, Stadium 4: *oben:* errechnetes Papillenbild, *mitte:* Foto derselben Papille, *unten:* Gesichtsfeldbefund desselben Auges.
b *Unten links:* Farbcodiertes Höhenbild der in **a** gezeigten Papille, dieses Bild wird auf dem Monitor dargestellt. Für eine Tiefenmessung wird vom Untersucher auf diesem errechneten Bild die gewünschte Meßposition markiert (hier: Markierung in Papillenmitte). Durch diesen Meßpunkt kann wahlweise ein vertikaler *(links oben)* oder ein horizontaler *(rechts unten)* Profilschnitt gelegt werden. *Rechts oben:* Bildausschnitt des Monitorbildes: der Meßpunkt wird in räumlichen Koordinaten (x, y, z) dargestellt. Der Z-Wert gibt den Tiefenwert der jeweiligen Meßposition an.
c *links oben:* Farbcodiertes Höhenbild der in **a** gezeigten Papille, dieses Bild wird auf dem Monitor dargestellt. Durch Bewegen des Meßpunktes mittels eines Scrollers wird der Papillenrand mit Hilfe der in **b** gezeigten Profilschnitte per Hand festgelegt und vom Computer als Konturlinie auf dem Papillenrand im Höhenbild dargestellt. *Rechts oben:* Der Papillenrand wird nicht durch eine Ebene festgelegt, sondern durch eine Konturlinie, die sich den Höhendifferenzen des Papillenrandes anpaßt. Der Höhenverlauf der Konturlinie, die *links oben* dargestellt ist, wird so als Profil dargestellt. Darüber sind die räumlichen Koordinaten (x, y, z) des in der Papille positionierten Cursors gezeigt. *Links unten:* Entlang der Konturlinie des Papillenrandes legt der Computer eine Referenzebene über die Papille, die durch die Unregelmäßigkeiten des Papillenrandes keine gerade Ebene ist, sondern sich den anatomischen Verhältnissen anpaßt. Der Computer kennzeichnet die Strukturen, die innerhalb des Papillenrandes oberhalb der Referenzebene liegen grün, die Strukturen, die unterhalb des Papillenrandes liegen, orange. *Rechts unten:* Papillenparameter des Lasertomographicscanners, die auf dem Monitor dargestellt werden

ebene liegen, die Bildpunkte oberhalb der Referenzebene werden hierbei ausgeschlossen (Abb. 5c, links unten). Diese ausgeschlossenen Flächen sind in Abb. 5c, links unten grün vom Computer auf dem Bildschirm markiert. Es verbleibt die sogenannte effektive Exkavationsfläche, orange dargestellt in Abb. 5c, links unten. Da das Papillengewebe ausgehend vom Papillenrand durch die größere der Dichte der Nervenfasern leicht ansteigt, bevor es nach hinten zum Niveau des Opticus umbiegt [4], fallen Papillenrand und Exkavationsrand in der Regel nicht zusammen.

Die mittlere Exkavationstiefe, vom Computer unter der Bezeichnung effektive mittlere Tiefe ausgedruckt (vgl. Abb. 5c, rechts unten), errechnet sich aus den Tiefenwerten innerhalb der effektiven Exkavationsfläche als der Mittelwert aus circa 10 000 unabhängigen Bildpunkten (Pixeln). Diejenigen 5% aller Bildpunkte der Exkavation, die bezogen zur Referenzebene am tiefsten liegen, werden zur Berechnung der maximalen Tiefe herangezogen. Der Mittelwert dieser 5% Bildpunkte ergibt den maximalen Tiefenwert [105].

Das Exkavationsvolumen, vom Computer unter der Bezeichnung effektives Volumen ausgedruckt (vgl. Abb. 5c, rechts unten), errechnet sich aus dem Volumen, das unterhalb der Referenzebene liegt (siehe abb. 5c).

Vom Papillenrand aus ansteigendes Gewebe, das oberhalb oder auf gleicher Höhe mit der Referenzebene liegt, wird zur Berechnung des oberen Volumens herangezogen (vgl. Abb. 5c, links unten grün markierter Bereich). Abbildung 6 zeigt die beschriebenen Papillenparameter nochmals schematisch auf.

Form der Papillenexkavation errechnet aus dem Verhältnis effektive mittlere Tiefe der Papillenexkavation (HE) zu maximaler Tiefe der Papillenexkavation (HM)

Für diese Studie soll aus den Tiefenwerten der Papillenexkavation ein Rückschluß auf die Steilheit der Exkavationsränder und der Form des Exkavationsbodens bei Glaucoma chronicum simplex und Glaukom ohne Hochdruck gezogen werden. Hierzu wird der maximale Tiefenwert und die mittlere effektive Tiefe der untersuchen Papille herangezogen. Die beiden Werte werden im Verhältnis

$$\frac{\text{effektive mittlere Tiefe HE}}{\text{maximaler Tiefe HM}}$$

betrachtet.

Um eine Aussage über die Form der Papillenexkavation machen zu können, werden die beiden Tiefenwerte der Papillenexkavation HE (effektive mittlere Tiefe) und HM (maximale Tiefe) zueinander in Beziehung gesetzt. Einzeln ermöglichen sie keine Aussage über die Form der Exkavation. Einerseits stellt die maximale Tiefe nur einen abstrakten Meßwert des

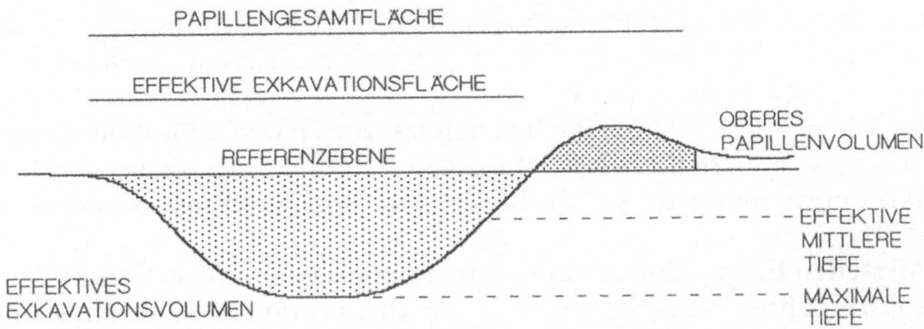

Abb. 6. Papillenparameter des Laser Tomographic Scanners: *Papillengesamtfläche:* Alle Bildpunkte innerhalb der Konturlinie, die den Papillenrand markiert. *Effektive Fläche:* Alle Bildpunkte innerhalb der Konturlinie (Papillenrand) die unterhalb der Referenzebene entlang der Konturlinie liegen. Sie entspricht etwa der ophthalmoskopisch sichtbaren Exkavationsfläche. *Effektives Volumen:* Exkavationsvolumen unterhalb der Referenzebene.
Oberes Volumen: Volumen aller Strukturen oberhalb der Referenzebene. *Effektive mittlere Tiefe:* Mittelwert aller Tiefenwerte unterhalb der effektiven Fläche. Sie gibt die mittlere Tiefe der Exkavation an. *Maximale Tiefe:* Mittelwert der 5% Bildpunkte mit den größten Tiefenwerte unterhalb der effektiven Fläche. Sie ist eine Maßzahl für die maximale Tiefe der Exkavation

Papillenbodens dar und bezieht weitere Meßpunkte nicht mit ein. Die effektive mittlere Tiefe andererseits erlaubt keinen Rückschluß auf den tiefsten Punkt des Papillenbodens, da in diesem Wert die Tiefenwerte gemittelt werden. In Abhängigkeit voneinander jedoch lassen sich Rückschlüsse auf die Steilheit der Exkavationsränder und den Verlauf des Exkavationsbodens ziehen:

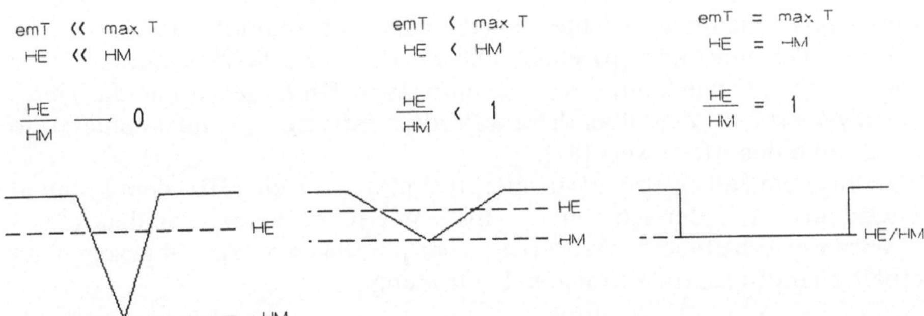

Abb. 7a–c. Das Verhältnis effektive mittlere Tiefe (HE) zu maximaler Tiefe (HM) bei unterschiedlichen Papillenformen. **a** Bei *steilen* Exkavationsrändern und *spitzem* Exkavationsboden geht das Verhältnis HE/HM gegen 0. **b** Bei *flachen* Exkavationsrändern und *spitzem* Exkavationsboden liegt das Verhältnis HE/HM zwischen 0 und 1. Dies entspricht der Form einer gesunden Papille bzw. einer Papille im Anfangsstadium der Glaucoma chronicum simplex. **c** Bei *steilen* Exkavationsrändern und *flachem* Exkavationsboden liegt das Verhältnis HE/HM bei 1. Dies entspricht der Form einer Papille im fortgeschrittenen Stadium der Glaukomerkrankung

Bei steilen Exkavationsrändern mit flachem Exkavationsboden geht das Verhältnis HE/HM gegen 1, da effektive mittlere Tiefe und maximale Tiefe sich einander annähern (Abb. 7c)

– Bei flachem Exkavationsrändern mit spitzem Exkavationsboden geht das rechnerische Verhältnis HE/HM gegen 0.3 bis 0.5, da die maximale Tiefe stets etwa doppelt so groß ist wie die effektive mittlere Tiefe (Abb. 7b).

– Bei steilen Exkavationsrändern mit einem spitzen Exkavationsboden geht das Verhältnis HE/HM gegen 0, da die maximale Tiefe stets um ein Vielfaches größer ist als die effektive mittlere Tiefe (Abb. 7a).

Mit Zunahme der Steilheit der Exkavationsränder und Abflachung des Exkavationsbodens, wie es mit Fortschreiten der Glaukomerkrankung bereits ophthalmoskopisch erkennbar ist, strebt das Verhältnis aus effektiver mittlerer Tiefe zu maximaler Tiefe gegen 1.

Form der Papillenexkavation errechnet aus dem dritten zentralen Moment

Ein weiterer Rückschluß auf die Exkavationsform ist durch das 3. zentrale Moment möglich, das in diesem Fall eine Aussage über die Häufigkeit von Tiefenwerten der Papille gibt.

Mathematische Grundlagen:

a) Moment 1. Ordnung = Erwartungswert = Mittelwert

$$\alpha_1 = \int\limits_{-\infty}^{+\infty} x^1 \, f(x) \, dx$$

Ein x-Wert wird mit der Dichte (f(x) dx = Dichtefunktion) multipliziert, die der Wahrscheinlichkeit (p) entspricht mit der der x-Wert an dieser Stelle vorkommt, d.h. wie häufig es zu jedem x-Wert (In dieser Studie die Tiefe) einen y-Wert gibt. Wird über diesem Produkt integriert (= aufsummiert), so erhält man den Mittelwert [87].

In unserem Fall entspricht die effektive mittlere Tiefe (HE) dem Moment 1. Ordnung. Der Bereich von $+\infty$ bis $-\infty$ entspräche der Papillentiefe.

Wird der erhaltene Mittelwert α_1 vom jeweiligen x-Wert abgezogen, so erhält man das zentrale Moment 1. Ordnung.

$$\mu_1 = \int\limits_{-\infty}^{+\infty} (x - \alpha_1)^1 \, f(x) \, dx$$

b) zentrales Moment 2. Ordnung = Varianz

$$\mu_2 = \int\limits_{-\infty}^{+\infty} (x - \alpha_1)^2 \, f(x) \, dx$$

Hierdurch wird gezeigt, wie die Werte der Verteilungsfunktion um den Mittelwert gestreut sind. Das Maß für die Streuung ist die Varianz. Bei der Verwendung des Moments 2. Ordnung (= Quadratmittel) würde man keine Aussage über die Verteilung bekommen. Es muß also vom jeweiligen x-Wert der Mittelwert α_1 abgezogen werden (= zentrales Moment 2. Ordnung) um eine Aussage über die Streuung der x-Werte um den Mittelwert α_1 zu erhalten [87].

c) Zentrales Moment 3. Ordnung = 3. Zentralmoment
   = Maßzahl für die Assymetrie = Schiefe

$$\mu_3 = \int_{-\infty}^{+\infty} (x - \alpha_1)^3 \, f(x) \, dx$$

Das zentrale 3. Moment gibt die Schiefe einer Dichtefunktion an, d.h. mit welcher Häufigkeit ein Tiefenwert in der Papillenexkavation zu erwarten ist [87].

Das zentrale 3. Moment läßt somit Rückschlüsse auf die Papillenform zu: Über die Dichtefunktion wird angegeben, wie häufig ein Tiefenwert in der Papillenexkavation vorkommt. Hierbei gibt es prinzipiell zwei Möglichkeiten:

– Bei flachen Exkavationsrändern mit relativ spitzen Exkavationsboden gibt es viele kleine Tiefenwerte und wenig große Tiefenwerte. Die Steigung der Geraden der Dichtefunktion wird somit negativ sein (Abb. 8, gestrichelte Gerade).

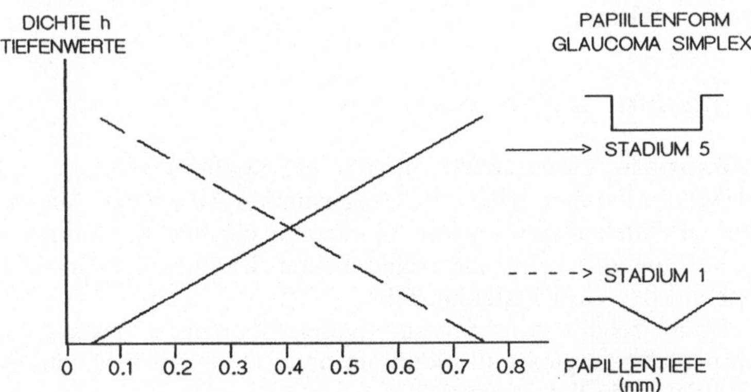

Abb. 8. Häufigkeitsverteilung der Tiefenwerte in Papillen bei unterschiedlicher Papillenform. *Rechts unten:* Papillenform im Anfangsstadium bei Glaucoma simplex. Diese weist viele kleine Tiefenwerte auf, aber nur wenig große, da der Exkavationsrand flach abfällt. Die Steigung der Geraden für die Dichtefunktion ist somit negativ *(gestrichelte Gerade).* *Rechts oben:* Papillenform im Endstadium der Glaukomerkrankung. Diese weist viele große Tiefenwerte auf, aber nur wenig kleine, da der Exkavationsrand steil abfällt. Die Steigung der Geraden für die Dichtefunktion ist somit positiv *(durchgezogene Gerade)*

– Bei steilen Exkavationsrändern mit flachem Exkavationsboden gibt es innerhalb einer Papille nur wenig kleine Tiefenwerte, aber dafür viele große Tiefenwerte. Die Steigung der Geraden der Dichtefunktion wird positiv sein (Abb. 8, durchgezogene Gerade).

Bei Gesunden und Patienten mit okulärer Hypertension und Glaukom mit bzw. ohne Augeninnendruckerhöhung im Anfangsstadium ist eine schiefe Grundsymmetrie mit einem negativen Vorzeichen zu erwarten, da normalerweise in einer gesunden Papille mit einer physiologischen Exkavation (vgl. Abb. 8, rechts unten) mehr geringe Tiefenwerte als große Tiefenwerte vorkommen. Mit zunehmender glaukomatöser Exkavation (vgl. Abb. 8, rechts oben) nimmt die Anzahl der kleinen Tiefenwerte ab und die großer Tiefenwerte zu. Es erfolgt im Laufe der Glaukomerkrankung ein Vorzeichenwechsel der schiefen Grundsymmetrie von negativ nach positiv.

Signifikanzberechnung

In dieser Studie erfolgte die Berechnung der Signifikanz zweier Stichproben, die unverbunden waren, nach dem U-Test von Wilcoxon, Mann und Whitney [87]. Ergebnisse der Signifikanzberechnung mit dem U-Test von Wilcoxon, Mann und Whitney [87], die eine Irrtumswahrscheinlichkeit $p \leq 0.05$ ergaben, wurden als signifikant gewertet.

Ergebnisse der Berechnung, die eine Irrtumswahrscheinlichkeit p größer/gleich 0.05 ergaben, wurden als nicht signifikant gewertet.

Ergebnisse

Tiefe der Papillenexkavation

Maximale Tiefe (HM). Tabelle 2a, Spalte 1 zeigt die maximale Tiefe (HM) der Papillenexkavation bei gesunden Augen und Augen von Patienten mit okulärer Hypertension, Glaucoma chronicum simplex und Glaukom ohne Hochdruck im unterschiedlichen Stadium der Erkrankung definiert anhand des Gesichtsfeldausfalls.

Dabei zeigt sich, daß beim stadienabhängigen Vergleich von Glaucoma chronicum simplex und Glaukom ohne Hochdruck für das Stadium 1 eine deutliche, für das Stadium 2, sowie den Vergleich der Stadien 3 bis 5 jeweils eine signifikant geringere maximale Tiefe (HM) der Papillenexkavation beim Glaukom ohne Hochdruck besteht ($p < 0.01$).

Der Vergleich der maximalen Tiefe (HM) der Papillenexkavation zwischen Augen im Stadium 1 der beiden Glaukomformen und gesunden Augen ergibt keinen signifikanten Unterschied in der maximalen Exkavationstiefe ($0.1 < p < 0.05$).

Tabelle 2a. Meßergebnisse für die maximale Tiefe der Papillenexkavation (*HM*), die effektive mittlere Tiefe der Papillenexkavation (*HE*), dem Verhältis *HE/HM* und des 3. Zentralmoments geordnet nach Diagnosegruppen (n = Anzahl der ausgewerteten Augen in einer Diagnosegruppe). Signifikante Unterschiede sind gekennzeichnet. Diese sind in der Tabelle 2b nochmals schematisch aufgezeigt

Diagnose	n	Maximale Tiefe HM (mm)		Effektive mittlere Tiefe HE (mm)		HE/HM		3. Zentralmoment	
Gesund	37	0.42 ± 0.14	] $p < 0.01$	0.16 ± 0.06	] $p < 0.01$	0.37 ± 0.06	] $0.2\ p < 0.64$	-0.16 ± 0.09	] $0.2 < p < 0.64$
Okuläre Hypertension	2	0.64 ± 0.03	]	0.25 ± 0.02	]	0.38 ± 0.02	]	-0.15 ± 0.03	]
Glaucoma chronicum simplex Stadium 1	26	0.53 ± 0.20	] $p > 0.1$	0.21 ± 0.10	] $p > 0.64$	0.39 ± 0.06	] $p < 0.0001$	-0.14 ± 0.07	] $p < 0.01$
Glaukom ohne Hochdruck Stadium 1	6	0.49 ± 0.20	]	0.24 ± 0.10	]	0.49 ± 0.07	]	-0.03 ± 0.08	]
Glaucoma chronicum simplex Stadium 2	3	0.59 ± 0.24	] $p < 0.01$	0.27 ± 0.17	] $0.01 < p < 0.05$	0.44 ± 0.09	] $p < 0.01$	-0.06 ± 0.13	] < 0.01
Glaukom ohne Hochdruck Stadium 2	2	0.31 ± 0.04	]	0.19 ± 0.07	]	0.61 ± 0.13	]	$+0.12 \pm 0.14$	]
Glaucoma chronicum simplex Stadium 3 bis 5	4	0.71 ± 0.32	] $p < 0.01$	0.36 ± 0.21	] $0.38 < p < 0.64$	0.60 ± 0.10	] $0.2 < p < 0.64$	$+0.12 \pm 0.09$	] $0.2 < p < 0.64$
Glaukom ohne Hochdruck Stadium 3 bis 5	2	0.55 ± 0.06	]	0.31 ± 0.05	]	0.59 ± 0.06	]	$+0.07 \pm 0.05$	]

Der Vergleich der maximalen Tiefe (HM) der Papillenexkavation zwischen Augen mit okulärer Hypertension und gesunden Augen ergibt einen signifikanten Unterschied (p < 0.01).

Bei Augen mit Glaukom ohne Hochdruck sind somit insgesamt betrachtet, als auch bei Betrachtung der Stadien im einzelnen geringere maximale Exkavationstiefen vorhanden als bei Augen mit Glaucoma chronicum simplex.

Mittlere Tiefe (HE). Die effektive mittlere Tiefe (HE) der Papillenexkavation bei gesunden Augen und Augen von Patienten mit okulärer Hypertension, Glaucoma chronicum simplex und Glaukom ohne Hochdruck im unterschiedlichen Stadium der Erkrankung definiert anhand des Gesichtsfeldausfalls zeigt Tabelle 2a, Spalte 2.

Augen mit Glaucoma chronicum simplex Stadium 1 und Glaukom ohne Hochdruck Stadium 1 zeigen keine signifikanten Unterschiede in der effektiven mittleren Tiefe (HE) (p > 0.64). Es besteht im Gegensatz zur maximalen Tiefe (HM) ein geringfügig höherer Wert bei Augen mit Glaukom ohne Hochdruck. Im Stadium 2 besteht ein signifikanter Unterschied mit einer geringeren effektiven mittlere Tiefe (HE) der Papillenexkavation beim Glaukom ohne Hochdruck (0.01 < p < 0.05). In den fortgeschrittenen Stadien 3 bis 5 bestehen keine signifikanten Unterschiede mehr zwischen Glaucoma chronicum simplex und Glaukom ohne Hochdruck (0.38 < p < 0.64).

Bei Augen mit Glaukom ohne Hochdruck ist die effektive mittlere Tiefe (HE) der Papillenexkavation signifikant größer als bei gesunden Augen (p < 0.01). Dies trifft auch für Augen mit Glaucoma chronicum simplex und okulärer Hypertension im Vergleich zu gesunden Augen zu (p < 0.01).

Form der Papillenexkavation

Verhältnis effektive mittlere Tiefe zu maximaler Tiefe (HE/HM). Dieser Verhältniswert erlaubt eine Aussage über die Exkavationsform bei Augen mit Glaucoma chronicum simplex und Glaukom ohne Hochdruck. Die Form der Papillenexkavation, berechnet aus dem Verhältnis effektive mittlere Tiefe der Papillenexkavation (HE) zu maximaler Tiefe der Papillenexkavation (HM), zeigt Tabelle 2a, Spalte 3.

Je größer der Quotient HE/HM ist, desto steiler sind die Exkavationsränder und umso größer ist der Exkavationsboden.

Das Glaukom ohne Hochdruck weist im Stadium 1 signifikant steilere Exkavationsränder und einen flacheren Exkavationsboden als das Glaucoma chronicum simplex Stadium 1 auf (p < 0.0001). Im Stadium 2 bestehen wiederum beim Glaukom ohne Hochdruck die signifikant steileren Exkavationsränder und der flachere Exkavationsboden (p < 0.01). In den fortgeschrittenen Stadien 3 bis 5 bestehen keine signifikanten Unterschiede zwischen Augen mit Glaucoma chronicum simplex und Glaukom ohne Hochdruck mehr (0.2 < p < 0.64). Tabelle 2b zeigt die signifikanten Unterschiede in der Form der Papillenexkavation bei den einzelnen Diagnosegruppen nochmals schematisch auf.

Keine signifikanten Unterschiede in der Steilheit der Exkavationsränder und der Form des Exkavationsbodens bestehen zwischen Augen mit Glaucoma chronicum simplex Stadium 1, okulärer Hypertension und gesunden Augen ($0.2 < p < 0.64$). Das Glaukom ohne Hochdruck zeigt jedoch signifikante Unterschiede in der Form der Exkavation zu diesen drei Diagnosegruppen ($p < 0.0001$) mit steileren Exkavationsrändern und einem flacheren Exkavationsboden (vgl. Tabelle 2b).

Die absoluten Zahlen beim Glaukom ohne Hochdruck zeigen nur eine geringgradige Zunahme der primär schon sehr steilen Exkavationsränder beim Vergleich der Stadien 1, 2 und 3 bis 5. Beim Glaucoma chronicum simplex tritt die Zunahme der Steilheit der Exkavationsränder kontinuierlich und langsam auf und erreicht in den Endstadien gleiche Werte wie beim Glaukom ohne Hochdruck.

Die Unterschiede in der Steilheit der Exkavationsränder und der Form des Exkavationsbodens liegen beim Glaukom ohne Hochdruck beim Übergang von gesund zu Stadium 1, während die Vergrößerung der Steilheit der Exkavationsränder beim Glaucoma chronicum simplex erst beim Übergang vom Stadium 1 in das Stadium 2 der Glaukomerkrankung erreicht wird. Bezogen auf den Gesichtsfeldausfall tritt die Änderung der Papillenform beim Glaucoma chronicum simplex ein Erkrankungsstadium später auf als beim Glaukom ohne Hochdruck.

Dies bedeutet, daß Patienten mit Glaucoma chronicum simplex im Anfangsstadium eine Exkavationsform zeigen, die sich nicht von der Gesunder oder Patienten mit okulärer Hypertension mit flachen Exkavationsrändern und einem relativ spitzen Exkavationsboden unterscheidet (vgl.

Tabelle 2b. Signifikante (∗) und nicht signifikante (ns) Unterschiede in der Form der Papillenexkavation bestimmt mit dem Verhältnis zwischen effektiver mittlerer Tiefe (HE) zu maximaler Tiefe der Papillenexkavation und bestimmt mit dem 3. Zentramoment zeigen ein übereinstimmendes Ergebnis. Die Ergebnisse von Tabelle 2a werden daher schematisch zusammengefaßt: Es zeigt sich ein *signifikanter Unterschied* in der Form der Papillenexkavation zwischen Augen mit Glaucoma chronicum simplex und Augen mit Glaukom ohne Hochdruck in den Stadien 1 und 2. In den Stadien 3 bis 5 ist dieser *nicht mehr signifikant*. Es findet sich *kein signifikanter* Unterschied in der Form der Papillenexkavation zwischen gesunden Augen, Augen mit okulärer Hypertension und Augen mit Glaucoma simplex Stadium 1

Gesichtsfeld-ausfall	Gesund	Okuläre Hypertension	Glaucoma simplex	Glaukom ohne Hochdruck
Kein	ns ————	ns		
Stadium 1		ns ————	ns ∗ ————	∗
Stadium 2			∗ ————	∗
Stadium 3 bis 5			ns ————	ns

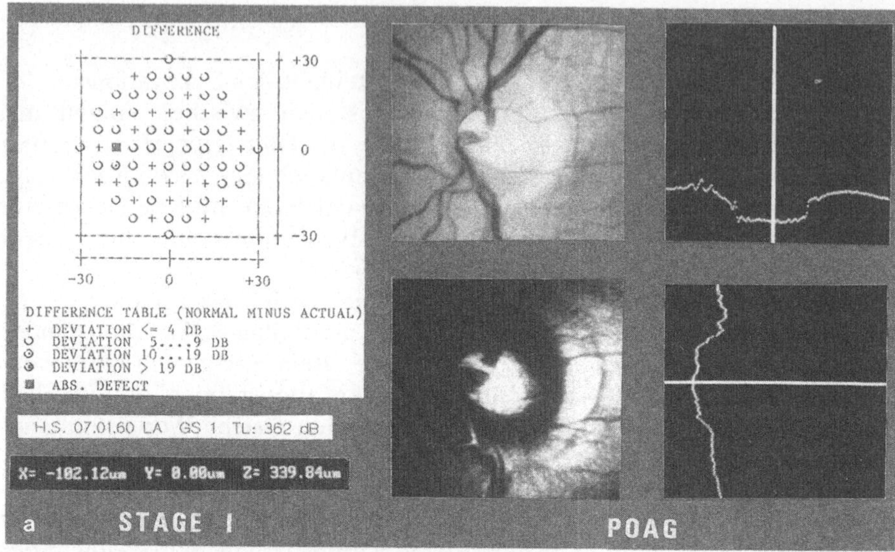

Abb. 9a. Papillenbefund des linken Auges einer 30jährigen Patientin mit Glaucoma chronicum simplex im Stadium 1 des Gesichtsfeldausfalls. *Links oben:* Gesichtsfeldbefund des linken Auges im Differenzwertausdruck des Programms 31 des Octopus Perimeters 201 mit ausschließlich relativen Skotomen. *Links unten:* Position des Meßpunktes in Papillenmitte. *Mitte oben:* Foto der Papille des linken Auges. *Mitte unten:* Vom Laser Tomographic Scanner errechnetes Papillenbild. *Rechts oben:* Horizontaler Profilschnitt durch die Papillenmitte. *Rechts unten:* Vertikaler Profilschnitt durch die Papillenmitte

Abb. 7b). Abbildung 9a zeigt den Papillen- und Gesichtsfeldbefund des linken Auges bei einer Patientin mit Glaucoma chronicum simplex im Stadium 1 der Erkrankung. Patienten mit Glaukom ohne Hochdruck – Abb. 9b zeigt den Papillen- und Gesichtsfeldbefund des linken Auges einer Patientin mit Glaukom ohne Hochdruck ebenfalls Stadium 1 des Gesichtsfeldausfalls. Bereits im Anfangsstadium zeigt die Patientin mit Glaukom ohne Hochdruck steilere Exkavationsränder und einen flacheren Exkavationsboden als die Patientin mit Glaucoma chronicum simplex. Die steileren Exkavationsränder beim Glaukom ohne Hochdruck im Stadium 1 sind auch in der dreidimensionalen Darstellungsweise der 3-D-Ausdrucke in Abb. 9c sichtbar.

Dieser Unterschied ist, wie in Tabelle 2a und 2b dargestellt, im fortgeschrittenen Stadium der Glaukomerkrankung nicht mehr vorhanden. So zeigt Abb. 9d die glaukomatöse Papille bei Glaucoma chronicum simplex Stadium 4 und Abb. 9e die Papillenexkavation bei Glaukom ohne Hochdruck Stadium 4 des Gesichtsfeldausfalls. Die Profilschnitte durch die Papillenexkavation in Abb. 9d und 9e lassen ebenso wie die dreidimensionale Darstellung der 3-D-Ausdrucke in Abb. 9f keine Unterschiede mehr erkennen.

Drittes zentrales Moment der Tiefenwerte. Dieser Wert erlaubt eine Aussage über Unterschiede in der Form der Papillenexkavation bei

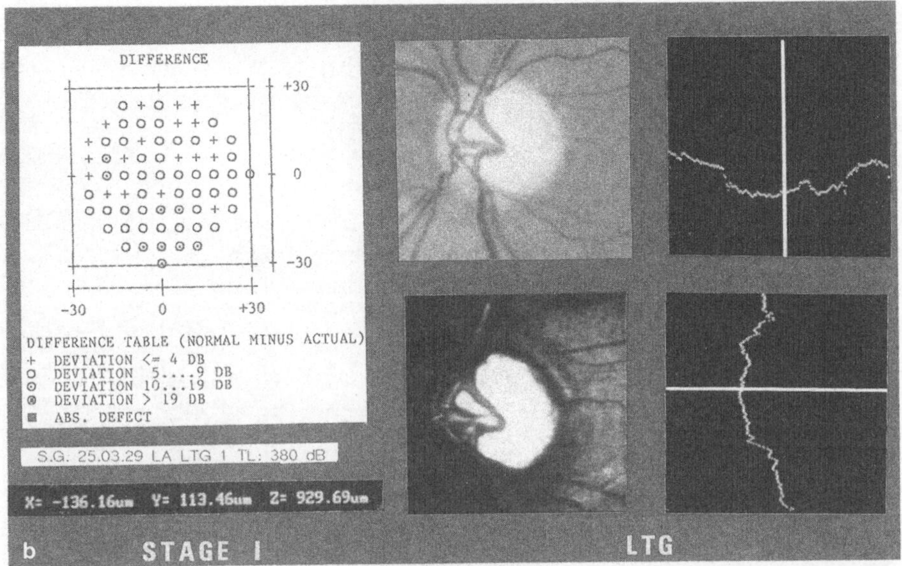

Abb. 9b. Papillenbefund des linken Auges einer 61jährigen Patientin mit Glaukom ohne Hochdruck im Stadium 1 des Gesichtsfeldausfalls. Die Anordnung der Befunde entspricht der **Abb. 9a.** Im Vergleich zur Papille mit Glaucoma chronicum simplex Stadium 1 (vgl. Abb. **9a**) zeigt sich eine deutlich größere Papillenexkavation. Beim Vergleich der Profilschnitte erscheinen hier bei Glaukom ohne Hochdruck die Exkavationsränder steiler und der Exkavationsboden flacher als in Abb. **9a** beim Glaucoma chronicum simplex bei gleichem Stadium des Gesichtsfeldausfalls. Obwohl sich der Gesichtsfeldbefund bei den beiden Augen entspricht (362 dB Total Loss bei Glaucoma chronicum simplex und 380 dB Total Loss bei Glaukom ohne Hochdruck) zeigt das Auge mit Glaukom ohne Hochdruck eine deutlich größere Papillenexkavation

gesunden Augen und Augen von Patienten mit okulärer Hypertension, Glaucoma chronicum simplex und Glaukom ohne Hochdruck. Das dritte zentrale Moment beschreibt die Form der Papillenexkavation nicht als ein Verhältnis von Tiefenwerten wie der HE/HM-Wert, sondern als eine Häufigkeitsangabe von Tiefenwerten in der Papillenexkavation (Vgl. Methodik, 7., vgl. Abb. 8). Dargestellt wird das 3. Zentralmoment der Tiefenwerte als Steigung der Geraden für die Dichtefunktion. Das 3. Zentralmoment der Tiefenwerte zeigt Tabelle 2a, Spalte 4 bei gesunden Augen und Augen von Patienten mit okulärer Hypertension, Glaucoma chronicum simplex und Glaukom ohne Hochdruck in unterschiedlichen Stadien der Erkrankung definiert anhand des Gesichtsfeldausfalls.

Je positiver (+) die Steigung der Geraden für die Dichtefunktion der Tiefenwerte ist, desto steiler sind die Exkavationsränder und desto flacher ist der Exkavationsboden.

Im Stadium 1 der Glaukomerkrankung weisen Augen mit Glaukom ohne Hochdruck eine signifikant flachere Steigung der Geraden für die Dichtefunktion der Tiefenwerte als Augen mit Glaucoma chronicum simplex

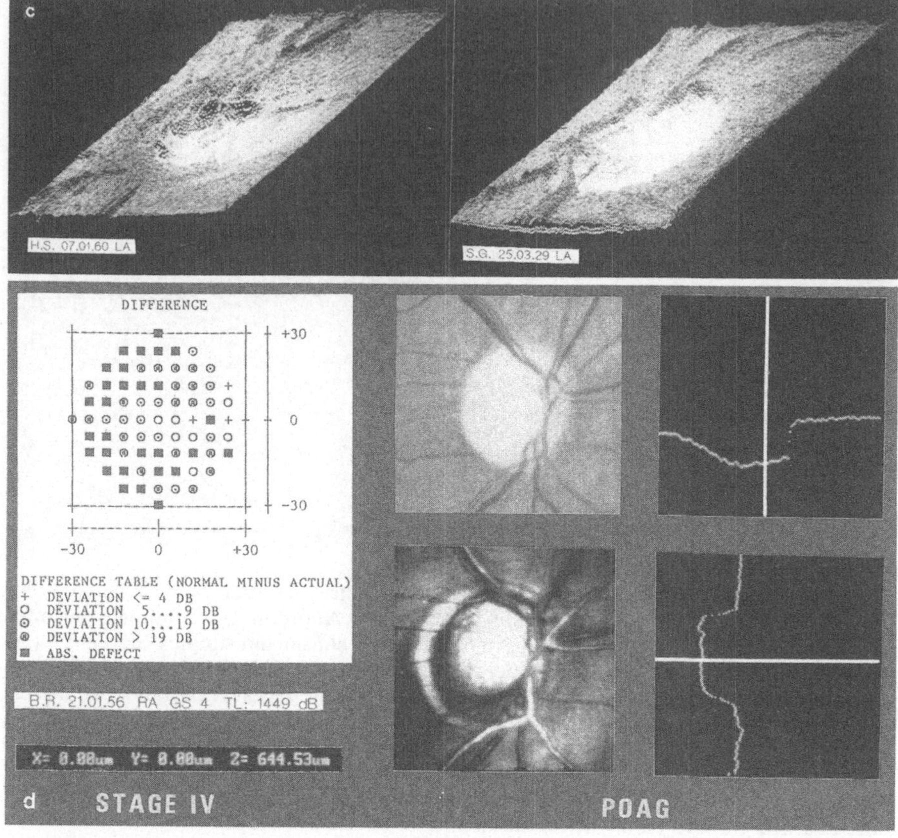

Abb. 9c. 3-D-Ausdrucke der in Abb. **9a** dargestellten Papille mit Glaucoma chronicum simplex *(links)* und der in Abb. **9b** dargestellten Papille mit Glaukom ohne Hochdruck *(rechts)* im Stadium 1 des Gesichtsfeldausfalls. In dieser dreidimensionalen Darstellung der Papille zeigt sich beim Vergleich der Papillen übereinstimmend die größere Papillenexkavation mit den steileren Exkavationsrändern und dem flacheren Exkavationsboden bei der Papille mit Glaukom ohne Hochdruck (rechts)

Abb. 9d. Papillenbefund des rechten Auges einer 34jährigen Patientin mit Glaucoma chronicum simplex im Stadium 4 des Gesichtsfeldausfalls (Gesamtverlust 1449 dB). Die Anordnung der Befunde entspricht der **Abb. 9a**

Stadium 1 auf (p < 0.01). Augen mit Glaukom ohne Hochdruck Stadium 1 haben somit steilere Exkavationsränder und einen flacheren Exkavationsboden als Augen mit Glaucoma chronicum simplex Stadium 1. Auch im Stadium 2 der Erkrankung sind die Exkavationsränder bei Glaukom ohne Hochdruck signifikant steiler als bei Glaucoma chronicum simplex (p < 0.01). In den fortgeschrittenen Stadien 3 bis 5 bestehen keine signifikanten Unterschiede zwischen Augen mit Glaucoma chronicum simplex und Glaukom ohne Hochdruck mehr (0.2 < p < 0.64), d.h. die Steigung der

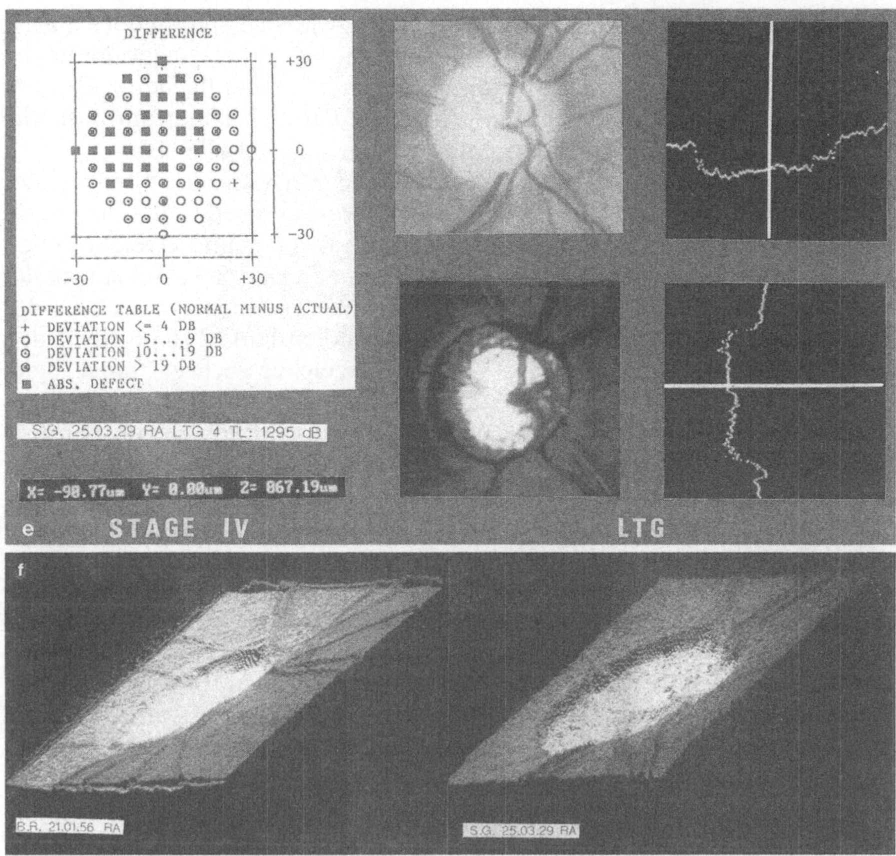

Abb. 9e. Papillenbefund des rechten Auges einer 61jährigen Patientin mit Glaukom ohne Hochdruck Stadium 4 des Gesichtsfeldausfalls (Gesamtverlust 1295 dB). Die Anordnung der Befunde entspricht der **Abb. 9a.** Im fortgeschrittenen Stadium der Glaukomerkrankung zeigt sich hier kein Unterschied in der Größe der Papillenexkavation und der Steilheit der Exkavationsränder (vgl. Profilschnitte rechts) zwischen Glaucoma chronicum simplex (vgl. **Abb. 9d**) und Glaukom ohne Hochdruck mehr

Abb. 9f. 3-D-Ausdrucke der in Abb. 9d dargestellten Papille mit Glaucoma chronicum simplex *(links)* und der in **Abb. 9b** dargestellten Papille mit Glaukom ohne Hochdruck *(rechts)* im Stadium 4 des Gesichtsfeldausfalls. In dieser dreidimensionalen Darstellung der Papille zeigt sich beim Vergleich der Papillen kein Unterschied in der Papillenform und der Exkavationsgröße mehr

Geraden für die Dichtefunktion der Tiefenwerte ist bei beiden Glaukomformen gleich (vgl. Tabelle 2b).

Keine signifikanten Unterschiede in der Steilheit der Exkavationsränder und der Form des Exkavationsbodens bestehen zwischen Augen mit Glaucoma chronicum simplex Stadium 1, okulärer Hypertension und gesunden Augen ($0.2 < p < 0.64$). Die Steigung der Geraden für die Dichtefunktion weist bei allen drei Diagnosegruppen einen gleich negativen

Wert auf. Das Glaukom ohne Hochdruck zeigt jedoch signifikante Unterschiede in der Form der Exkavation zu diesen drei Diagnosegruppen ($p < 0.001$) mit steileren Exkavationsrändern und einem flacheren Exkavationsboden. Ausgedrückt wird dies durch die deutlich näher am positiven Bereich gelegene Steigung der Dichtefunktion (vgl. Tabelle 2b).

Beim Glaucoma chronicum simplex tritt die Zunahme der Steilheit der Exkavationsränder, ausgehend von einem Wert, der mit dem gesunder Augen übereinstimmt, kontinuierlich und langsam auf und erreicht in den Endstadien gleiche Werte wie das Glaukom ohne Hochdruck. Bei Augen mit Glaucoma chronicum simplex zeigt sich ein Wechsel des Vorzeichens der Geradensteigung von negativ in den Anfangsstadien 1 und 2 zu positiv in den fortgeschrittenen Stadien 3 bis 5. Der Vorzeichenwechsel findet beim Übergang vom Stadium 2 in die Stadien 3 bis 5 statt (Abb. 10).

Die absoluten Zahlen beim Glaukom ohne Hochdruck zeigen nur eine geringgradige Zunahme der primär schon sehr steilen Exkavationsränder beim Vergleich der Stadien 1, 2 und 3 bis 5. Der Vorzeichenwechsel der Geradensteigung findet beim Übergang vom Stadium 1 in das Stadium 2 statt (vgl. Abb. 10).

Beim Glaukom ohne Hochdruck liegen beim Übergang von Gesund zum Stadium 1 bereits steile Exkavationsränder vor, während beim Glaucoma chronicum simplex erst beim Übergang vom Stadium 1 in das Stadium 2 eine vergleichbare Steilheit der Exkavationsränder vorliegt. Bezogen auf den Gesichtsfeldausfall tritt die Änderung der Papillenform beim Glaucoma chronicum simplex ein Erkrankungsstadium später auf als beim Glaukom ohne Hochdruck.

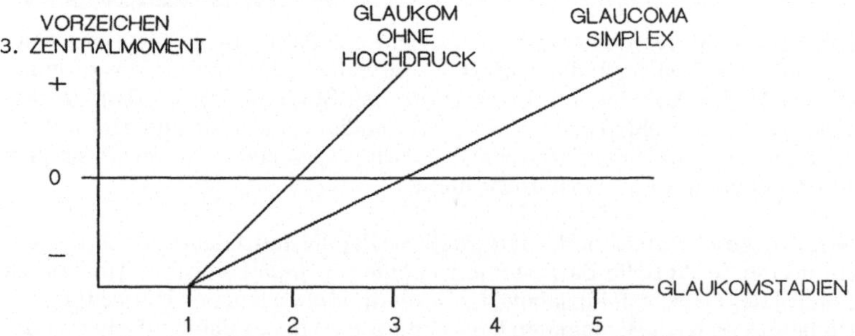

Abb. 10. Vorzeichen der Geraden für die Dichtefunktion des 3. Zentralmoments (Maßzahl für die Steilheit der Exkavationsränder) bei Glaukom ohne Hochdruck und Glaucoma chronicum simplex in den Stadien 1 bis 5. Augen mit Glaukom ohne Hochdruck weisen im Anfangsstadium der Erkrankung steilere Exkavationsränder und einen flacheren Exkavationsboden als Augen mit Glaucoma chronicum simplex auf. Beim Glaukom ohne Hochdruck erfolgt der Vorzeichenwechsel von negativ nach positiv beim Übergang vom Stadium 1 in das Stadium 2, während beim Glaucoma chronicum simplex der Vorzeichenwechsel beim Übergang vom Stadium 2 in das Stadium 3 erfolgt. Bezogen auf den Gesichtsfeldausfall tritt beim Glaucoma chronicum simplex die Änderung der Papillenform, also die Zunahme der Steilheit der Exkavationsränder ein Gesichtsfeldstadium später auf als beim Glaukom ohne Hochdruck

Papillenparameter

Exkavationsvolumen. Das effektive Exkavationsvolumen zeigt Tabelle 3a, Spalte 1 bei gesunden Augen und Augen von Patienten mit okulärer Hypertension, Glaucoma chronicum simplex und Glaukom ohne Hochdruck im unterschiedlichen Stadium der Erkrankung definiert anhand des Gesichtsfeldsausfalls.

Augen mit Glaukom ohne Hochdruck weisen im Stadium 1 ein signifikant größeres effektives Exkavationsvolumen als Augen mit Glaucoma chronicum simplex Stadium 1 auf ($p < 0.05$). Im Stadium 2 ($0.1 < p < 0.64$) und in den fortgeschrittenen Stadien 3 bis 5 der Glaukomerkrankung ($0.2 < p < 0.64$) bestehen keine signifikanten Unterschiede im effektiven Exkavationsvolumen zwischen Augen mit Glaukom mit bzw. ohne Augeninnendruckerhöhung. Im Vergleich zu gesunden Augen zeigen sowohl Augen mit okulärer Hypertension als auch Augen mit Glaucoma chronicum simplex Stadium 1 einen signifikanten Unterschied im Exkavationsvolumen ($p < 0.05$) (Tabelle 3b).

Die absoluten Zahlen beim Glaukom ohne Hochdruck zeigen nur eine geringgradige Zunahme der primär schon großen Exkavationsvolumina beim Vergleich der Stadien 1, 2 und 3 bis 5.

Beim Glaucoma chronicum simplex tritt die Zunahme der Exkavationsvolumina kontinuierlich und langsam auf und erreicht in den Endstadien gleiche Werte wie beim Glaukom ohne Hochdruck (vgl. Tabelle 3b).

Die Unterschiede im Exkavationsvolumen liegen beim Glaukom ohne Hochdruck beim Übergang von gesund zu Stadium 1, während die Vergrößerung des Exkavationsvolumens beim Glaucoma chronicum simplex erst beim Übergang vom Stadium 1 in das Stadium 2 der Glaukomerkrankung erreicht wird.

Exkavationsfläche. Die effektive Fläche bezeichnet die Fläche der Exkavation innerhalb der Papille (vgl. Abb. 5c und Abb. 6). Die effektive Exkavationsfläche zeigt Tabelle 3a, Spalte 2 bei gesunden Augen und Augen von Patienten mit okulärer Hypertension, Glaucoma chronicum simplex und Glaukom ohne Hochdruck im unterschiedlichen Stadium der Erkrankung definiert anhand des Gesichtsfeldausfalls.

Augen mit Glaukom ohne Hochdruck weisen eine signifikant größere Exkavationsfläche als Augen mit Glaucoma chronicum simplex Stadium 1 auf ($p < 0.02$), was sich auch im Stadium 2 fortsetzt ($p < 0.05$). In den fortgeschrittenen Stadien 3 bis 5 der Glaukomerkrankung ist kein signifikanter Unterschied in der Exkavationsfläche zwischen Augen mit Glaucoma chronicum simplex und Augen mit Glaukom ohne Hochdruck zu finden ($0.37 < p < 0.64$). Im Vergleich zu gesunden Augen zeigen sowohl Augen mit okulärer Hypertension und Augen mit Glaucoma chronicum simplex Stadium 1 einen signifikanten Unterschied in der Exkavationsfläche ($p < 0.02$).

Tabelle 3a. Meßergebnisse für den Mittelwert des Exkavationsvolumens, der Exkavationsfläche und des Verhältnisses von Exkavationsfläche zu Papillengesamtfläche geordnet nach Diagnosegruppen (n = Anzahl der ausgewerteten Augen in einer Diagnosegruppe)

Diagnose	n	Exkavationsvolumen (mm^3)		Exkavationsfläche (mm^2)		$\dfrac{\text{Exkavationsfläche}}{\text{Papillengesamtfläche}}$	
Gesund	37	0.18 ± 0.13		1.01 ± 0.52		0.55 ± 0.29	
			$p < 0.05$		$p < 0.02$		$0.1 < p < 0.2$
Okuläre Hypertension	2	0.30 ± 0.09		1.25 ± 0.38		0.66 ± 0.15	
Glaucoma chronicum simplex Stadium 1	26	0.28 ± 0.29		1.20 ± 0.49		0.64 ± 0.14	
			$p < 0.05$		$p < 0.02$		$p < 0.01$
Glaukom ohne Hochdruck Stadium 1	6	0.41 ± 0.19		1.67 ± 0.39		0.71 ± 0.07	
Glaucoma chronicum simplex Stadium 2	3	0.48 ± 0.37		1.62 ± 0.26		0.73 ± 0.10	
			$0.1 < p < 0.64$		$p < 0.05$		$p < 0.05$
Glaukom ohne Hochdruck Stadium 2	2	0.42 ± 0.29		2.04 ± 0.79		0.83 ± 0.17	
Glaucoma chronicum simplex Stadium 3 bis 5	4	0.70 ± 0.48		1.97 ± 0.26		0.86 ± 0.06	
			$0.2 < p < 0.64$		$0.37 < p < 0.64$		$p > 0.64$
Glaukom ohne Hochdruck Stadium 3 bis 5	2	0.55 ± 0.25		1.96 ± 0.54		0.85 ± 0.07	

Tabelle 3b. Signifikante (∗) und nicht signifikante (ns) Unterschiede im Exkavationsvolumen zwischen gesunden Augen, Augen mit okulärer Hypertension und Augen mit Glaucoma chronicum simplex und Glaukom ohne Hochdruck. Ein *signifikanter* Unterschied besteht im Exkavationsvolumen bei Augen mit Glaucoma chronicum simplex und Glaukom ohne Hochdruck nur im Stadium 1 mit dem größeren Exkavationsvolumen bei Augen mit Glaukom ohne Hochdruck. Im Stadium 2 und 3 bis 5 besteht kein *signifikanter* Unterschied zwischen den beiden Glaukomformen mehr. Im Vergleich zu gesunden Augen weisen Augen mit okulärer Hypertension ein *signifikant* größeres Exkavationsvolumen auf. Augen mit okulärer Hypertension zeigen im Vergleich zu Augen mit Glaucoma chronicum simplex Stadium 1 *keine signifikanten* Unterschiede

Gesichtsfeld-ausfall	Gesund	Okuläre Hypertension	Glaucoma simplex	Glaukom ohne Hochdruck
Kein	∗ ——— ∗			
Stadium 1		ns ——— ns	∗ ——— ∗	
Stadium 2			ns ——— ns	
Stadium 3 bis 5			ns ——— ns	

Tabelle 3c. Signifikante (∗) und nicht signifikante (ns) Unterschiede in dem Verhältnis Exkavationsfläche zu Papillengesamtfläche bei gesunden Augen, Augen mit okulärer Hypertension und Augen mit Glaucoma chronicum simplex und Glaukom ohne Hochdruck. Ein *signifikanter* Unterschied in der Exkavationsfläche besteht bei Augen mit Glaucoma simplex und Glaukom ohne Hochdruck im Stadium 1 und Stadium 2 mit der größeren Exkavationsfläche bei Augen mit Glaukom ohne Hochdruck. Im Stadium 3 bis 5 besteht *kein signifikanter* Unterschied zwischen den beiden Glaukomformen mehr. Zwischen gesunden Augen, Augen mit okulärer Hypertension und Augen mit Glaucoma chronicum simplex Stadium 1 besteht *kein signifikanter* Unterschied in der Exkavationsfläche

Gesichtsfeld-ausfall	Gesund	Okuläre Hypertension	Glaucoma simplex	Glaukom ohne Hochdruck
Kein	ns ——— ns			
Stadium 1		ns ——— ns	∗ ——— ∗	
Stadium 2			∗ ——— ∗	
Stadium 3 bis 5			ns ——— ns	

Betrachtet man die Größenzunahme der Exkavationsfläche für jede Glaukomform getrennt, so findet man bei Augen mit Niederdruckglaukom eine relativ kleine Steigerung des Wertes von 1.67 mm^2 im Anfangsstadium auf 1.96 mm^2 im Endstadium der Erkrankung (14.8%). Bei Augen mit

Glaucoma chronicum simplex steigert sich die Exkavationsfläche ausgehend von Werten mit 1.20 mm^2, die nahe bei denen der Patienten mit okulärer Hypertension liegen, bis zu Werten von 1.97 mm^2 im Mittel, die mit den Werten im Endstadium der Augen mit Glaukom ohne Hochdruck identisch sind, was einer Steigerung um 39.1% entspricht.

Verhältnis der Exkavationsfläche zur Papillengesamtfläche.
Der Wert für die Papillenexkavationsfläche (vgl. Abb. 5c, Abb. 6) zeigt große individuelle Schwankungen, die eine Zuordnung des erhaltenen Wertes zu einem Gesichtsfeldbefund erschweren. Daher wird die Exkavationsfläche zur Papillengesamtfläche in Beziehung gesetzt.

Die Werte für das Verhältnis Exkavationsfläche zu Papillengesamtfläche zeigt Tabelle 3a, Spalte 3 bei gesunden Augen und Augen von Patienten mit okulärer Hypertension, Glaucoma chronicum simplex und Glaukom ohne Hochdruck im unterschiedlichen Stadium der Erkrankung definiert anhand des Gesichtsfeldausfalls.

Im Stadium 1 der Glaukomerkrankung findet sich bei Augen mit Glaukom ohne Hochdruck ein signifikant größerer Wert für das Verhältnis Exkavationsfläche zu Papillengesamtfläche als bei Augen mit Glaucoma chronicum simplex (p < 0.01). Auch im Stadium 2 ist der Wert beim Glaukom ohne Hochdruck signifikant größer (p < 0.05). In den fortgeschrittenen Stadien 3 bis 5 der Glaukomerkrankung findet sich kein signifikanter Unterschied zwischen den beiden Glaukomformen mehr (p > 0.64) (Tabelle 3c).

Die drei Diagnosegruppen Gesund, okuläre Hypertension und Glaucoma chronicum simplex Stadium 1 zeigen keine signifikanten Unterschiede in dem Wert für das Verhältnis Exkavationsfläche zu Papillengesamtfläche (0.1 < p < 0.2). Man sieht eine deutliche Steigerung des Wertes bei Augen mit okulärer Hypertension im Vergleich zu gesunden Augen, die jedoch nicht signifikant ist (vgl. Tabelle 3c).

Auch dieser Papillenparameter weist beim Glaucoma chronicum simplex eine erheblich größere Zunahme ausgehend vom Anfangsstadium (0.64) bis zum Endstadium (0.86) auf (25.6%) als das Glaukom ohne Hochdruck, das ausgehend von einem relativ hohen Wert (0.71) nur einen geringen Anstieg des Verhältnisses bis zum Endstadium (0.85) zeigt (16.5%).

Diskussion

Mit dem Laser Tomographic Scanner (LTS) oder dem Optic Nerve Head Analyzer wurde es möglich, mit Einsatz der Computertechnik Papillenparameter zu quantifizieren [35, 41, 43, 45, 56, 60, 61, 62, 69, 80, 89, 91, 92, 93, 100, 102, 104, 105, 106]. Auf diese Weise können computerperimetrisch quantifizierte Gesichtsfeldausfälle [9, 10, 24, 25, 26, 27, 28, 31, 32, 36, 42, 43, 46, 47, 54, 55, 74, 75, 78] mit Meßwerten der Papille korreliert werden. Es stellt sich dabei die Frage, welcher der angegebenen Papillenmeßwerte die beste Übereinstimmung mit dem Gesichtsfeldausfall liefert. Wünschenswert wären Papillenparameter, die den Glaukomschaden schon im Vorfeld von Gesichtsfeldausfällen erfassen können, so daß eine morphologische Frühdiagnose erfolgt.

Frühere eigene Studien [37, 38, 39] zeigten ophthalmoskopische Unterschiede der Größe der Papillenexkavation zwischen Augen mit Glaucoma chronicum simplex und Glaukom ohne Hochdruck, die später mit quantifizierenden Untersuchungsmethoden von Papille und Gesichtsfeld bestätigt wurden (11, 28, 30, 43, 45, 103). In einem 3-D-Videofilm mit dem LTS wurde dies für einzelne Papillen demonstriert (49, 50). Ziel der vorliegenden Studie ist es, die neuen Papillenparameter des LTS zur Größe des Gesichtsfeldausfalls in Beziehung zu setzen, um mit Hilfe des konfokalen Prinzips des LTS Unterschiede in der Morphologie der Papille zwischen Augen mit Glaucoma chronicum simplex und Glaukom ohne Hochdruck erneut zu untersuchen.

Tiefe der Papillenexkavation

In dieser Studie werden die Meßwerte für die maximale und effektive mittlere Tiefe der Papillenexkavation bei Augen mit Glaukom mit bzw. ohne Augeninnendruckerhöhung stadienabhängig definiert nach der Größe des Gesichtsfeldausfalls betrachtet.

> Augen mit Glaucoma chronicum simplex zeigen in allen Stadien der Glaukomerkrankung die größeren maximalen und mittleren Tiefenwerte der Papillenexkavation als Augen mit Glaukom ohne Hochdruck. Nur im Stadium 1 ist die mittlere Tiefe bei Augen mit Glaukom ohne Hochdruck geringfügig größer.

Will man eine Aussage über das Stadium der Erkrankung machen, ist es nicht sinnvoll, die Werte für die maximale Tiefe und effektive mittlere Tiefe gesondert zu betrachten. Beide Werte müssen zusammen zur Papillenbeurteilung herangezogen werden, da sie so im Verhältnis zueinander eine Aussage über die Form der Papillenexkavation erlauben. Ansonsten erhält man bei der Angabe der maximalen Tiefe der Papillenexkavation nur eine Aussage über einen einzigen Meßwert der Exkavationstiefe, bei der Angabe der effektiven mittleren Tiefe der Papillenexkavation keine Aussage über die maximale Tiefe der Papillenexkavation.

Sowohl die Betrachtung des Exkavationsvolumens und der Exkavationsfläche, als auch der Vergleich der maximalen Tiefe (HM) und der effektiven mittlere Tiefe (HE) der Papillenexkavation bei allen Diagnosegruppen zeigen, daß durch Einzelparameter allein nicht auf die Größe des Gesichtsfeldsausfalls zurückgeschlossen werden kann. Dies ist unabhängig von der Aufnahmetechnik. Die Tiefe der Papillenexkavation läßt sowohl bei Untersuchung der Papille mit dem LTS als auch mit dem ONHA beim einzelnen Patienten wegen der großen individuellen Variabilität aller Papillenparameter keinen sicheren Rückschluß auf die Größe des Gesichtsfeldausfalls zu.

Form der Papillenexkavation

Form der Papillenexkavation bei Augen mit Glaucoma chronicum simplex und Glaukom ohne Hochdruck bei gleichem Stadium des Gesichtsfeldsausfalls. Durch ophthalmoskopische Untersuchungen [37, 38, 39] und Untersuchungen mit dem Optic Nerve Head Analyzer (ONHA) ist durch verschiedene Studien gesichert, daß es signifikante Unterschiede bei Augen mit Glaucoma chronicum simplex und Glaukom ohne Hochdruck bei gleichem Stadium des Gesichtsfeldausfalls in der Größe der Papillenexkavation und in der Fläche der neuroretinalen Randzone gibt [11, 41, 44, 45, 90, 91, 99]: Es findet sich eine signifikant kleinere neuroretinale Randzone bei Augen mit Glaukom ohne Hochdruck im Vergleich zu Augen mit Glaucoma chronicum simplex bei gleichem Stadium des Gesichtsfeldausfalls.

Eine Definition des Stadiums der Erkrankung muß daher anhand des Gesichtsfeldausfalls erfolgen, und nicht, wie in früheren Studien zum Teil erfolgt, anhand der Größe der Papillenexkavation [45].

Für das Verhältnis zwischen effektiver mittlere Tiefe (HE) zu maximaler Tiefe der Papillenexkavation zeigen sich sowohl im Stadium 1 des Gesichtsfeldausfalls als auch im Stadium 2 bei Augen mit Glaukom ohne Hochdruck für das Verhältnis HE/HM jeweils höhere Werte (vgl. Tabelle 2a, Spalte 3, Tabelle 2b, rechts oben und rechts mitte).

Beim 3. Zentralmoment ist die Steigung der Geraden der Dichtefunktion für die Tiefenwerte der Papillenexkavation bei Augen mit Glaukom ohne Hochdruck signifikant flacher als bei Augen mit Glaucoma chronicum simplex. Die Progredienz derErkrankung ist an der Zunahme der größeren Tiefenwerte in den weiter fortgeschrittenen Glaukomstadien zu sehen. Dies drückt sich in einem Annähern des Wertes an 0 und dem Übergang zu einer positiven Steigung der Geraden der Dichtefunktion für die Tiefenwerte aus (vgl. Abb. 8). Während im Stadium 2 des Gesichtsfeldausfalls beim Glaucoma chronicum simplex noch ein negatives drittes Zentralmoment (-0.06) gefunden wird, weisen Augen mit Glaukom ohne Hochdruck bereits eine positive Steigung ($+0.12$) auf (vgl. Tabelle 2a, Spalte 4, Tabelle 2b, rechts oben und rechts mitte). Dies belegt somit unsere im 3-D-Videofilm dokumentierten Unterschiede der Papillenform bei Augen mit Glaukom ohne Hochdruck und Glaucoma chronicum simplex jetzt quantitativ [49, 50].

In den fortgeschrittenen Stadien 3 bis 5 der Erkrankung finden sich in der dreidimensionalen Darstellung keine Unterschiede mehr in der Papillenform bei Glaukom mit bzw. ohne Augeninnendruckerhöhung ([49, 50], vgl. Abb. 9d und Abb. 9e). Dies wird durch die Angleichung des Verhältnisses zwischen effektiver mittlerer Tiefe (HE) zu maximaler Tiefe (HM) der Papillenexkavation und die Angleichung der Steigung der Geraden des 3. Zentralmoments der Tiefenwerte bei Augen mit Glaucoma chronicum simplex und Glaukom ohne Hochdruck im gleichen Stadium des Gesichtsfeldausfalls quantitativ bestätigt (vgl. Tabelle 2a, Spalte 3 und 4, Tabelle 2 b, rechts unten).

Die Untersuchungen mittels der quantitativen Papillenanalyse mit dem LTS und dem ONHA zeigen, daß Gruppen von Patienten mit Glaucoma chronicum simplex und Glaukom ohne Hochdruck im Papillenbefund [38, 38, 39] Unterschiede aufweisen. Die Papillenexkavation der Augen mit Glaukom ohne Hochdruck Stadium 1 zeigt eine *flache, schüsselförmige Papillenexkavation mit steilen Exkavationsrändern und einem flachen Exkavationsboden* (Abb. 11, rechts oben). Die Papillenexkavation der Diagnosegruppen gesund, okuläre Hypertension und Glaucoma chronicum simplex im Stadium 1 zeigt eine *tiefe Papillenexkavation mit flachen Exkavationsrändern und einem spitzen Exkavationsboden* (Abb. 11, mitte rechts oben).

Inwieweit aus dem Wert Total Loss (TL) im Gesichtsfeld und dem Wert für das 3. Zentralmoment bzw. dem Verhältnis HE/HM für den einzelnen Patienten die Diagnosestellung Glaukom ohne Hochdruck möglich ist, kann in diesem Zusammenhang nicht beantwortet werden. Dies erfordert weitere Studien, die die Trennschärfe zwischen gesund und pathologisch anhand dieser neuen Meßwerte prüfen. Für einzelne Meßwerte wie die Fläche der neuroretinalen Randzone hat sich keine ausreichende Trennschärfe ergeben [41]. Eine Diagnosestellung erscheint anhand dieser neuen, komplexeren Meßwerte derzeit nicht ausgeschlossen. Eine solche Untersuchung erscheint notwendig, da dann aufgrund morphologischer Kriterien die Diagnose

GESICHTSFELD AUSFALL	GESUND	OKULÄRE HYPERTENSION	GLAUCOMA SIMPLEX	GLAUKOM OHNE HOCHDRUCK
KEIN				
STADIUM 1				
STADIUM 2				
STADIUM 3 BIS 5				

Abb. 11. Papillenexkavation bei gesunden Augen, Augen mit okulärer Hypertension und Augen mit Glaucoma chronicum simplex und Glaukom ohne Hochdruck. Es zeigt sich *kein signifikanter* Unterschied in der Form der Papillenexkavation bei gesunden Augen, Augen mit okulärer Hypertension und Augen mit Glaucoma chronicum simplex Stadium 1: Die Papillenexkavation weist flache Exkavationsränder und einen relativ spitzen Exkavationsboden auf. *Signifikant* ist der Unterschied in der Form der Papillenexkavation beim Vergleich dieser drei Diagnosegruppen mit Augen mit Glaukom ohne Hochdruck Stadium 1: Augen mit Glaukom ohne Hochdruck zeigen schon im Stadium 1 *steilere* Exkavationsränder und einen *flacheren* Exkavationsboden. Augen mit Glaucoma chronicum simplex zeigen in den Stadien 1 und 2 des Gesichtsfeldausfalls nur eine geringe Formänderung und erst in den fortgeschrittenen Stadien 3 bis 5 eine deutliche Zunahme der Steilheit der Exkavationsränder. Augen mit Glaukom ohne Hochdruck weisen *bereits primär* steile Exkavationsränder bei flachem Exkavationsboden auf, die sich in den fortgeschrittenen Stadien der Glaukomerkrankung 3 bis 5 nur noch geringfügig ändern kann. Dies spricht für Unterschiede in den Schädigungswegen im Anfangsstadium der Erkrankung

Glaukom ohne Hochdruck möglich wäre. Bisher stellt die Diagnose eine Ausschlußdiagnose aufgrund der Druckmessung dar und ist somit erst nach langer Beobachtungszeit mit hinreichender Wahrscheinlichkeit möglich.

Die gute Reproduzierbarkeit der Papillenbefunde bei Untersuchung mit bildgebenden Methoden [12, 19, 41, 60, 62, 69, 71, 72, 73, 76, 91, 92, 96, 97, 98] erlaubt im Vergleich zur Ophthalmoskopie eine bessere Langzeitbeobachtung der Patienten. In der verbesserten Langzeitbeobachtung könnte daher ein Anwendungsbereich der quantitativen Bildanalyse liegen. Langzeitstudien werden zeigen können, ob die Papillenanalyse oder die Computerperimetrie sensitiver ist. Vermutlich werden beide Untersuchungen benötigt, da sich der durckabhängige Schaden eher im Gesichtsfeld, der druckunabhängige Schaden eher an der Papille zeigen wird.

Form der Papillenexkavation bei gesunden Augen, Augen mit okulärer Hypertension und Glaucoma chronicum simplex Stadium 1. Augen mit Glaucoma chronicum simplex Stadium 1 zeigen im Verhältnis HE/HM und dem 3. Zentralmoment keine signifikante Änderung im Vergleich zu gesunden Augen und Augen mit okulärer Hypertension (vgl. Tabelle 2a, Spalte 3 und 4, Tabelle 2b, oben). Somit findet sich bei den drei Diagnosegruppen gesunde Augen, Augen mit okulärer Hypertension und Glaucoma chronicum simplex Stadium 1 *kein signifikanter* Unterschied in der Form der Papillenexkavation. Allen gemeinsam sind die flachen Exkavationsränder und ein spitzer Exkavationsboden. Deshalb bietet die quantitative Papillenanalyse keine weitere Differenzierungsmöglichkeit zwischen einem Normalbefund und einer Papille bei Glaucoma chronicum simplex im Stadium 1 des Gesichtsfeldausfalls (vgl. Abb. 11).

Änderung der Form der Papillenexkavation in den fortgeschrittenen Stadien Glaukomerkrankung. Die Form der Papillenexkavation, ausgedrückt durch das Verhältnis zwischen effektiver mittlere Tiefe (HE) zu maximaler Tiefe der Papillenexkavation und das 3. Zentralmoment, ändert sich in den fortgeschrittenen Stadien der Glaukomerkrankung 3 bis 5 im Vergleich zu den Stadien 1 und 2 bei Augen mit Glaucoma chronicum simplex *signifikant*, bei Augen mit Glaukom ohne Hochdruck *nicht signifikant* (vgl. Tabelle 2a, Spalte 3 und 4, Tabelle 2b, Spalte 3 und 4, vgl. Abb. 11).

Somit ist es nicht möglich, bei Augen mit Glaukom ohne Hochdruck das Stadium der Glaukomerkrankung aus der Form der Papillenexkavation abzuleiten. Bei Augen mit Glaucoma chronicum simplex ändert sich die Form der Papillenexkavation ausgehend von einer Form in den Stadien 1 und 2, die der gesunder Augen mit flachen Exkavationsrändern entspricht, hin zur Form einer Papille mit steilen Rändern und einem flachen Exkavationsboden in den Stadien 3 bis 5 (vgl. Abb. 11), wodurch ein Rückschluß auf das Stadium der Erkrankung gezogen werden kann. Eine Stadieneinteilung anhand der Papillenmorphologie ist jedoch aufgrund der großen individuellen Variabilität nicht sinnvoll [45]. Hierfür eignet sich der Gesichtsfeldbefund mittels computergesteuerter Perimetrie besser [26, 27, 36, 47, 54, 55].

Papillenparameter – Exkavationsvolumen, Exkavationsfläche und Verhältnis Exkavationsfläche zu Papillengesamtfläche

Für das effektive Exkavationsvolumen und die effektive Exkavationsfläche finden sich im Anfangsstadium der Erkrankung größere Werte bei Augen mit Glaukom ohne Hochdruck als bei Glaucoma chronicum simplex. Mit Fortschreiten der Glaukomerkrankung gleichen sich die Meßwerte der beiden Glaukomformen an. Zwischen Augen mit Glaukom ohne Hochdruck und Glaucoma chronicum simplex finden sich – anders als beim Verhältnis effektive mittlere Tiefe zu maximaler Tiefe oder beim 3. zentralen Moment – bereits im Stadium 2 der Erkrankung keine signifikanten Unterschiede der genannten Papillenparameter mehr.

Dies ist durch die große individuelle Variabilität der Papillenmorphologie, für das effektive Exkavationsvolumen und die effektive Exkavationsfläche, zu erklären: Die Werte für das effektive Volumen schwanken in dieser Studie individuell zwischen 0.1 mm^3 und 2.3 mm^3 sowohl bei Augen mit Glaucoma chronicum simplex als auch bei Glaukom ohne Hochdruck im Stadium 1. Durch diese Schwankungen treten auch bei einem fortgeschrittenen Gesichtsfeldausfall von mehr als 1000 dB effektive Exkavationsvolumina von z.B. 0.35 mm^3 auf, die nur gering über dem mittleren Wert für Gesunde liegen. Aus diesem Grund läßt die Angabe der effektiven Exkavationsvolumina keine Aussage über den Gesichtsfeldausfall zu. Dies wurde auch für die mit dem ONHA errechneten Exkavationsvolumina festgestellt [41, 45, 91].

Eine einzelne Messung des effektiven Exkavationsvolumens läßt somit keinen Rückschluß auf das Stadium des Gesichtsfeldausfalls zu. Man muß die Größe der Exkavation immer in Abhängigkeit von der Papillenfläche sehen, um scheinbar normale und scheinbar glaukomatöse Papillen voneinander unterscheiden zu können [41, 45, 58, 91].

Gemäß der Definition dürften Augen mit okulärer Hypertension an der Papille keine Veränderungen aufweisen. Bei einer früheren Studie mit dem ONHA fanden wir einen größeren mittleren Blässewert bei Augen mit okulärer Hypertension im Vergleich zu gesunden Augen [94]. In dieser Studie wird besonders beim Exkavationsvolumen ein deutlicher Unterschied zwischen Augen mit okulärer Hypertension und gesunden Augen gefunden. Das größere Exkavationsvolumen und der größere mittlere Blässewert bei Augen mit okulärer Hypertension zeigen, daß eine ophthalmoskopisch als normal eingestufte Papille häufig doch Befundabweichungen aufweist, die nur mittels quantifizierender Papillenanalyse aufdeckbar sind. Diese Verfahren zeigen die Unterschiede zwischen gesunden Augen und Augen mit okulärer Hypertension jedoch nur bei Gruppen von Patienten als signifikante Unterschiede, nicht jedoch für den einzelnen Patienten.

Auch die Werte für die Exkavationsfläche erlauben, wie das Exkavationsvolumen, keinen Rückschluß auf die Größe des Gesichtsfeldausfalls. Es läßt sich schon wegen der großen individuellen Schwankungsbreite für die Papillengesamtfläche (Airaksinen fand eine Variabilität von 1.10 mm^2 bis

4.09 mm^2 bei gesunden Augen [3]) und den geringen Unterschieden in der Exkavationsfläche zwischen den drei Diagnosegruppen Gesund, Patienten mit okulärer Hypertension und Glaucoma chronicum simplex Stadium 1 einerseits und der geringen Änderung der Exkavationsfläche im Krankheitsverlauf bei Augen mit Glaukom ohne Hochdruck andererseits keine Zuordnung eines Meßwertes zur Größe des Gesichtsfeldausfall treffen.

Die große individuelle Variabilität der Papillengröße zeigte sich auch in anderen Studien z.B. mit dem ONHA [7, 9, 12, 45, 58, 93] oder im histologischen Vergleich der Papillengröße verschiedener Diagnosegruppen [20].

Beim direkten Vergleich der Meßwerte des LTS mit den Meßwerten des gleichen Auges mit dem ONHA zeigten sich Unterschiede in den Meßergebnissen beider Geräte [70]. Ursächlich dafür ist die unterschiedliche Definition der Papillenexkavation bei beiden Geräten. Beide Methoden der quantifizierenden Papillenanalyse – beim LTS das konfokale Prinzip mit 32 transversalen Schichtbildern, beim ONHA die simultanen Stereobilder – liefern mit dem Exkavationsvolumen und der Exkavationsfläche keine Papillenparameter, die aus den Papillenparametern eines einzelnen Patienten einen Rückschluß auf die Größe des Gesichtsfeldausfalls, also eine Bestimmung des Erkrankungsstadiums, erlauben.

Unterschiede in der Pathogenese bei Glaucoma chronicum simplex und Glaukom ohne Hochdruck

Unterschiede in der Steilheit der Exkavationsränder, der Form des Exkavationsbodens und die zeitliche Dynamik der Änderung der Form der Papillenexkavation weisen auf Unterschiede in den Schädigungswegen bei Augen mit Glaucoma chronicum simplex und Glaukom ohne Hochdruck in den Anfangsstadien hin. Diese Untersuchung der Papillenform mit dem LTS hat – wie bereits zuvor die quantitativen Untersuchungen im Gesichtsfeld mit dem Octopus Perimeter 201 [31, 32, 38, 43] und die Unterschiede in der Papillenexkavation und der Fläche der neuroretinalen Randzone mit dem ONHA [11, 45, 90, 91] – einen weiteren Hinweis auf eine unterschiedliche Pathogenese bei Glaukom ohne Hochdruck und Glaucoma chronicum simplex im Anfangsstadium der Erkrankung gegeben.

Beim Glaukom ohne Hochdruck zeigen sich bereits im Stadium 1 der Erkrankung steilwandige Papillenformen, wie sie beim Glaucoma chronicum simplex erst in den fortgeschrittenen Stadien der Erkrankung definiert nach dem Gesichtsfeldausfall gefunden werden. In früheren Untersuchungen haben wir gezeigt, daß bei gleichem Stadium des Gesichtsfeldausfalls beim Glaukom ohne Hochdruck größere Papillenexkavationen und kleinere Flächen der neuoretinalen Randzone bei gleicher Papillengröße im Vergleich zum Glaucoma chronicum simplex mit hohen intraokularen Druckwerten vorlagen [45]. Das konfokale Untersuchungsprinzip ergänzt diese Aussage dahingehend, daß auch die Steilheit der Exkavationsränder bei gleichem

Stadium des Gesichtsfeldausfalls beim Glaukom ohne Hochdruck signifikant größer ist im Vergleich zum Glaucoma chronicum simplex.

Die flachen, schüsselförmigen Papillenexkavationen der Augen mit Glaukom ohne Hochdruck mit steilen Exkavationsrändern und einem flachen Exkavationsboden können nicht allein durch den Untergang von Nervengewebe bedingt sein, da sonst der Gesichtsfeldausfall größer sein würde. In einer früheren Studie mit dem ONHA wurde für Augen mit Glaukom ohne Hochdruck im Anfangsstadium eine kleinere neuroretinale Randzone als für Augen mit Glaucoma chronicum simplex gefunden [45]. Daraus wurde geschlossen, daß bei Augen mit Glaukom ohne Hochdruck mehr intakte Nervenfasern pro Flächeneinheit der neuroretinalen Randzone vorhanden sein müssen als bei Augen mit Glaucoma chronicum simplex bei gleichem Stadium des Gesichtsfeldausfalls. Beim Glaukom ohne Hochdruck geht die Zunahme der Papillenexkavation durch den Verlust an Stützgewebe – hier gezeigt durch ein größeres Verhältnis HE/HM und dem früheren Wechsel des Vorzeichens des 3. Zentralmoments im Vergleich zu Augen mit Glaucoma chronicum simplex – einer Schädigung der Nervenfaserschicht möglicherweise voraus.

Bei eigenen Untersuchungen mit dem Laser Tomographic Scanner findet sich kein signifikanter Unterschied in der Maßzahl für die Nervenfaserschichtdicke bei Augen mit Glaucoma chronicum simplex und Glaukom ohne Hochdruck Stadium 1 der Erkrankung [69, 95]. Die Maßzahl für die Nervenfaserschichtdicke war bei den beiden Glaukomformen auch in unterschiedlichen Stadien der Erkrankung, definiert anhand des Gesichtsfeldausfalls nicht signifikant unterschiedlich. Die Grenzen dieser erstmals in vivo angewandten Methode eine Maßzahl für die Nervenfaserschichtdicke zu errechnen, sind bisher nicht bekannt. Die Maßzahl für die Nervenfaserschichtdicke könnte jedoch in der Frühdiagnostik – wie das Gesichtsfeld – im Gegensatz zu den Papillenparametern das Stadium der Erkrankung besser bestimmen, da Augen mit Glaucoma chronicum simplex als erstes Veränderungen an der Nervenfaserschicht zeigen [2, 3, 4, 7, 52, 59, 82, 83, 84, 85]. Mit Hilfe der computergesteuerten quantitativen Papillenanalyse mit dem LTS [6, 69, 95, 10,, 101], dem Optic Nerve Head Analyzer (ONHA) [8, 9] oder monochromatischen rotlichtfreien Fundusaufnahmen [1, 77] lassen sich Rückschlüsse auf die Nervenfaserschicht ziehen. Voraussetzung ist, daß die Methoden sensitiv genug sind.

Quigley fand bei histologischer Untersuchung von Augen mit Glaukom ohne Hochdruck weniger bindegewebige Querverbindungen und Bindegewebsfasern im Bereich der Lamina cribrosa, wodurch die Augen kostitutionell bedingt eine geringere Drucktoleranz als Augen mit Glaucoma chronicum simplex aufweisen könnten [81]. Hierdruch könnte bereits ein normaler Augeninnendruck, der bei Augen mit Glaukom ohne Hochdruck im Mittel an die obere Grenze der Norm verschoben ist [38], zu einem Glaukomschaden führen. Die Augen der Patienten mit Glaukom ohne Hochdruck werden zudem durch große Druckschwankungen geschädigt [48], die in einer Studie von Gramer und Mitarbeitern 8.09 ± 2.42 mmHg [48] im Vergleich zu

3.7 ± 1.8 mmHg bei Gesunden [16, 17] in der Tagesdruckkurve ohne Medikation betrugen.

Das Vorhandensein von weniger neuralem Stützgewebe wurde in früheren Arbeiten von uns als hypothetischer Risikofaktor für Glaukom ohne Hochdruck beschrieben [30, 39, 45]. Bei Vorliegen von weniger neuralem Stützgewebe kann ein normaler oder nur leicht erhöhter intraokularer Druck zu Kompression und Kollaps der Kapillaren führen [30, 39], was die verminderte Tensionstoleranz des Sehnerven bei Glaukom ohne Hochdruck erklären könnte.

Dies erklärt dann auch die beim Glaukom ohne Hochdruck häufigeren lokalisierten, primär bereits tiefen Gesichtsfeldausfälle und die sonstigen quantitativen Unterschiede im Gesichtsfeldausfall im Vergleich von Augen mit Glaucoma chronicum simplex und Glaukom ohne Hochdruck und Pigmentglaukom [33].

Die Gesichtsfeldausfälle der Augen mit Glaukom ohne Hochdruck sind wie beim Glaucoma chronicum simplex in der oberen Gesichtsfeldhälfte häufiger [31, 43, 51]. Bei Augen mit Glaukom ohne Hochdruck finden sich häufiger bereits primär tiefe, lokalisierte Skotome, die näher an das Gesichtsfeldzentrum heranreichen. Beim Glaukom ohne Hochdruck und Glaucoma chronicum simplex sind nasale Gesichtsfeldausfälle häufiger als beim Pigmentglaukom, was für vaskuläre Risikofaktoren spricht [22, 31, 43]. Die Lage des Gesichtsfeldausfalls ist dabei abhängig vom Ort der ischämischen Schädigung [29]. Die Lage der Gesichtsfeldausfälle beim Glaucoma chronicum simplex ist abhängig vom intraokularen Druck, da mit zunehmender Höhe des maximalen intraokularen Drucks eine zunehmende Gleichverteilung der Skotome in oberer und unterer Gesichtsfeldshälfte gefunden wird [33, 43, 44, 51]. Dies spricht für die schädigende Wirkung des intraokularen Drucks [14, 48, 64, 65, 66], der zu einem diffusen Gesichtsfeldausfall führt.

In der Pathogenese des Glaukoms ohne Hochdruck wird neben diesem hypothetischen konstitutionellen Risikofaktor (weniger neurales Stützgewebe) auch die vaskuläre Situation der Patienten als Ursache für den Glaukomschaden der Papille angesehen. In einer experimentellen Studie fanden Hayreh und Mitarbeiter, daß eine Erniedrigung des systemischen Blutdrucks die gleiche schädigende Wirkung auf das Auge haben kann wie eine Erhöhung des intraokularen Drucks [53]. Patienten mit Glaukom ohne Hochdruck zeigten in einer früheren Studie in 59% der Fälle einen niedrigen systolischen Blutdruck [33, 38]. Auf den Risikofaktor Hypotonie wurde auch von anderen Untersuchern hingewiesen [16, 17, 18, 23, 57, 86, 88].

Die mittels Laser Tomographie ermittelten Papillenparameter 3. Zentralmoment und das Verhältnis zwischen effektiver mittlerer Tiefe (HE) zu maximaler Tiefe (HM) der Papillenexkavation erlauben eine Aussage über die Form der Papillenexkavation bei Augen mit Glaucoma chronicum simplex und Glaukom ohne Hochdruck. Bei Augen mit Glaucoma chronicum simplex zeigt sich im Stadium 1 keine signifikante Veränderung der Steilheit der Exkavationsränder und der Form des Exkavationsbodens, die im Vergleich zu gesunden Augen durch quantitative Papillenanalyse sicher zu bestimmen sind. Hier ist die Änderung Gesund zu Glaucoma chronicum simplex nur am *Gesichtsfeldausfall* zu diagnostizieren [27, 47, 54, 55], während beim Glaukom ohne Hochdruck die Papillenparameter wie beim ONHA signifikante Unterschiede zu gesunden Augen zeigen.

Es zeigt sich bei Augen mit Glaukom ohne Hochdruck bereits im Stadium 1 eine primäre Änderung an der *Papillenexkavation* mit steileren Exkavationsrändern und flacherem Exkavationsboden als bei gesunden Augen und Augen mit Glaucoma chronicum simplex, an der sich im weiteren Krankheitsverlauf nur wenig ändert. Somit ist die Änderung Gesund zu Glaukom ohne Hochdruck mit der quantitativen Papillenanalyse besser erfaßbar als bei Glaucoma chronicum simplex. Die Gesichtsfelduntersuchung ist bei druckabhängigen Glaukomen und die quantitative Papillenanalyse bei Glaukom ohne Hochdruck möglicherweise die sensitivere Methode.

Die Diagnose Glaukom ohne Hochdruck ist unverändert eine Ausschlußdiagnose bei Auftreten eines glaukomatösen Gesichtsfeldausfalls mit glaukomatöser Papillenexkavation bei Augeninnendruckwerten im statistischen Normbereich. Durch die mit dem LTS zusätzlichen quantifizierenden Papillenparameter 3. Zentralmoment und Verhältnis zwischen effektiver mittlerer Tiefe (HE) zu maximaler Tiefe (HM) der Papillenexkavation ist es zusammen mit dem Total Loss (TL) im Gesichtsfeld möglich, anhand der Steilheit der Exkavationsränder und der Form des Exkavationsbodens möglicherweise auch beim Einzelpatienten einen zusätzlichen Hinweis für die Diagnose Glaukom ohne Hochdruck zu erhalten (vgl. Abb. 11).

Ob und inwieweit aus der papillenanalytisch quantifizierten Steilheit der Exkavationsränder und der Form des Exkavationsbodens und dem aktuellen intraokulären Druck die Diagnose Glaukom ohne Hochdruck besser eingegrenzt werden kann, müssen prospektive Studien zeigen, die den Rückschluß von der Papillenexkavation ziehen, was nicht Ziel dieser Studie war.

Mit neuen Papillenparametern konnte hier erstmals gezeigt werden, daß Unterschiede in der Steilheit der Exkavationsränder bei Glaukom ohne Hochdruck und Glaucoma chronicum simplex bei gleichem Stadium des Gesichtsfeldausfalls bestehen. Dies steht in Übereinstimmung mit unseren früheren Studien, die erstmals quantifizierend Unterschiede im Gesichtsfeldausfall [28, 31, 43], in der ophthalmoskopisch bestehenden Papillenexkavation [37, 38, 39] und der Fläche der neuroretinalen Randzone [45, 91] zwischen Glaukom ohne Hochdruck und Glaucoma simplex zeigten. Die Unterschiede in der Steilheit der Exkavationsränder und der Form des Exkavationsbodens sind somit weitere Parameter, die auf unterschiedliche Schädigungswege im Anfangsstadium der Glaukomerkrankung hinweisen. Eine Therapie entsprechend der Unterschiede in den Risikofaktoren ist somit erforderlich.

Die Therapie eines Glaukoms ohne Hochdruck muß somit u. a. neben der augeninnendrucksenkenden Therapie auch eine zusätzliche Behandlung der kardiovaskulären Risikofaktoren, sowie die Therapie einer arteriellen Hypotonie, die Verbesserung der Fließeigenschaften des Blutes und eine ausreichende Digitalisierung berücksichtigen.

Danksagung. Für die Mithilfe bei der statistischen Auswertung bedanken wir uns bei Frau Dr. Imme Haubitz, Rechenzentrum der Universität Würzburg und bei Dr. Gerhard Zinser, Heidelberg Engeneering, Heidelberg.

Literatur

1. Airaksinen PI, Nieminen H (1985) Retinal nerve fiber photography in glaucoma. Ophthalmology 92: 877–879
2. Airaksinen PI, Mustonen E, Alanko HI (1981) Optic disc hemorrhages precede retinal nerve fiber layer defects in ocular hypertension. Acta Ophthalmol 59: 627–641
3. Airaksinen PI, Tuulonen A, Werner EB (1989) Clinical evaluation of the optic disc and retinal nerve fiber layer. In: Ritch R, Shields MB, Krupin T eds. The Glaucomas. CV Mosby, St. Louis, pp 467–493
4. Armaly MF (1969) The correlation between appearance of the optic cup and visual function. Trans Am Acad Ophthalmol Otolaryngol 73: 898–913
5. Aulhorn E, Harms H (1960) Papillenveränderung und Gesichtsfeldstörung bei Glaukom. Ophthalmologica 139: 279–285
6. Bille IF, Dreher A, Reiter K, Weinreb RN (1989) Nerve fiber thickness with the Laser Tomographic Scanner presented on the first international symposium on Scanning Laser Ophthalmoscopy and Tomography, July, 7–8, 1989, Vortragsabstract.
7. Caprioli J (1989) Correlation of visual function with optic nerve and nerve fiber layer structure in glaucoma. Survey of Ophthalmol 33: 319–330
8. Caprioli J (1989) Image analysis of the optic disc and nerve fiber layer. Presented on the Second International Glaucoma Symposium, new trends in the detection and management of glaucoma, Nov. 1989, Tokyo, Japan
9. Caprioli I, Miller JM (1988) Correlation of structure and function in glaucoma. Quantitative measurements of disc and field. Ophthalmology 95: 723–737
10. Caprioli I, Spaeth GL (1984) Comparison of visual field defects in the low-tension glaucomas with those in the high-tension glaucoma. Am J Ophthal 97: 730–737
11. Caprioli I, Spaeth GL (1985) Comparison of the optic nerve head in high- and low-tension glaucoma. Arch ophthalmol 103: 1145–1149
12. Caprioli I, Klingbeil U, Sears M, Pope B (1986) Reproducibility of optic disc measurements with computerized analysis of stereoscopic video images. Arch ophthalmol 104: 1035–1039
13. Caprioli I, Miller JM, Oritz-Colberg R, Tressler C (1989) Profiles of the peripapillary nerve fiber layer in glaucoma. Invest Ophthalmol Vis Sci (suppl) 30: 430
14. David R, Livingston DG, Luntz MH (1977) Ocular hypertension. A long term follow up of treated and untreated patients. Br J Ophthalmol 61: 668–674
15. Douglas GR (1990) Topographic analysis of the optic nerve head using automated equipment. In: Gramer E (Hrsg) Glaukom – Diagnostik und Therapie Enke, Stuttgart, S 120–145
16. Drance SM (1960) The significances of the diurnal tension variations in normal and glaucomatous eyes. Arch Ophthalmol 64: 494–501
17. Drance SM (1972) Some factors in the production of low-tension glaucoma. Br J Ophthalmol 56: 229–242
18. Drance SM, Sweeny VP, Morgan RW, Feldman F (1973) Studies of factors involved in the production of low-tension glaucoma. Arch Ophthalmol 89: 457–465

19. Dreher A, Shaw B, Weinreb RN (1989) Reproducibility and accuracy of optic nerve head topography with the laser tomographic scanner, presented on the first international symposium of Scanning Laser Ophthalmoscopy and Tomography, July, 7–8, 1989. Vortragsabstract

20. Fernandez MC, Jonas JB, Naumann GOH (1990) Größe und Form der Papilla nervi optici als Parameter für die Diagnose und Pathogenese von Nervus-Opticus-Erkrankungen. Tagung der bayrischen Augenärzte, 18.–19. 05. 1990 München

21. Frohn A, Jean B, Zinser, G, Thiel HJ (1990) The problem of reference plane definition for cup volume measurements. In: Nasemann JF, Burk ROW (editors): Scanning Laser Ophthalmoscopy and Tomography. Quintessenz-Verlag, Berlin, 1990, pp 207–214

22. Glicklich RE, Steinmann WC, Spaeth GI (1989) Visual field change in low-tension glaucoma over a five year follow up. Ophthalmology 96: 316–320

23. Golberg I, Hollows FC, Kass MA, Becker B (1982) Systemis factors in patients with low-tension glaucoma. Br J Ophthalmol 65: 56

24. Gramer E (1982) Der Informationsgehalt der computergesteuerten Perimetrie für die Diagnostik und Verlaufskontrolle von Augenkrankheiten. Habil Schrift, Würzburg

25. Gramer E (1982) Computerperimetrie bei Glaukom. In: Leydhecker W, Krieglstein GK (editors): Programmgesteuerte Perimetrie, Kaden Verlag, Heidelberg. pp 99–120

26. Gramer E (1987) Gesichtsfeldveränderungen bei Glaukom. In: Krieglstein GK (editor): Das chronische Glaukom – zeitgemäße Diagnostik und Therapie. Augenspiegel-Verlag, Ratingen, pp 19–60

27. Gramer E (1990) Test pattern in computer perimetry of glaucoma. Second International Glaucoma Symposium, new trends in the detection and management of glaucoma. November 1989, Tokyo, Japan. Journal of the Eye, Vol 7, Suppl 1, p 69–85 (Atarashii Ganka)

28. Gramer E (1991) Low tension glaucoma. A synopsis of various clinical studies concerning the optic nerve lesions, in low tension glaucoma. Ophthalmologia, Vol 3, No 4, p 356–361 (Organon of the Panhellenic Opthalmological Society)

29. Gramer E (1991) Perimetrie bei Glaukom ohne Hochdruck. In: Gloor B (editor): Perimetrie, Enke Verlag Stuttgart (im Druck)

30. Gramer E, Althaus G (1987) Risikofaktoren bei Niederdruckglaukom. Klinische Studie zur Gesichtsfeldverschlechterung bei Glaukom ohne Hochdruck und Glaucoma simplex mit reguliertem intraokularen Druck mit dem Programm Delta des Octopus Perimeters 201. Z prakt Augenheilk 8: 388–399

31. Gramer E, Althaus G (1988) Quantifizierung und Progredienz des Gesichtsfeldschadens bei Glaukom ohne Hochdruck, Glaucoma simplex und Pigmentglaukom. Eine klinische Studie mit dem Programm Delta des Octopus Perimeters 201. Klin Mbl Augenheilkd 191: 184–198

32. Gramer E, Althaus G (1988) Progredienz des glaukomatösen Gesichtsfeldschadens. Eine klinische Studie mit dem Programm Delta des Octopus Perimeters 201 zum Einfluß des Vorschadens auf die Gesichtsfeldverschlechterung beim Glaucoma simplex. Fortschritte Ophthalmol 85: 620–625

33. Gramer E, Althaus G (1990) Bedeutung des erhöhten intraokulären Drucks für den glaukomatösen Gesichtsfeldschaden. Eine klinische Studie. Klin Mbl Augenheilkd 197: 1–7

34. Gramer E, Cunha L (1989) Quantitative differences in location, size depth and progression of visual field defects in glaucoma with different intraocular pressure. Chibret International Journal of Ophthalmol vol 6, No 1, pp 22–36

35. Gramer E, Klingbeil U (1986) Quantitative Papillenanalyse mit dem Optic Nerve Head Analyzer. Z prakt Augenheilkd 7: 30–36

36. Gramer E, Knauth-Spaeth M (1990) Glaukomspezifische Untersuchung des Gesichtsfeldes. Eine klinische Studie zum Informationsgehalt der Prüfungsraster der ProG1 und 31 des Octopus Perimeters 201. In: Gramer E (Hrsg): Glaukom – Diagnostik und Therapie. Ferdinand Enke Verlag, Stuttgart, 38–59

37. Gramer E, Leydhecker W (1984) Risikofaktoren glaukomatöser Gesichtsfeldausfälle bei Glaukom ohne Hochdruck und Glaucoma simplex mit niedrigem und hohem intraokularen Druck (Vortragsabstract). 25. Tagung der österreichischen Ophthalmol. Gesellschaft, Wien, 2. 6. 1984
38. Gramer E, Leydhecker W (1985) Glaukom ohne Hochdruck. Eine klinische Studie. Klin Mbl Augenheilkd 186: 262–267
39. Gramer E, Leydhecker W (1985) Zur Pathogenese des Glaukoms ohne Hochdruck. Z prakt Augenheilkd 6: 329–333
40. Gramer E, Leydhecker W (1985) Papillendiagnostik bei Glaukom. Z prakt Augenheilkd 6: 294–302
41. Gramer E, Siebert M (1989) Optic Nerve Head Measurements. The Optic Nerve Head Analyzer – its advantages and its limitations. International Ophthalmology, Kluwer Academic Publishers, Dordrecht, 13: 3–13 and 13: 235
42. Gramer E, Althaus G, Leydhecker W (1986) Die Bedeutung der Rasterdichte bei der computergesteuerten Perimetrie. Eine klinische Studie. Z prakt Augenheilkd 7: 197–202
43. Gramer E, Althaus G, Leydhecker W (1986) Lage und Tiefe glaukomatöser Gesichtsfeldausfälle in Abhängigkeit von der Fläche der neuroretinalen Randzone der Papille bei Glaukom ohne Hochdruck, Glaucoma simplex, Pigmentglaukom. Eine klinische Studie mit dem Octopus Perimeter 201 und dem Optic Nerve Head Analyzer. Klin Mbl Augenheilkd 189: 190–198
44. Gramer E, Althaus G, Leydhecker W (1987) Topography and progression of visual field damage in low tension glaucoma, open angle glaucoma and pigmentary glaucoma with the programm Delta of the Octopus Perimeter 201. A clinical study. In: Greve EL, Heijl A (editors): Seventh International Visual Field Symposium, Amsterdam, September 1986, Dordrecht, Martinus Nijhoff/Dr W Junk Publishers, pp 349–363
45. Gramer E, Bassler M, Leydhecker W (1987) Cup/disc ratio, excavation volume, neuroretinal rim area of the optic disc in correlation to computer-perimetric quantification of visual field defects in glaucoma with and without pressure. A clinical study with the Rodenstock Optic Nerve Head Analyzer and programm Delta of the Octopus Perimeter 201. In: Greve EL and Heijl A (editors): Seventh International Visual Field Symposium, Amsterdam, Dordrecht, Martinus Nijhoff/Dr W Junk Publishers, pp 329–346
46. Gramer E, Gerlach R, Krieglstein GK, Leydhecker W (1982) Zur Topographie früher glaukomatöser Gesichtsfeldausfälle bei der Computerperimetrie. Klin Mbl Augenheilkd 180: 515–523
47. Gramer E, Gerlach R, Krieglstein GK, Leydhecker W (1982) Zur Sensitivität des Computerperimeters Competer bei frühen glaukomatösen Gesichtsfeldausfällen. Eine kontrollierte klinische Studie. Klin Monatsbl Augenheilkd 180: 203–209
48. Gramer E, Mohamed J, Krieglstein GK (1982) Der Ort von Gesichtsfeldausfällen bei Glaucoma simplex, Glaukom ohne Hochdruck und ischämischer Neuropathie. Indikationen zur vasoaktiven Therapie. In: Krieglstein GK, Leydhecker W (editors): Medikamentöse Glaukomtherapie. JF Bergmann Verlag, München, pp 59–72
49. Gramer E, Kampik, A, Maier H, Siebert M (1990) Optic disc and visual field in patients with low-tension glaucoma (LTG) and primary open angle glaucoma (POAG). Video Film, Internatinal Congress of Ophthalmology – Glaucoma Symposium 16.–17. 03. 90, Singapore
50. Gramer E, Kampik, A, Maier, H, Siebert M, Lau, H-J, Zinser G (1989) Die Papille bei Glaukom mit und ohne Augeninnendruckerhöhung. Eine 3-D-Dokumentation mit dem Laser Tomographic Scanner. Video Film bei der Deutschen Ophthalmologischen Gesellschaft, Heidelberg, Sept. 1989, Zentralblatt Ophthalmologie, Springerverlag
51. Greve EL, Geijssen HC (1983) Comparison of glaucomatous visual field defects in patients with high and with low intraocular pressure. In: Greve EL, Heijl A (editors): 5th International Visual Field Symposium, Dr W Junk Publishers, Dordrecht, pp 101–105
52. Hart WM, Yablonski M, Kass MA, Becker B (1978) Quantitative visual field and optic disc correlates early in glaucoma. Arch Ophthalmol 96: 2209–2211

53. Hayreh SS, Revie, IHS, Edwards J (1970) Vasogenetic origin of visual field defects and optic nerve changes in glaucoma. Br J Ophthalmol 54: 461
54. Heijl A (1989) Test point density and early detection of glaucomatous visual field. Invest Ophthalmol Vis Sci (suppl.) 30: 55
55. Heijl A (1989) Glaucoma follow-up with automated perimetry. Presented on the Second International Glaucoma Symposium, new trends in the detection and management of glaucoma, November 1989, Tokyo, Japan
56. Jester JV, Cavanagh HD, Lemp MA (1988) In vivo confocal imaging of the eye using tandem scanning confocal microscopy. Proc SPIE vol. 1028: 122–126
57. Johnson DG, Drance SM (1968) Some studies on the circulation in patients with advanced open angle glaucoma. Canad J Ophthalmol 3: 149–153
58. Jonas JB, Königsreuther KA, Naumann, GOH (1990) Histomorphometrie der normalen und glaukomatösen Papilla nervi optici. Tagung der bayrischen Augenärzte, 18.–19. 05. 90, München
59. Katsumori N, Mizokami K (1989) Clinicopathological studies of the retinal nerve fiber layer in early glaucomatous visual field damage. In Heijl A, editor: Perimetry update 1988/89, Kugler & Ghedini Publications, Amsterdam 1989, pp 289–295
60. Kruse FE, Burk, ROW, Völcker HE, Zinser G, Harbarth U (1988) Laser Tomographic Scanning of the Optic Nerve Head. Ophthalmology Vol 95: 165
61. Kruse FE, Völcker HE, Burk ROW, Zinser G, Harbarth U (1988) Laser Tomographic Scanning of the optic nerve head. Poster at the 92nd annual meeting of the AAO in Las Vegas
62. Kruse FE, Burk ROW, Völcker HE, Zinser G, Harbarth U (1989) Zur dreidimensionalen Biomorphologie der Papille mit dem Laser Tomographic Scanverfahren – erste Erfahrungen an pathologischen Papillenbefunden. Fortschr Ophthalmol 86: 710–713
63. Kruse FE, Burk ROW, Völcker HE, Zinser G, Harbarth U (1989) Reproducibility of topographic measurements of the optic nerve head with Laser Tomographic Scanning. Ophthalmology 96: 1320–1324
64. Leibowitz HM, Krueger DE, Muender LR, Milton RD, Kini MM, Kahn HA, Nickerson RJ, Pool J, Colton TL, Ganley JP, Loewenstein JI, Dawber TR (1980) The Framingham eye study monography. An Ophthalmological and epidemiological study of cataract, glaucoma diabetic retinopathy, macular degeneration, and visual acuity in a general population of 2631 adults. 1973–1975. Survey Ophthalmol Suppl 24: 335–610
65. Leydhecker W (1983) Eine neue Definition der okulären Hypertension. Z prakt Augenheilkd 4: 173–176
66. Leydhecker W, Akiyama K, Neumann HG (1958) Der intraokulare Druck gesunder menschlicher Augen. Klin Mbl Augenheilkd 133: 662–670
67. Littmann H (1982) Zur Bestimmung der wahren Größe eines Objektes auf dem Augenhintergrund des lebenden Auges. Klin Mbl Augenheilkd 180: 286–289
68. Littmann H (1988) Zur Bestimmung der wahren Größe eines Objektes auf dem Augenhintergrund eines lebenden Auges. Klin Mbl Augenheilkd 192: 66–67
69. Maier H, Siebert M, Gramer E, Kampik A (1990) Eine Maßzahl für die Nervenfaserschichtdicke. Messungen mit dem Laser Tomographic Scanner. In: Gramer E (editor): Glaukom – Diagnostik und Therapie. Ferdinand Enke Verlag, Stuttgart, pp 120–145
70. Maier H, Siebert M, Gramer E (1992) Vergleich der Meßwerte des Laser Tomographic Scanners und des Optic Nerve Head Analyzers: Eine vergleichende klinische Studie. Klin Mbl Augenheilk (im Druck)
71. Miller KN, Shields MB, Ollie A (1988) Reproducibility of pallor measurements with the Optic Nerve Head Analyzer. Invest Ophthalmol Vis Sci (suppl.) 29: 352
72. Minkleberg FS, Douglas GR, Drance SM, Schulzer M, Wijsman K (1988) Reproducibility of computerized pallor measurements obtained with the Rodenstock Disc Analyzer. Graefe's Arch Clin Exp Ophthalmol 226: 269–272

73. Minkleberg FS, Douglas SM, Schulzer, Cornsweet TN,Wijsman K (1984) Reliability of optic disc topographic measurements recorded with a video-ophthalmolgraph. Am Journal of Ophthalmol 98: 98–102
74. Motolko M, Drance SM, Douglas GR (1982) Visual field defects in low-tension glaucoma. Arch Ophthalmol 100: 1074–1078
75. Motolko M, Drance SM, Douglas GR (1983) The visual field defects of low-tension glaucoma. In: Greve EL, Heijl A (editors): 5th International Visual Field Symposium. Dr W Junk Publishers, Dordrecht, pp 107–111
76. Nagin P, Schwartz B, Nanba K (1985) The reproducibility of computerized boundary analysis for measuring optic disc pallor in the normal optic disc. Ophthalmology 92: 243–251
77. Peli E, Hedges TR, McInnes T (1987) Nerve fiber layer photography, a comparative study. Acta Ophthalmol 65: 71–80
78. Phelps CD, Hayreh SS, Montague PR (1983) Visual fields in low-tension glaucoma, primary open angle glaucoma and anterior ischemic neuropathy. In: Greve EL, Heijl A (editors): 5th International Visual Field Symposium. Dr W Junk Publishers, Dordrecht, pp 113–124
79. Phelps CD, Hayreh SS, Montague PR (1984) Comparison of visual field defects in low-tension glaucomas with those in the high-tension glaucomas, letter. Am J Ophthalmol 98: 823–825
80. Plesch A, Klingbeil U (1988) Konfokales Laser-Scann-System zur Darstellung und Analyse des Fundus. Fortschritte der Ophthalmologie 85: 565–568
81. Quigley HA, Addicks EM, Green WR, Maumenee AE (1981) Optic nerve damage in human glaucoma. II. The site of injury and susceptibility to damage. Arch Ophthalmol 99: 635–649
82. Quigley HA, Addicks EM, Green WR (1982) Optic nerve damage in human glaucoma. III. Quantitative correlation of nerve fiber loss and visual field defects in glaucoma, ischemic neuropathy, papilledema, and toxic neuropathy. Arch Ophthalmol 100: 135–146
83. Quigley HA, Miller NR, George T (1980) Clinical evaluation of nerve fiber atrophy as an indicator of glaucomatous optic nerve damage. Arch Ophthalmol 98: 1564–1571
84. Radius LR (1989) Anatomy and pathophysiology of the retina and the optic Nerve. In: Ritch, R, Shields MB, Krupin T (editors): The Glaucomas, The CV Mosby Company, St. Louis Missouri 1989, pp 89–132
85. Read RM, Spaeth GL (1974) The practical clinical appraisal of the optic disc in glaucoma: The natural history of cup progression and some specific disc-field correlations. Trans Am Acad Ophthalmol Otolaryngol 78: 255–274
86. Richler M, Werner EB, Thomas D (1982) Risc factors for progression of visual field defects in medically treated patients with glaucoma. Canad J Ophthalmol 17: 245–248
87. Sachs L (1984) Angewandte Statistik, Anwendung statistischer Methoden. 6. Aufl., Springer Verlag, Berlin, Heidelberg, New York, Tokio 1984.
88. Sachsenweger R (1963) Der Einfluß des Blutdrucks auf die Prognose des Glaukoms. Klin Mbl Augenheilkd 142: 625–633
89. Shields MB, Martone JF, Shelton AR, Ollie AR, MacMillan J (1987) Reproducibility of topographic measurements with the Optic Nerve Head Analyzer. Am Journal of Ophthalmol 104: 581–586
90. Shirato S (1989) Optic disc findings of low-tension glaucoma. Presented of the Second International Glaucoma Symposium, new trends in the detection and management of glaucoma, November 1989, Tokyo, Japan
91. Siebert M, Gramer E (1990) Reproduzierbarkeit und klinische Anwendbarkeit der Meßergebnisse mit dem Optic Nerve Head Analyzer. In: Gramer E (Hrsg): Glaukom – Diagnostik und Therapie. Ferdinand Enke Verlag, Stutgart, pp 96–107
92. Siebert M, Gramer E, Leydhecker W (1988) Die Reproduzierbarkeit der Papillen-meßwerte mit dem Optic Nerve Head Analyzer. Spektrum Augenheilkd 2/4: 167–176

93. Siebert M, Gramer E, Leydhecker W (1988) Papillenparameter bei Gesunden – Quantifiziert mit dem Optic Nerve Head Analyzer. Klin Mbl Augenheilkd 92: 302–310
94. Siebert M, Gramer E, Leydhecker W (1989) Papillenabblassung – ein Frühzeichen des Glaukoms. Eine klinisch kontrollierte Untersuchung von Papillenblässe und Papillenexkavation bei Glaucoma simplex, okulärer Hypertension und gesunden Augen mit dem Optic Nerve Head Analyzer. Klin Mbl Augenheilkunde 194: 433–436
95. Siebert M, Maier H, Gramer E (1990) Bestimmung einer Maßzahl für die Nervenfaserschichtdicke mit dem Laser Tomographic Scanner. Eine Pilotstudie. Tagung der bayrischen Augenärzte 18.–19. 05. 90, München.
96. Stodtmeister R, Pillunat L (1989) Reproducibility of optic nerve head topographic measurements with a new laser tomographic scanning system. Invest Ophthalmol Vis sci (suupl) 30: 429
97. Takamoto T, Schwartz B (1985) Reproducibility of photogrammetric optic disc cup measurements. Invest Ophthalmol Vis Sci 26: 814
98. Tomita G, Goto Y, Yamada T, Kitazawa Y (1986) Reliability of optic disc measurement with computerized stereoscopic video image analyzer. Acta Soc Ophthalmol Jpn 90 (11): 1317–1321
99. Tomita G, Takamoto T, Schwartz B (1988) Optic disc changes over time in glaucoma like discs without increased intraocular pressure of visual field loss. Invest Ophthalmol Vis Sci (suppl) 29: 352
100. Weinreb RN, Dreher AW, Bille JF (1989) Quantitative assessment of the optic nerve head with the LTS Laser Tomographic Scanner. Int Ophthalmol 13: 25–29
101. Weinreb RN, Dreher A, Coleman, AL, Quigley HA (1989) Histopathologic validation of Fourier-ellipsometric measurements of monkey nerve fiber layer. Presented on the first international symposium on Scanning Laser Ophthalmoscopy and Tomography, July, 7–8, 1989. Vortragsabstract
102. Wilson T, Sheppard C (1984) Theory and practice of scanning optical microscopy. Academic press, London
103. Yamagami I, Shirato S, Araie M (1989) Differences in neuroretinal rim area between low tension glaucoma and primary open angle glaucoma. Jpn J Ophthalmol 43 (9): 1391–1394
104. Zinser G, Wijnaendts-van-Resandt RW, Ihrig C (1988) Confocal Laser Scanning Microscopy for Ophthalmology. Proc. SPIE Vol 1028: 127–132
105. Zinser G, Harbarth U, Schröder H (1990) Formation and Analysis of threedimensional data of the Laser Tomographic Scanner LTS. In: Nasemann JF, Burk ROW (editors): Scanning Laser Ophthalmoscopy and Tomography. Quintessenz-Verlag, Berlin, 1990, pp 243–252
106. Zinser G, Wijnaendts-van-Reandt RW, Dreher AW, Weinreb RN, Harbarth U, Schröder H, Burk ROW (1989) Confocal Laser Tomographic Scanning of the eye. Proc. SPIE Vol 1161: 337–339

Korrespondenzadresse
Professor Dr. med. Dr. jur. Eugen Gramer
Universitätsaugenklinik Würzburg, Josef-Schneider-Straße 11, D-8700 Würzburg

Optic Disc Findings and Disc Hemorrhages in Low-Tension Glaucoma and Their Therapeutical Suggestion

S. Shirato, M. Adachi, N. Koseki, and J. Yamagami

Summary

Fifty-eight eyes of 29 patients with low-tension glaucoma were followed monthly for 5.5 to 7.5 years (mean: 6.8 years) to determine if there were any connection between hemorrhaging and the progression of field defects. Disc hemorrhages were found in 19 eyes of 15 patients and the remaining 28 eyes of 14 patients (28 eyes) never experienced hemorrhaging in either eye throughout the follow-up. The progression of visual field defects was confirmed in 75% of bilateral bleeders (4 cases), 81% of the hemorrhagic eyes and 73% of the nonhemorrhagic eyes of the unilateral bleeders (11 cases), but the progression was observed in only 46% of the nonbleeders (14 cases). Furthermore, the hemifield corresponding to the bleeding side showed the deterioration frequency of 47%, while the hemifield corresponding to the nonbleeding side showed the frequency of 78% in the same disc. These results indicate that the fact that a low-tension glaucoma patient is a bleeder might be associated with the progression of the visual field defects.

Thirty low-tension glaucoma patients who had asymmetric intraocular pressure and visual field defects in both eyes were studied to investigate if there were any relationships between intraocular pressure and visual field defects. No patients had any disc hemorrhages during the 2-year follow-up. Twelve (80%) of 15 patients whose mean follow-up intraocular pressure was higher than 15 mmHg in both eyes, had more advanced field defects in the eye with higher intraocular pressure. On the other hand, in 14 patients whose intraocular pressure was equal to or lower than 15 mmHg in both eyes, 6 patients (42%) had greater defects in the eye with higher intraocular pressure. The results of this suggest that risk factors rather than intraocular pressure contribute to visual field defects progression in low-tension glaucoma patients whose intraocular pressure is lower than 15 mmHg.

Introduction

Despite the important advances made in glaucoma research in the last decades, the pathogenesis of glaucoma, especially of low-tension glaucoma

Gramer/Kampik (Hrsg.) Pharmakotherapie am Auge
© Springer-Verlag Berlin Heidelberg 1992

(LTG), remains controversial. There is no uniform opinion about the effects of treatment on the progression of LTG.

Gasser et al. [1] and Shirai et al. [2] reported the effectiveness of the Ca^{++} antagonist on the improvement of the visual field defects in LTG patients who showed improvement of the recovery rate of the skin temperature of their hands soaked in cold water. However, Abedin et al. [3] and de Jong et al. [4] reported that a stable and low intraocular pressure, as obtained by filtering surgery, may be beneficial to retain the visual field in LTG. These results suggest that in LTG there are at least two pathogenetic mechanisms, i.e., some kind of vascular insufficiency and intraocular pressure.

We herein report the results of our recent studies regarding these two pathogenetic mechanisms in LTG, i.e., the relationship between disc hemorrhages and the progression of field defects and the relationship between the IOP and the visual field defects.

Materials and Methods

Disc Hemorrhage Study

One hundred and thirteen eyes of 58 patients with LTG were followed from 1981 to 1989 to determine if there were any relationship between the hemorrhages and the progression of visual field defects (VFD). We examined the optic disc monthly using a direct ophthalmoscope with a fully dilated pupil, and recorded the position of the disc hemorrhages on the disc chart. Fifty-eight eyes of 29 patients, were successfully followed monthly until the end of 1989. The period of follow-up from 1981 ranged between 5.5 and 7.5 years (mean 6.8 years).

The identification criteria for LTG are:

1) the presence of typical glaucomatous field defects associated with glaucomatous optic disc changes not attributable to other ocular and systemic pathology,
2) peak intraocular pressure (IOP) equal to or lower than 21 mmHg including 24-hour diurnal curve, and
3) normal open angle.

All patients in this study have VFD in both eyes and have been followed since 1981 with no medication. Since the visual field examination was performed with the Goldmann perimeter before 1984 and with the Humphrey perimeter for more recent cases, the degree of the VFD was classified by the Aulhorn's classification with Greve's modification. The cases indicating the progression of more than one stage between the initial and the latest field examination were considered to show deterioration of the VFD.

IOP Study

To study the effect of the IOP on the VFD in LTG, the IOP level and the degree of VFD were compared in LTG patients who met the following criteria.

1) identification criteria for LTG were the same as above,
2) patients who had never had disc hemorrhages during the 2-year monthly follow-up,
3) patients who had differences between both eyes of more than one stage of the VFD classified by Aulhorn's classification with Greve's modification,
4) patients who had a difference between both eyes in mean follow-up IOP (As IOP data, the mean of IOPs measured at each visit to our outpatient clinic during the 2-year follow-up without medication was used).

Thirty patients with LTG were selected from our computer data base system which includes over 200 LTG patients. Eight of these 30 patients were among the nonbleeders of the disc hemorrhage study just mentioned above.

Results

Disc Hemorrhage Study

Prevalence of Disc Hemorrhages. Disc hemorrhages were found in 19 eyes of 15 patients during the entire period of follow-up. There were 4 bilateral bleeders and 11 unilateral bleeders. The remaining 14 patients (28 eyes) had never had disc hemorrhages in either eye throughout the 5- to 8-year follow-up started in 1981.

Progression of Visual Field Defects (VFD). The progression of the VDF was found in 79% of eyes with hemorrhages, and in 54% of eyes without hemorrhages. The frequencies were not significantly different between the two groups (P > 0.10, Table 1). When the patients were subdivided into three

Table 1. Frequency of progression of visual field defect in eyes with or without disc hemorrhage. VFD, visual field defects, DH, disc hemorrhage

Type of patients	Progression of VFD	
	+	−
Bilateral bleeder (4 cases)		
Unilateral bleeder (11 cases)		
Eyes with DH	9	2
Eyes without DH	8	3
Nonbleeder (14 cases)	13	15
		(Number of eyes)

groups, i.e., bilateral bleeders, unilateral bleeders and nonbleeders, deterioration was found in 75% of the bilateral bleeders, 81% of the hemorrhagic eyes and 73% of nonhemorrhagic eyes of the unilateral bleeders, but the deterioration was observed in 46% of the nonbleeders (Table 1).

Comparing the frequency of the deterioration of the upper or lower hemifields, which corresponded to either the upper or lower halves of the optic disc with or without disc hemorrhages (17 cases), the hemifield corresponding to the bleeding side showed the deterioration frequency of 47%, while the hemifield corresponding to the nonbleeding side showed the frequency of 78%.

The data of visual field classification, refraction at the initial examination and the intraocular pressure during the follow-up were not statistically different between the hemorrhagic eyes and nonhemorrhagic eyes (Table 2).

IOP Study

There were two groups of LTG patients. The first group was the 18 patients whose VFD were more advanced in the eye with higher IOP (IOP-dependent group), and the second group consisted of the 11 patients whose VFD were less advanced in the eye with higher IOP in comparison with the fellow eye (IOP-independent group). Even though the difference in the IOP in both eyes of each patient was small, the IOP-dependent group had higher IOP levels in

Table 2. Data at the initial examination and intraocular pressure during the follow-up. DH, disc hemorrhage

Follow-up IOP (mmHg)	Eyes with DH (19 eyes)	Eyes without DH (39 eyes)
Mean	15.4 ± 1.8	15.6 ± 1.8
Max.	19.1 ± 1.0	20.0 ± 0.9
Min.	11.9 ± 1.5	11.7 ± 1.3
		(Mean ± SD)
Visual field classification		
0	7	10
I–II	6	10
III–IV	3	10
V–VI	3	9
		(Number of eyes)
Refraction (D)		
0 < < +3	0	3
−3 < 0	8	13
−6 < < −3	11	23
		(Number of eyes)

Table 3. Mean follow-up intraocular pressure (IOP) in eyes with asymmetric visual field defect (VFD), (mean ± SD)

	IOP (mmHg)	
	Higher side	Lower side
Patients with greater VFD in higher IOP eye n = 18	15.9 ± 1.5	15.3 ± 1.3
greater VFD in lower IOP eye n = 12	14.4 ± 2.2	13.9 ± 2.0
	P < 0.05	P < 0.05

both eyes (15.9 ± 1.5 mmHg for the higher IOP side, 15.3 ± 1.3 mmHg for the lower IOP side) compared to the IOP-independent group (14.4 ± 2.2 mmHg for the higher IOP side, 13.9 ± 2.0 mmHg for the lower IOP side; Table 3).

Therefore it was suggested that the IOP level of 15 mmHg is the critical level to separate these IOP-dependent and -independent groups. Then the frequencies of the IOP-dependent or -independent patients were calculated based on their mean IOP levels. Since mean IOP of one patient were 15.6 mmHg in the higher side and 14.4 mmHg in the lower side, this patient was excluded. Twelve (80%) of 15 patients whose mean follow-up IOPs were higher than 15 mmHg in both eyes, had more advanced VFD in the higher IOP side. On the other hand, in 14 patients whose follow-up IOPs were equal to or lower than 15 mmHg in both eyes, 6 patients (42%) had the greater VFD in the higher IOP side (Table 4). However the difference was not statistically significant. There were no significant differences in the age, refraction and the degree of VFD in both groups (Table 5).

Table 4. Frequency of patients with asymmetric visual field defect (VFD)

	IOP in both eyes	
	< = 15 mmHg	> 15 mmHg
Patients with greater VFD in higher IOP eye n = 18	6	12
greater VFD in lower IOP eye n = 11	8	3
		X2-test: P < 0.10

Table 5. Data at initial examination of patients with asymmetric visual field defect (VFD)

| | Patients with greater VFD | | |
	in higher IOP eye n = 18	in lower IOP eye n = 12	
Age (years)	62.3 ± 13.5	59.3 ± 10.0	NS
Refraction (D)	− 2.0 ± 3.4	− 2.4 ± 3.3	NS
Variation of IOP (mmHg)	0.6 ± 1.2	0.7 ± 1.0	NS
		(Mean ± SD)	
VFD (worse side)			
0	0	0	
I	2	0	
II	4	2	
III	5	4	
IV	7	4	
V	0	2	
		(Number of eyes)	

Discussion

The results of the present study indicated that even after a 5- to 8-year follow-up, not all LTG patients develop disc hemorrhages, and that disc hemorrhages might not be a precursor to the progression of VFD in LTG. Furthermore, it was also suggested that the IOP level of 15 mmHg or more may contribute to VFD in LTG.

In the previous study of 0.5 to 3 years follow-up of LTG, we reported that the ultimate incidence of disc hemorrhages in LTG was 25 (43%) in 58 LTG patients and the remaining 33 (57%) did not show disc hemorrhages [5]. The present study, a subsequent 5-year follow-up of 29 LTG patients, also showed that 14 patients (48%) have had no hemorrhage during the entire period of follow-up of 5 to 8 years by monthly examination of the optic disc. The results agree with Airaksinen [6] that some glaucoma patients show disc hemorrhages, while other show none.

Disc hemorrhages have been emphasized as an important sign of the development and progression of glaucomatous VFD in ocular hypertension and primary open angle glaucoma [7, 8, 9, 10, 11, 12, 13]. However, the present study shows that in LTG, the progression of the VFD was prevalent in bilateral bleeders, but also frequent in nonhemorrhagic eyes of unilateral bleeders and in the nonhemorrhagic side of the same disc. On the other hand, the progression of VFD was less frequent in both eyes of the nonbleeder. Therefore, it seems to be difficult to suggest that the disc hemorrhage itself is responsible for the progression of the VFD. The present study indicates that the important factor in the progression of the VFD might be if the patient is a bleeder or not.

Airaksinen suggested that the pathologic diurnal variation of intraocular pressure seems more important than mean intraocular pressure in the development of hemorrhage [14]. It was pointed out by Poinooswamy et al [15] that the patients with disc hemorrhages had a higher incidence of abnormal glucose tolerance. However, we could not find any significant differences in the ophthalmological and the systemic findings between bleeders and nonbleeders. The identification of the systemic factors related to the bleeders would help us understand the pathogenesis of LTG and find a way of the treatment for LTG.

The role of IOP in the development of optic nerve damage in LTG is still controversial. Cartwright et al [16] reported that in 12 of 14 cases of LTG with asymmetric IOP, the glaucomatous cupping and field loss was greater in the eye with higher pressure. Abedin et al. [3] and de Jong et al. [4] reported that a stable and low intraocular pressure as obtained by filtering surgery may contribute to the retention of the visual field in LTG. These results indicate that the IOP contributes in some manner in the development of optic nerve damage in LTG. However, as shown above, the fact that the patient is bleeder or not might affect the progression of the VFD.

In our IOP study, all patients were confirmed by monthyl examination not to have had disc hemorrhages during the 2-year follow-up. As a result, it was shown that the patients whose IOPs were equal to or higher than 15 mmHg in both eyes frequently had more advanced VFD in the eye with higher IOP. On the other hand, contrary cases (more advanced VFD in the eye with lower pressure) were found in the patients whose IOP was lower than 15 mmHg. Even though it has been suggested that pressure variation might play an important role in the development or the progression of VFD, in our study the asymmetry of IOP in both eyes was similar in the two groups. Since the damaged disc may become more vulnerable to the IOP, from the viewpoint of treatment, the IOP level of 15 mmHg may be too high to retared the progression of VFD in LTG. However, our results suggested that risk factors rather than IOP contribute to the progression of VFD in LTG patients whose IOP is lower than 15 mmHg.

References

1. Gasser P, Flammer J, Guthause U et al (1990) Do vasospasms provoke ocular diseases? Angiology 41: 213–220
2. Shirai H, Asano K, Kitazawa Y et al (1988) The effect of Ca^{2+} antgonist on visual field in low tension glaucoma. Acta Soc Ophthalmol Jpn (Nihon Gankagakkai Zassi) 92: 729–797
3. Abedin S, Simmons RJ, Grant WM (1982) Progressive low-tension glaucoma: Treatment to stop glaucomatous cupping and field loss when these progress despite normal intraocular pressure. Ophthalmology 89: 1–6
4. de Jong N, Greve EL, Hoyng PF et al (1989) Results of a filtering procedure in low tension glaucoma. Int Ophthalmol 13: 131–138

5. Kitazawa Y, Shirato S, Yamamoto T (1986) Optic disc hemorrhage in low-tension glaucoma. Ophthalmology 93: 853–857
6. Airaksinen PJ (1984) Are optic disc hemorrhages a common finding in all glaucoma patients? Acta Ophthalmol 62: 193–196
7. Drance SM, Begg IS (1970) Sector hemorrhage – a probable acute ischemic disc change in chronic simple glaucoma. Can J Ophthalmol 5: 137–141
8. Airaksinen PJ et al (1981) Optic disc hemorrhages precede retinal nerve fiber layer defects in ocular hypertension. Acta Ophthalmol (Copenh) 59: 627–641
9. Airaksinen PJ, Tuulonen A (1984) Early glaucoma changes in patients with and without an optic disc hemorrhage. Acta Ophthalmol 62: 197–202
10. Chumbley LC, Brubaker RF (1976) Low-tension glaucoma. Br J Ophthalmol 81: 761–763
11. Drance SM (1989) Disc hemorrhages in the glaucomas. Survey Ophthalmol 33: 331–337
12. Shihab ZM et al (1982) The significance of disc hemorrhages in open angle glaucoma. Ophthalmology 89: 211–213
13. Susanna R et al (1979) Disc hemorrhages in patients with elevated intraocular pressure. Arch Ophthalmol 97: 284–285
14. Airaksinen PJ (1981) Optic disc hemorrhage – Analysis of stereophotographs and clinical data of 112 patients. Arch Ophthalmol 99: 1795–1801
15. Poinooswamy D et al (1986) Association between optic disc hemorrhages in glaucoma and abnormal glucose tolerance. Br J Ophthalmol 70: 599–602
16. Cartwright MJ, Anderson DR (1988) Correlation of asymmetric damage with asymmetric intraocular pressure in normal-tension glaucoma (low-tension glaucoma). Arch Ophthalmol 106: 898–900

Corresponding Address
Professor S. Shirato, M.D.
Department of Ophthalmology, School of Medicine, University of Tokyo,
7-3-1 Hongo, Bunkyo-ku, Tokyo 113, Japan

Ocular Microvascular Vasoconstriction Following Topical Adrenergic Therapy

E. M. Van Buskirk, D. R. Bacon, and K. Sugiyama

Our group has been interested in examining the anatomy of the uveal microvasculature and in measuring the regulatory response of ocular vessels to physiologic and pharmacologic stimuli [1–3]. We have used a methacrylate intraluminal microvascular corrosion casting model. We have examined the ciliary microvasculature of 10 different mammalian species [4–6]. Although the old world cynomolgus monkey or the baboon most completely resemble the human ciliary vasculature, the rabbit also provides a suitable experimental model. Of all the species examined, only the rabbit and the primate have a dual arterial supply to each ciliary process. Unlike the primate, the very rudimentary ciliary muscle of the rabbit affords some advantage for measurement and statistical analysis of changes in ciliary process arterial diameters in response to experimental manipulation. The ciliary process arteriolar diameters of the rabbit however can be directly measured at the scanning electron microscope with a minimum of ciliary muscle dissection required.

Over the past few years we have worked to develop a method for production of castings under physiologic conditions that replicates the microvascular luminal changes in responses to physiologic variables such as intraocular pressure and to pharmacologic influences with adrenergic drugs.

Recently we have begun expansion of these studies to include the microvasculare of the optic nerve head (optic disk) of the rabbit, studies that will eventually include other non-primate mammals and primates. Like the primate, the rabbit has a vascularized retina supplied by a central retinal artery and the optic disk vasculature has retinal, ciliary or choroidal components. Unlike the primate, the rabbit retinal vasculature supplies only two wing-like portions of the retina. The ocular vasculature derives mainly from the external carotid artery by way of the external ophthalmic artery that, in turn, gives off both the ciliary and the central retinal arteries. In a minority of rabbits, the central retinal artery derives from the internal ophthalmic, a branch of the internal carotid artery [7]. The rabbit possesses virtually no lamina cribrosa [8, 9].

Gramer/Kampık (Hrsg) Pharmakotherapıe am Auge
© Springer-Verlag Berlın Heıdelberg 1992

Techniques

Materials and Methods

Castings of the rabbit ocular microvasculature were obtained under maximal physiologic injection condition as described elsewhere [10]. Every effort was made to maintain physiologic hemostasis of the animal by mechanical respiration with a Harvard small animal respirator and maintenance of normal blood gases. Batson's #17 methacrylate injection media was modified to reduce the viscosity to 11 centipoise, only slightly more viscous than mammalian blood. The animals were maintained at physiologic temperature (37 degrees). The injection pressure was maintained at physiologic perfusion pressure (100–120 mmHg) until the plastic polymerized in about 15 minutes. The eyes were not manipulated.

Two hours after injection the eyes were enucleated, stored overnight in warm formalin to complete polymerization and corroded in potassium hydroxide. The resultant castings of the ocular vasculature were rinsed in running water and air dried.

The rabbit eyes were hemisected at the equator. The anterior segments and posterior segments were mounted separately on large stubs for scanning electron microscopic examination.

Analysis of Data

Ciliary Body

The major circle of the iris was exposed for its entire circumference. Each anterior and posterior radial arteriole branching from the major circle and supplying the ciliary processes were measured at the constricted zonen ear the branching point from the major arterial circle. A second measurement was then taken at a reference point 50 microns downstream from the posterior end of the constricted zone as previously reported [10]. The relative constriction at the constricted zone was determined as: % of constriction = (constricted diameter/downstream diameter) × 100) – 100.

Optic Nerve

The optic nerve microvasculature has been examined only qualitatively to date. The posterior segment castings were examined from either the anterior or posterior aspects by the sequential microdissection technique [11]. For posterior dissections, an initial scanning electron micrograph of the posterior view of the optic nerve was taken, and the vessel wall of the pial system removed. The specimen was then recoated and photographed again. After removing some of the capillaries within the optic nerve we were able to photograph and investigate previously inaccessible vessels and to identify sites crucial to optic nerve head perfusion. From the anterior aspect, we dissected the retinal vasculature at the edge of the optic disk and examined the vascular communications between the disk and the choroid. Finally, we bisected the optic nerve castings longitudinally to investigate the relationships between the optic disk and retinal vasculature.

Drug Effects

In previous reported studies, adult, normal, nonpigmented rabbits received one drop of the test drug centrally on the cornea of the left eye approximately one hour before microvascular casting [3]. The three drugs tested were phenylephrine hydrochloride, timolol maleate 0.5%, and betaxolol hydrochloride ß.5%. Each eye was compared to the fellow, untreated eye.

Other rabbits underwent unilateral, long-term therapy (one drop daily) with one of the three vasoconstrictive drugs, phenylephrine, timolol or betaxolol, for 30–50 days. Seven rabbits were treated with phenylephrine hydrochloride, two rabbits were treated with timolol maleate, and two rabbits were treated with betaxolol hydrochloride. Optic nerves were evaluated only in phenylephrine treated eyes to date.

Results

Rigid whole eye luminal castings of the entire ocular microvasculature are produced with the "physiologic technique". These have a clean surface, show minimal or no extravasation and exhibit better replication of focal alterations in luminal diameter. Replication of the nuclear imprint differentiates arteries and veins.

Ciliary Process Microvasculature

The rabbit possesses some similarities in anatomy to the primate and some important differences. There are no anterior ciliary arteries in the rabbit eye; the entire anterior segment including the iris and ciliary processes receives its arterial supply from the two long posterior ciliary arteries. The ciliary muscle is very rudimentary and the major circle of the iris lies at the peripheral extreme of the iris near the surface. Anterior and posterior arteriole branches from the major circle of the iris supply anterior and posterior portions of the ciliary or irido-ciliary processes (the anterior portion of the ciliary process in the rabbit extends well on to the posterior surface of the iris) [5].

Like the primate, focal constrictions were observed in arterial branches from the major circle that supply the ciliary processess [1, 2, 3, 10]. These focal constrictions occur with equal frequency in the arterial supply to the anterior and the posterior portion of the process, an important difference from the primate.

Optic Nerve Vasculature

From the posterior aspect, three short posterior ciliary arteries contrive to from an incomplete vascular ring corresponding to the circle of Zinn-Haller of other mammals. Most of the efferent vessels of this circle pass to the choroid; however, several pial branches pass posteriorly from it (arrow). These branches penetrate the nerve centripetally to nourish the optic nerve head capillaries. By the same token, numerous septal veins inside the optic nerve head are seen to drain to the pial system (Fig. 1).

Identifying the choroidal blood supply to the optic nerve head required the removal of the circle of Zinn-Haller. This revealed many venous connections between the choroid vessels and the optic nerve head vasculature along the optic nerve head margin (Fig. 2) except in the inferior quadrant of the optic nerve head, where no connections to the choroid are observed.

The retinal vasculature is continuous with the superficial optic nerve head

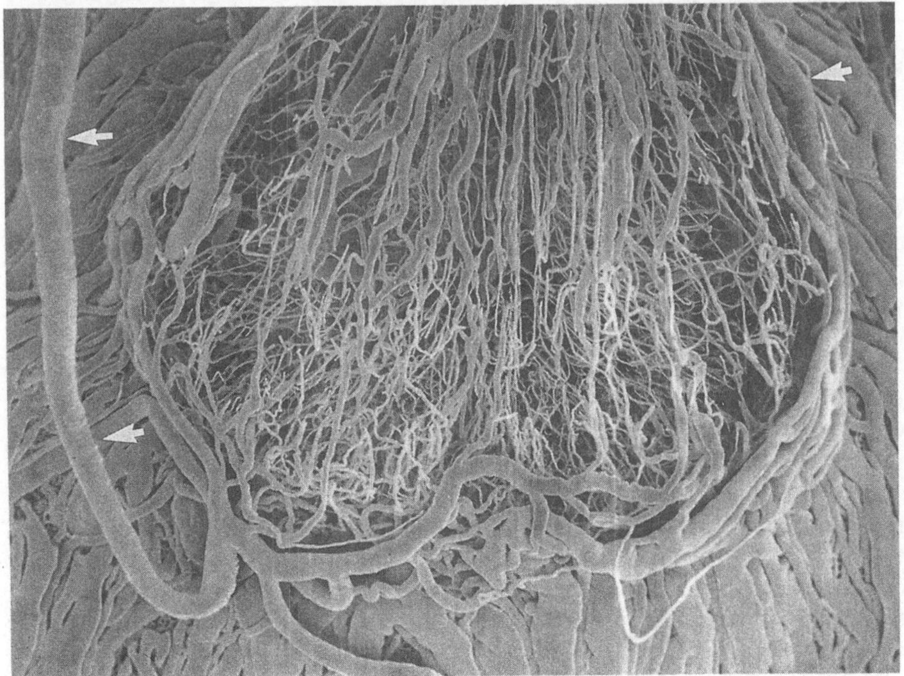

Fig. 1. Posterior view of rabbit optic nerve showing posterior ciliary arterial supply to Zinn-Haller circle that provides arterial supply to the posterior aspect of the optic nerve head (33×)

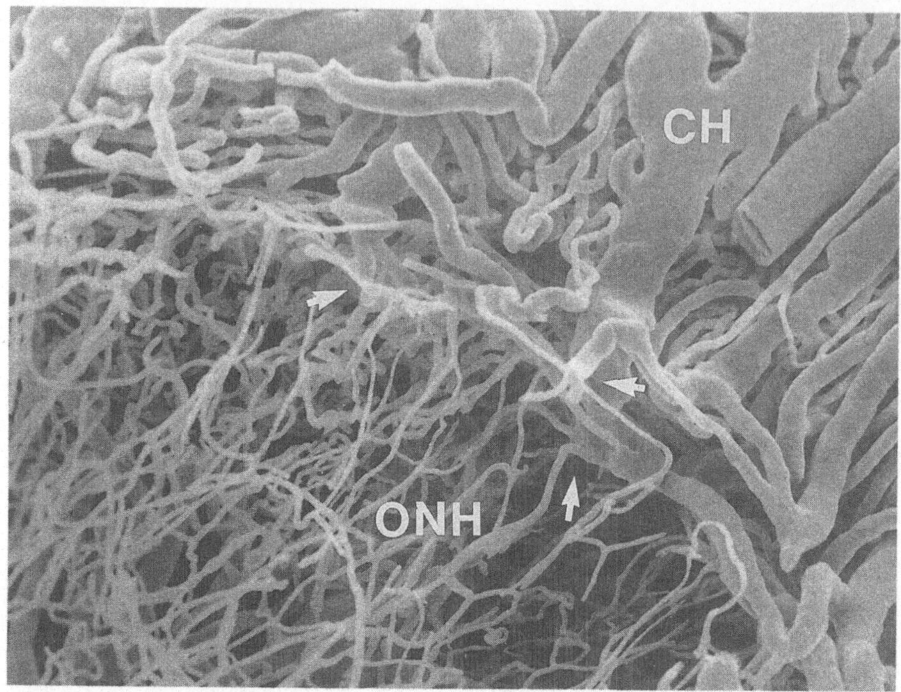

Fig. 2. Posterior view of optic nerve head (ONH) vasculature showing choroidal (CH) communications which are primarily venous (116×)

vessels. Longitudinally, small vessels from the optic nerve head surface are continuous with these counterparts in the intraorbital portion of the optic nerve (Fig. 3). The retinal artery gives off branches to the superficial vasculature of the optic nerve head, the venous drainage of which empties into the retinal veins.

In order to visualize both the retinal artery and veins it was necessary to remove the interior capillaries within the "retrolaminar" optic nerve head. Occasionally, one of the principal retinal arterial branches derives not from the central retinal artery, but directly from a short posterior ciliary artery, similar to the cilio-retinal arteries seen in man. More often, each wing of retinal vasculature is nourished by branches of the central retinal artery. Occasionally, branches from the central retinal artery make a direct connection with the circle of Zinn-Haller. The retinal artery usually gives off a few branches which have an intraneural distribution within the anterior optic nerve head. Two large retinal veins pass from lateral and medial wings of retinal vasculature through the optic nerve head to drain the pial system of the optic nerve. In addition, two small separate retinal veins drain the anterior vasculature of the optic nerve head and peripapillary retina independently and then join the pial venous drainage system.

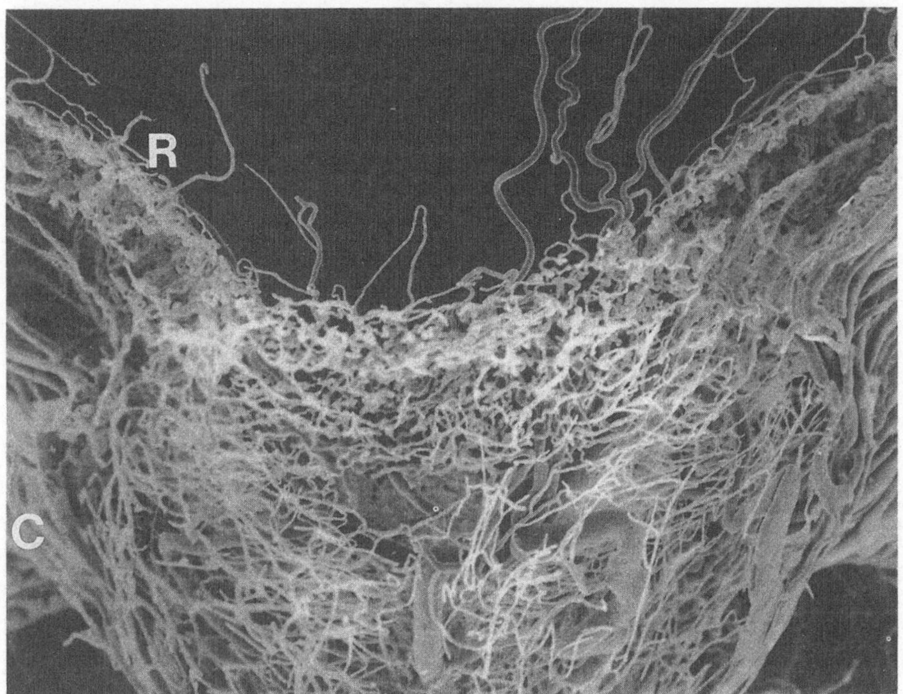

Fig. 3. Cross sectional view of the rabbit optic nerve head vasculature showing retinal (R) supply to anterior nerve head vasculature and choroidal (C) supply to posterior nerve head vasculature (78×)

Experimental Alterations of the Ciliary Vasculature

Drugs

In the ciliary processes the adrenergic drugs tested produced no alteration in downstream diameter compared to untreated controls or to each other ($p > 0.5$ for each of the three drugs compared to each other or to control) [3].

In contrast to the downstream diameters, however the eyes treated with vasoconstricting, alpha agonist or beta antagonist, drugs regularly showed marked focal constriction at the branch point. The phenylephrine treated eyes exhibited 32% constriction, the timolol treated eyes 23%, and the betaxolol 30% after single dose administration. The constriction of these arteriolar cuffs after each drug was highly significant ($p < 0.001$) compared to controls (Fig. 4) [3].

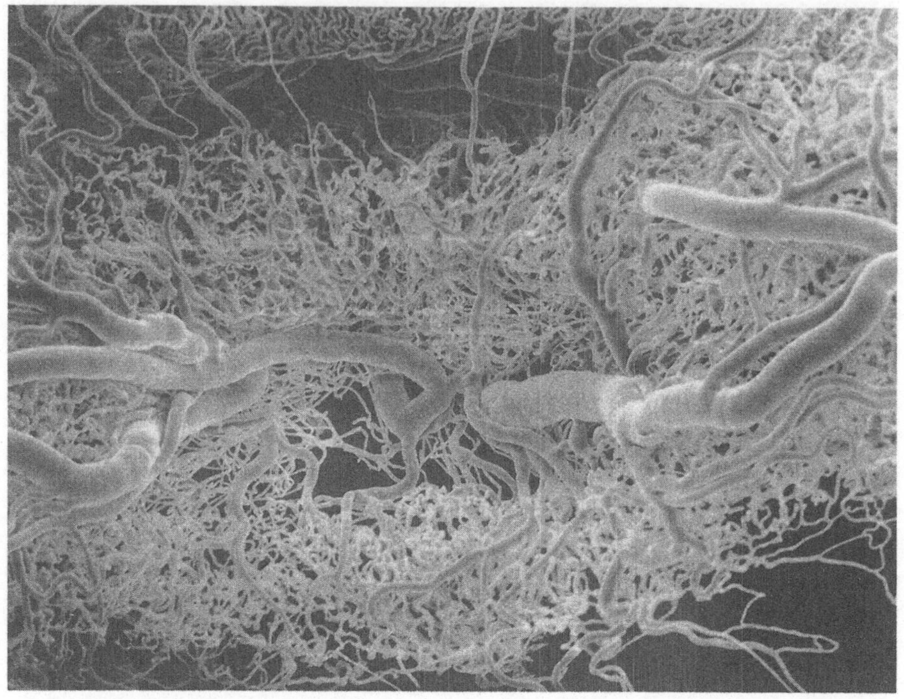

Fig. 4. Scanning electron micrograph of the rabbit peripapillarly retinal vasculature showing wing-shaped area of retinal vasculature (72×)

Chronic Administration

Eyes treated for a minimum of five weeks with timolol maleate continued to show focal constriction comparable to those receiving only a single dose with the constriction measuring 21.5%. There was no statistically significant difference between the per cent constriction following acute or chronic timolol. In contrast, the betaxolol treated eyes showed no significant focal vasoconstriction after chronic therapy (15.8%) compared to 15.2% for controls (Fig. 5). Phenylephrine treated eyes continued to show ciliary vasoconstriction after chronic therapy (20.0%), but to a considerably less degree than following single dose therapy (Fig. 6).

Adrenergic Vasoconstriction Effect
on Optic Disc Microvasculature

Preliminary studies of phenylephrine treated rabbit eyes qualitatively show very little of any effect of single drop exposure of phenylephrine on the optic disc vasculature. However, eyes treated for 30 days with one daily exposure

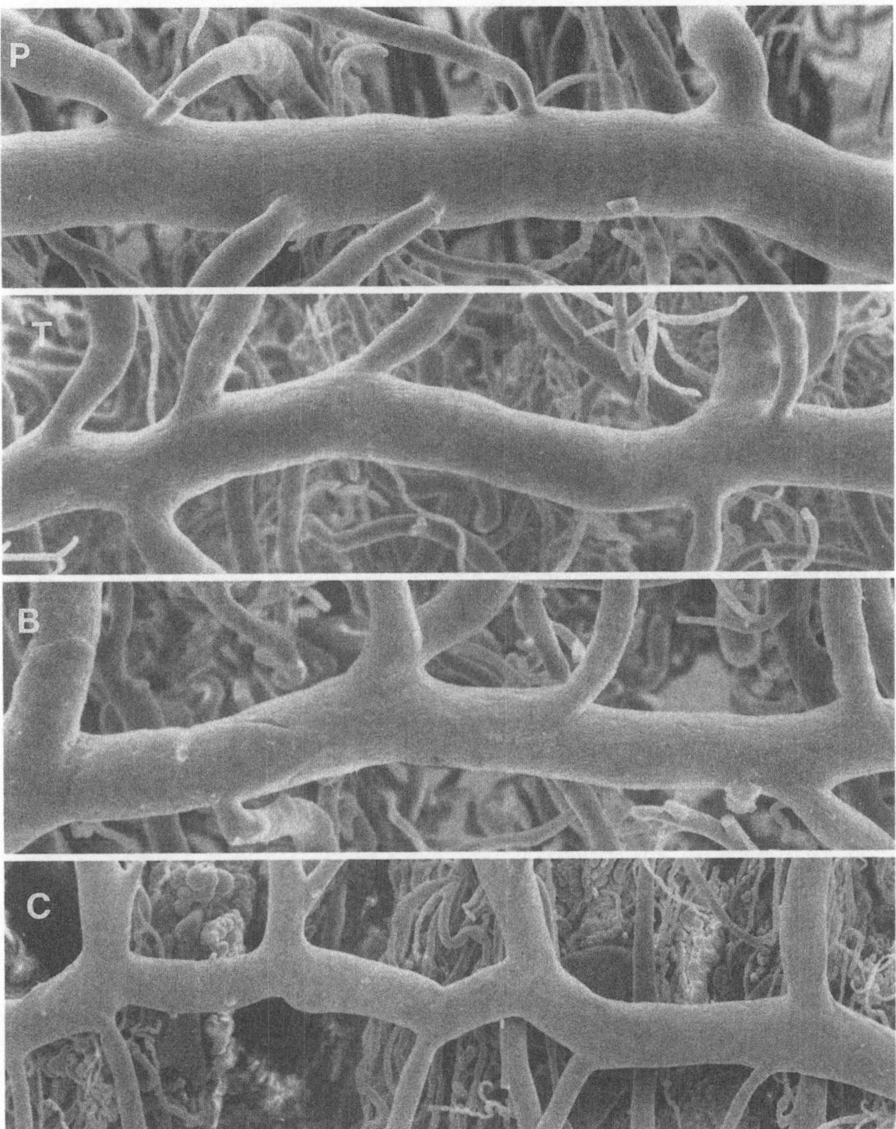

Fig. 5. Major circle of the iris and branch arterials to the ciliary processes showing increased branch point constriction after chronic topical phenylephrine (P) (150×) and timolol therapy (T) (160×), but not after betaxolol therapy (B) (190×) in control (C) (after no treatment). (Reproduced with permission of the Ophthalmic Publishing Company, American Journal of Ophthalmology)

showed marked multiple focal constrictions within the anterior optic disc vasculature. The constrictions seemed primarily in the choroidal component, (branch of the Zinn-Haller) but no quantitative studies have yet been

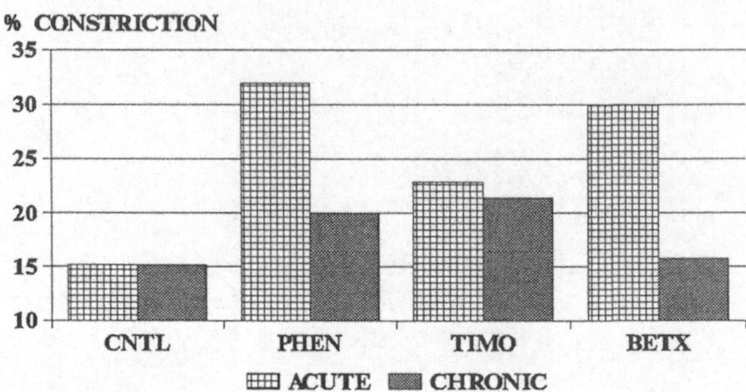

Fig. 6. Histogram showing effects of acute and chronic drug therapy on mean relative vasoconstriction at the branch point of ciliary process arterials from the major circle of the iris (histogram)

completed. In some eyes, the optic disc vasculature was virtually unfilled except for the retinal component. Others showed partial filling of the ciliary component, but the retinal arteries and retinal contribution to the optic disc vasculature appeared relatively unaffected. The vessels that were filled, particularly those branching from the perineural vascular circle showed multiple segmental constricted zones lending a sausage-like configuration not seen in the untreated rabbits (Fig. 7).

In contrast to the anterior segment studies where the fellow untreated eyes showed no vasoconstriction after contralateral adrenergic therapy, the untreated eyes also demonstrate some evidence of vasoconstriction after chronic phenylephrine therapy to the contralateral eye.

Discussion

Our studies described here and elsewhere have demonstrated focal vasoconstrictor zones in the arterioles supplying the ciliary processes of the rabbit eye [1, 2, 3, 10]. The use of physiologic injection techniques has permitted documentation of activity of these vasoconstrictor zones when exposed to alpha adrenergic agonists or beta adrenergic antagonist drugs.

Originally, we could not rule out vasoconstrictor activity in methacrylate itself or that it derived from agonal vasoconstriction produced by autonomic stimulation in response to the stress of the procedure. However, with refinement of the injection technique to include maintenance of physiologic conditions up to the moment of injection, we observe only minimal vasoconstriction in control eyes. Further, this vasoconstriction is neither accentuated nor diminished by paracentesis and reduction of intraocular pressure to zero, a procedure known to disrupt the blood aqueous barrier [10]. Any vasoconstriction beyond this minimal amount can only be

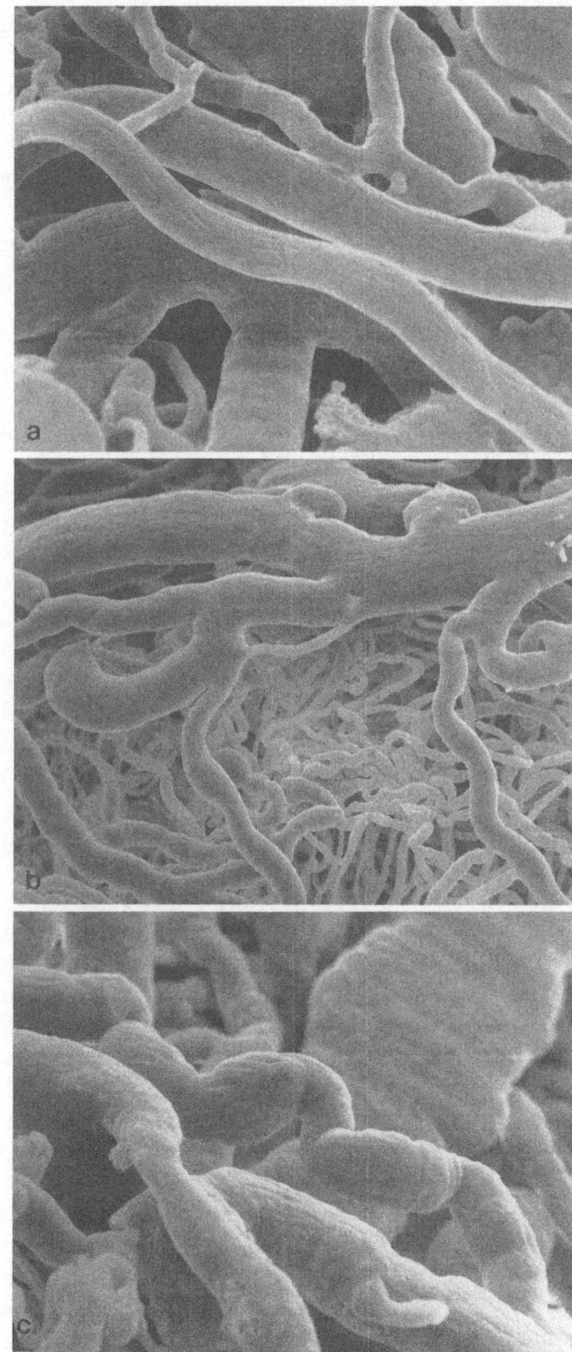

Fig. 7a–c. Arteriolar branches from the circle of Zinn-Haller to the posterior optic disc head vasculature of the rabbit after chronic phenylephrine therapy. **a** Control (240×); **b** ipsilateral (252×); **c** contralateral eye (264×). The figures show multiple focal constrictions in the treated eye and to a lesser degree in the untreated, control eye

experimentally produced by the release of endogenous neural hormones or from exogenously administered pharmacologic drugs such as we have employed. All of the durgs studied selectively contracted the pre-capillary arteriolar "sphincter" zones but produced no diffuse narrowing of down-stream arterioles.

As expected, we observe focal constriction in response to the direct alpha adrenergic agonist phenylephrine. Further, we observed such constriction following administration of beta adrenergic antagonists presumably through blockade of beta 2 receptors leading to relative dominance of endogenous alpha adrenergic activity. Although the relative beta 2 selective antagonist betaxolol produced vasoconstriction after a single dose to the rabbit eye, but this effect was diminished to insignificant levels after chronic exposure [3].

With these studies, we have extended our examinations of the rabbit ocular microvasculature from the ciliary body to the optic nerve. Although the rabbit posterior segment microvasculature possesses many important differences from primate, enough important fetures are shared to make it a valid model. In particular, both rabbit and primate have a retinal vasculature that contributes to the optic disk blood supply and that is served by a central retinal artery. In contrast, some mammals lack a retinal vasculature altogether, while the retinal arteries in others, such as dog and cat, are entirely branches from the ciliary system. The rabbit optic disc receives arterial contributions from both the retinal and ciliary supplies, as in the primate. The capillary supplies appear not only contiguous with occasional, venous interconnections.

Chronic topical therapy with the adrenergic agonist phenylephrine seems to have produced significant segmental vasoconstriction in the optic disc, particularly in the *choroidal vasculature constriction*. In contrast to the studies of the ciliary microvasculature, chronic therapy produced a much greater effect than did single dose therapy where virtually no discernible effect was observed. Moreover, a lessor but also obvious vasoconstrictor response occurred in the fellow untreated eye. This suggests, that, in contrast to ciliary process microvasculature drug adrenergic effects on the nerve derive not from intraocular drug transport but from systemic exposure possibly reaching the neural tissue by way of the peripapillary choroid. Other studies have demonstrated increased permeability of intravascular material into the optic nerve head from the perineural choroid in both monkey and rabbit [12].

By using these techniques to study eyes exposed to various physiological and pharmacological stimuli we hope to understand better the regional vasomoter abilities of the optic nerve head vasculature, its response to physiologic and pharmacologic stimuli, and the prospects for agents that may improve perfusion and thus protect the glaucomatous optic nerve.

References

1. Van Buskirk EM (1988) The ciliary vasculature and its perturbation with drugs and surgery. Tr Am Ophthalmol Soc 86: 794–841
2. Van Buskirk EM, Bacon DR, Fahrenbach WH (1989) Replication of vasomotor effects with controlled intravascular corrosion casting. Tr Am Ophthalmol Soc 87: 125–142
3. Van Buskirk EM, Bacon DR, Fahrenbach WH (1990) Ciliary vasoconstriction after topical adrenergic drugs. Am J Ophthalmol 109: 511–517
4. Morrison JC, Van Buskirk EM (1984) Ciliary process microvascular of the primate eye. AM J Ophthalmol 97: 372–373
5. Morrison JC, DeFrank MP, Van Buskirk EM (1987) Regional microvascular anatomy of the rabbit ciliary body. Invest Ophthalmol Vis Sci 28: 1314–1340
6. Morrison JC, DeFrank MP, Van Buskirk EM (1987) Comparative microvascular anatomy of mammalianciliary processes. Invest Ophthalmol Vis Sci 28: 1325–1340
7. Ruskell GL (1964) Blood vessels of the orbit and globe. In: Prince JH (ed) The rabbit in eye research. Thomas, Springfield, pp 514–553
8. Prince JH, Diesem CD, Eglitis I, Ruskell GL (1960) The rabbit, optic nerve. In: Anatomy and histology of the eye and orbit in domestic animals. Thomas, Springfield, pp 277–278
9. Prince JH, McConnell DG (1964) Retina and optic nerve. In: Prince JH (ed) The rabbit in eye research. Thomas, Springfield, pp 385–449
10. Fahrenbach WH, Bacon DR, Van Buskirk EM (1988) Controlled vascular corrosion casting of the rabbit eye. J Electron Microscopy Tech 10: 15–26
11. Morrison JC, Van Buskirk EM (1984) Sequential microdissection and scanning electron microscopy of ciliary microvascular castings. Scanning Electron Microscopy II: 857–865
12. Flage T (1977) Permeability properties of the tissues in the optic nerve head region in the rabbit and the monkey. Acta Ophthalmologica 55: 652–664

Corresponding Address

Professor E. M. van Buskirk, M.D.
Chairman, Devers Eye Institute / Good Samaritan Hospital and Medical Center,
1040 N.W. 22nd Ave, N 320, Portland, Oregon 97210, USA

Morphologische Veränderungen des Ziliarkörpers nach Langzeitbehandlung mit Timolol und Adrenalin

E. Lütjen-Drecoll

Abstrakt

Die morphologischen Veränderungen des vorderen Anteils des Ziliarfortsatzes nach Langzeitbehandlung mit Timolol (ca. 3, 6 und 7 Monate) werden beschrieben und die funktionelle Bedeutung der Befunde diskutiert.

Nach Langzeitbehandlung mit Timolol weisen die morphologischen wie die physiologischen Veränderungen auf eine Reduktion der Kammerwassersekretion hin: die Gefäße sind eng und das Epithel enthält wenig Mitochondrien und Membraneinfaltungen. Nach Adrenalinbehandlung sind die morphologischen Veränderungen heterogen. In einigen Teilen der Zirkumferenz sind die Gefäße erweitert und die Mitochondrien vermehrt, Zeichen einer Hypersekretion. In anderen Teilen sind die Fortsätze geschwollen und das Epithel degenerativ verändert. In diesen Teilen der Zirkumferenz könnte die Sekretion negativ sein. Die Veränderungen nach Adrenalin weisen große Ähnlichkeit mit Veränderungen nach Behandlung mit Prostaglandinen auf.

Einleitung

Medikamente, die in der Glaukomtherapie zur Senkung des intraokulären Drucks (IOP) eingesetzt werden, wirken entweder durch Erhöhung der Abflußrate des Kammerwassers (KaWa) oder durch Senkung der Sekretionsrate. Der Wirkungsmechanismus der einzelnen Pharmaka ist jedoch bisher noch keineswegs eindeutig geklärt.

Prof. Funk zeigt im nachfolgenden Beitrag, daß die Gefäßreaktionen des Ziliarkörpers nach Applikation verschiedener Pharmaka bei Albinokaninchen mit unserer mikroendoskopischen Methode direkt in vivo untersucht werden können. Diese Gefäßreaktionen lassen jedoch primär nur Rückschlüsse über Volumenänderungen der Fortsätze zu. Für die Kammerwassersekretionsrate ist die Durchblutung der Ziliarfortsätze jedoch nicht allein ausschlaggebend. Der größte Teil des Flüssigkeitstransportes erfolgt durch aktive energiefordernde Prozesse des Ziliarepithels.

Gramer/Kampik (Hrsg) Pharmakotherapie am Auge
© Springer-Verlag Berlin Heidelberg 1992

Sekretionsvorgang

Die Gefäße sind vor allem an dem passiven Prozeß der Ultrafiltration beteiligt. Abhängig vom hydrostatischen Druck in den Gefäßen können Flüssigkeit, teilweise auch Proteine, aus den dünnwandigen, stark gefensterten Kapillaren der Ziliarfortsätze in das Stroma zwischen Kapillaren und Ziliarepithel austreten. Von hier aus dringt die Flüssigkeit bis zu den Zonulae occludentes vor, die die apikalen Zellmembranen des unpigmentierten Ziliarepithels (UPE) miteinander verbinden. Die Zonulae occludentes bilden den wesentlichen Teil der Blutkammerwasserschranke. Der weitere Transport der Flüssigkeit erfolgt aktiv. In den basolateralen Membraneinfaltungen der Ziliarepithelzellen (ZE) sind Enzyme vorhanden, wie z.B. die Na-Ka-ATPase und die Carboanhydrase, die bestimmte Ionen (vor allem Na^+) aktiv in das Labyrinth der Membraneinfaltungen und Interdigitationen zwischen den benachbarten UPE-Zellen pumpen. Durch diese Ionen wird ein osmotischer Gradient aufgebaut. Da die Zonulae occludentes wasserdurchlässig sind, kann Wasser durch die Zellhaften hindurchtreten und dadurch dem Ionengradienten folgen (Abb. 1). Das Zytoplasma der UPE-Zellen zeichnet sich durch den Besitz zahlreicher Mitochondrien aus, die die Energie für die Aktivität dieser Pumpsysteme bereitstellen. Da Eiweiß nicht durch die Zellhaften hindurchtreten kann, wird im Strom andererseits ein onkotischer Druck aufgebaut. Dieser wirkt dem osmotischen Druck entgegen. Theoretisch ist es also vorstellbar, daß bei erhöhtem onkotischen und vermindertem osmotischen Druck Kammerwasser sogar rückwärts in Richtung Stroma in den Ziliarkörper zurückfließen, d.h. Kammerwasser von den Ziliarfortsätzen auch resorbiert werden kann (Abb. 1).

In der Glaukomtherapie spielen die Medikamente Timolol und Adrenalin heute eine wesentliche Rolle. Timolol, ein nicht selektiver β-adrenerger Antagonist senkt den IOP durch Verminderung der Kammerwassersekretionsrate [1, 2]. Die Wirkung des Adrenalins, eines kombinierten α- und

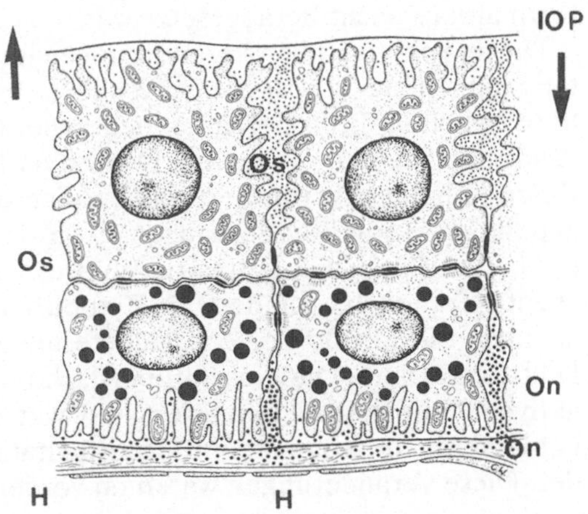

Abb. 1. Schematische Darstellung der Prozesse, die an der Kammerwasserproduktion beteiligt sind: Hydrostatischer Druck (H) und osmotischer Druck (Os) fördern die Sekretionsrate; intraokularer Druck (IOP) und onkotischer Druck (On) wirken diesem Sekretionsdruck entgegen

β-adrenergen Agonisten, wird in der Literatur unterschiedlich beschrieben. Nach Kolker und Hetherington sowie nach früheren Untersuchungen von Sears soll Adrenalin die Kammerwassersekretionsrate senken [3, 4]. Neuere fluorophotometrische Untersuchungen an menschlichen Augen weisen hingegen daraufhin, daß die Sekretionsrate nach Adrenalingabe erhöht ist [5, 6].

Methoden

Um der Frage nach dem Wirkungsmechanismus dieser Medikamente weiter nachzugehen und um zu untersuchen, welche der obengenannten Systeme durch Langzeitbehandlung mit diesen Medikamenten beeinflußt werden, haben wir vor einigen Jahren die morphologischen Veränderungen des Ziliarkörpers bei Macaca fascicularis nach Langzeitbehandlung (2,5 und 6 Monate) mit Timolol und Adrenalin untersucht [7, 8]. Die Versuche sowie die ophthalmologischen Kontrollen der Tiere wurden von Prof. Kaufman am Institut für Ophthalmologie der Universität Madison/Wisconsin/USA durchgeführt. Die genannten Medikamente wurden in der Regel 4mal täglich lokal appliziert, wobei die Dosierung der beim Menschen angewandten entsprach (180 μg Timolol und 540–600 μg Adrenalin/Dosis). Nach Abschluß der Behandlung wurden die Augen für die morphologischen Untersuchungen in Epon eingebettet und die gesamte Zirkumferenz des Auges licht- und elektronenmikroskopisch untersucht.

Ergebnisse und Diskussion

Timolol

Die physiologischen und ophthalmologischen Untersuchungen zeigten, daß auch nach 6monatiger Behandlung noch die Kammerwassersekretionsrate der Timolol-behandelten Tiere gegenüber einer Gruppe unbehandelter Normaltiere leicht herabgesetzt war.

Die morphologischen Veränderungen im Bereich des Ziliarkörpers stimmten weitgehend mit diesen physiologischen Befunden überein. Schon im histologischen Bild fiel eine deutliche Hyalinisierung des Stromas der Ziliarfortsätze auf, d.h. die Diffusionsstrecke zwischen Kapillaren und Ziliarepithel war verbreitert und verdichtet. Der Durchmesser der Stromakapillaren war deutlich geringer als in der unbehandelten Kontrollgruppe (Abb. 2). Auch die Ultrastruktur des Ziliarepithels dieser Region war ebenfalls deutlich verändert. Im Zytoplasma des UPE war sowohl die Anzahl als auch die Größe der energieliefernden Mitochondrien nahezu um die Hälfte reduziert. Die Gesamtoberfläche der Zellmembranen, in denen die aktiven Pumpsysteme lokalisiert sind, war signifikant verringert. Basolaterale Membraneinfaltungen und -Interdigitationen waren kaum noch ausgebildet. Diese Veränderungen waren im vorderen Teil der pars plicata, der nicht

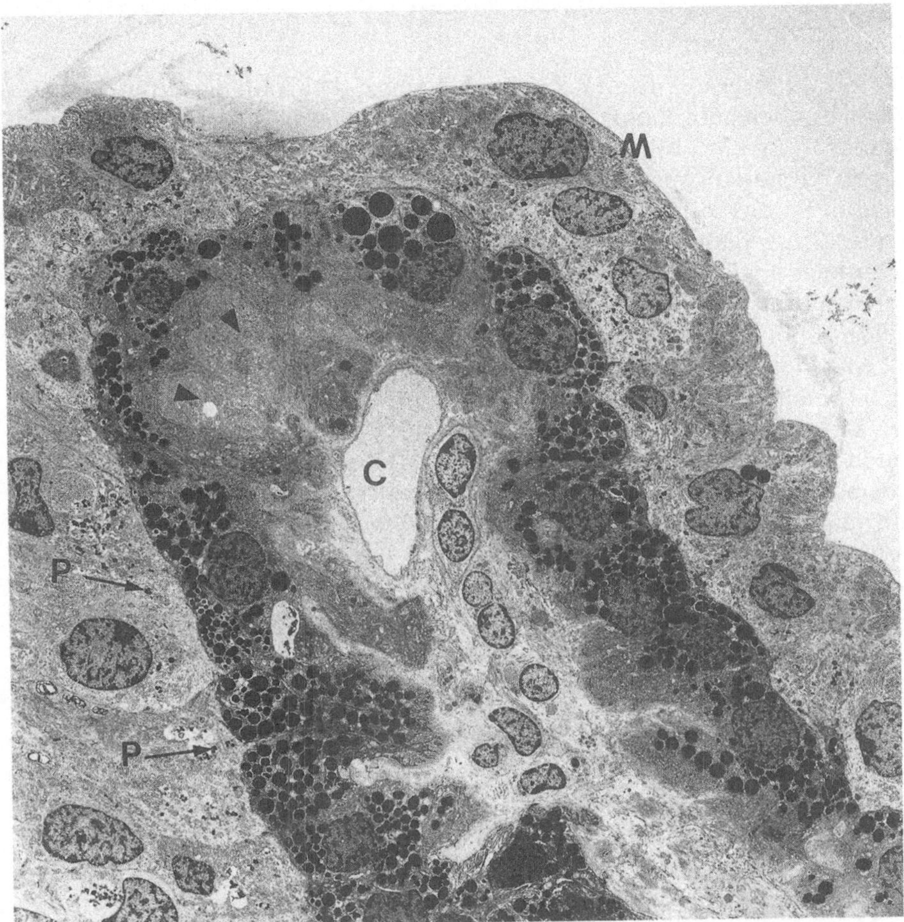

Abb. 2. Elektronenmikroskopische Übersichtsaufnahme aus dem vorderen Anteil eines Ziliarfortsatzes nach 6monatiger Behandlung mit Timolol (Cynomolgusaffe × 2400). Die Kapillaren (C) sind durch die Hyalinisierung des angrenzenden Stromas (Pfeilköpfe) eingeengt. Die unpigmentierten Ziliarepithelzellen zeigen kaum basolaterale Einfaltungen und wenig kleine Mitochondrien (M). *P* = Pigmentgranula

von Zonula bedeckt ist und frei in die mit KaWa gefüllte hintere Augen-kammer hineinragt, besonders deutlich ausgeprägt. Ultrastrukturelle und enzymhistochemische Untersuchungen weisen daraufhin, daß im genannten Teil der pars plicata der größte Teil der KaWa-Sekretion erfolgt. Allerdings waren nicht alle Fortsätze an der Zirkumferenz des Auges gleichmäßig betroffen. In einigen der untersuchten Augen waren 10–50% der Fortsätze morphologisch weitgehend unverändert.

Eine Praeferenz der genannten Veränderungen in bestimmten Quadranten des Auges war nicht zu erkennen. Die Ursache dieser Zirkumferenzunter-schiede ist bisher nicht geklärt.

Adrenalin

Interessanterweise wies der ZK nach Langzeitbehandlung mit Adrenalin deutlich andere morphologische Veränderungen auf als nach Behandlung mit Timolol (Abb. 3a, b). Im vorderen Anteil der Ziliarfortsätze waren die Kapillaren stark erweitert. Das Stroma der Fortsätze war lockermaschig und zellarm. Es wies keine Hyalinisierungen des Bindegewebes auf. Die angrenzenden ZE zeigten ultrastrukturell ausgeprägte Membraneinfaltungen und -interdigitationen. Im Zytoplasma der NPE-Zellen waren Anzahl und Volumen der Mitochondrien gegenüber der Kontrollgruppe deutlich vermehrt (Abb. 3a). Diese morphologischen Veränderungen weisen insgesamt auf eine Steigerung der sekretorischen Aktivität des Ziliarepithels hin. Aber auch bei den Versuchen mit Adrenalin zeigte sich, daß die Veränderungen in der Zirkumferenz des Auges unterschiedlich waren. In einigen Regionen waren die Gefäße so stark dilatiert, daß es in den Ziliarfortsätzen zu einer Ödembildung gekommen war. In diesen Bereichen war das Ziliarepithel weit von den Stromakapillaren getrennt und wies deutliche Zeichen degenerativer Veränderungen auf (Abb. 3b). Es ist vorstellbar, daß in diesen Abschnitten des Ziliarkörpers nicht nur die Sekretionsleistung des Ziliarepithels reduziert wurde, sondern daß auch noch durch den erhöhten onkotischen Druck im Stroma Kammerwasser resorbiert worden ist und damit die KaWa-Produktionsrate hier sogar negativ wird.

Wiederum andere Teile der Zirkumferenz der behandelten Augen erschienen dagegen morphologisch unverändert. Die Heterogenität der morphologischen Befunde könnte die in der Literatur beschriebenen unterschiedlichen Messungen der Kammerwassersekretionsrate nach Adrenalingabe erklären: abhängig von der Ausprägung der jeweiligen Veränderungen kann die Sekretionsrate erhöht, normal oder auch verringert sein.

Wie lassen sich jedoch diese morphologischen Befunde mit der Tatsache in Einklang bringen, daß Adrenalingabe auch in den Ziliarkörperarteriolen eine deutliche Gefäßkontraktion und nicht wie in unseren Langzeitversuchen eine -dilation hervorruft. Die Klärung dieser Frage hat Prof. Funk im nachfolgenden Beitrag gegeben.

Nur im Akutversuch tritt nach Applikation von Adrenalin eine kurzfristige Vasokonstriktion auf. Die Dauer dieser Konstriktionsphase ist konzentrationsabhängig, aber immer etwa 4mal kürzer als die anschließende Phase der Vasodilatation.

Abb. 3a, b. Elektronenmikroskopische Übersichtsaufnahmen des vorderen Anteils eines Ziliarfortsatzes nach 6monatiger Behandlung mit Adrenalin (Cynomolgusaffe × 2400). Die morphologischen Veränderungen des Ziliarkörpers nach Adrenalinbehandlung zeigen deutliche regionale Unterschiede; in einigen Bereichen der Zirkumferenz des Auges (**a**) sind die Stromakapillaren (C) erweitert und die unpigmentierten Ziliarepithelzellen enthalten zahlreiche große Mitochondrien (M). In anderen Bereichen (**b**) ist es durch Ruptur der Fenestrationen der Kapillaren zur Ödembildung gekommen und das Ziliarepithel ist degenerativ verändert

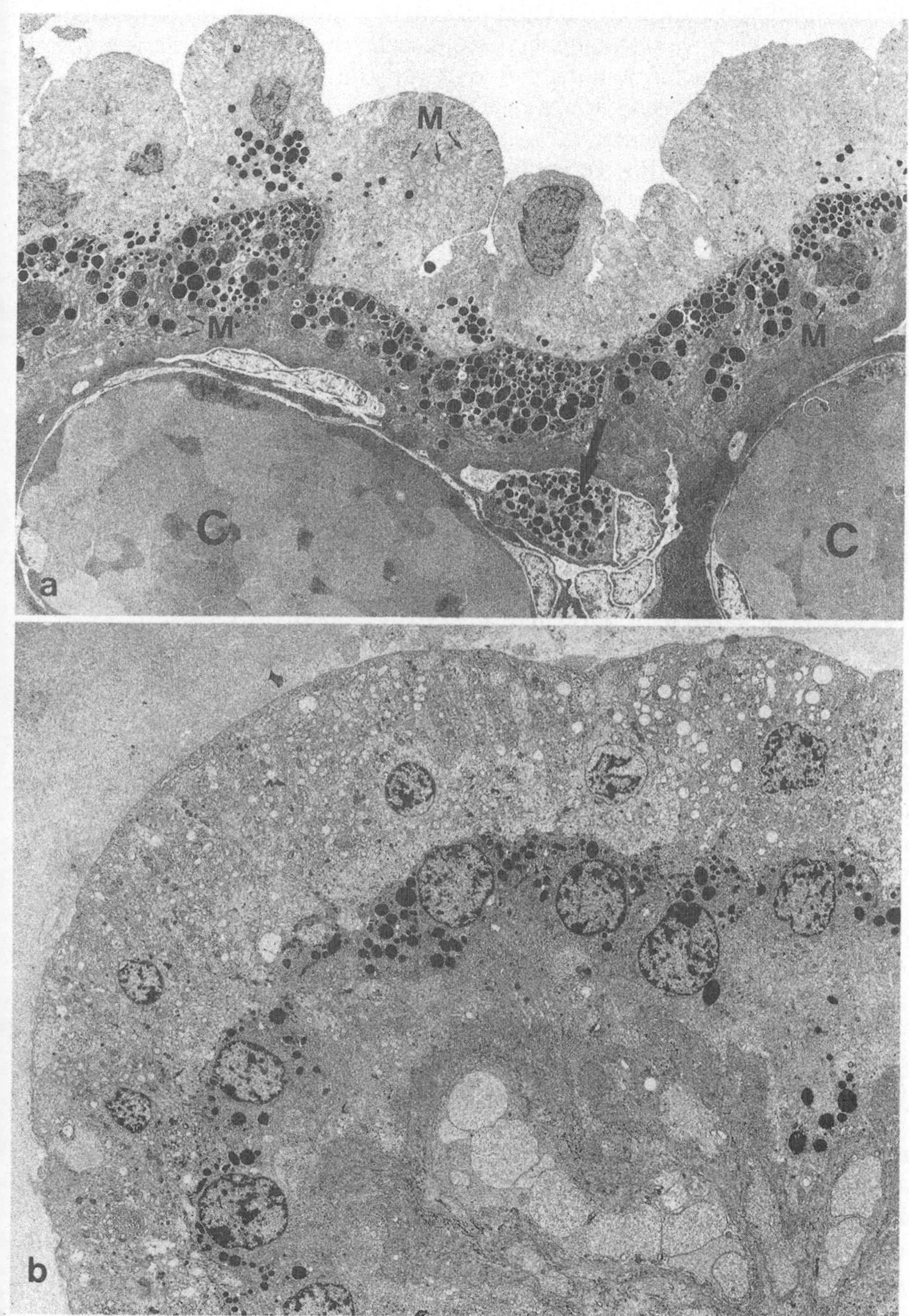

Interessanterweise ließ sich die Dilatation der Gefäße durch Indomethazin verhindern, ist also wahrscheinlich sekundär durch Prostaglandinwirkung induziert. Da auch nach 6monatiger Behandlung mit Adrenalin die Kapillaren noch erweitert waren, könnte die Langzeitwirkung von Adrenalin, zumindest teilweise, auf einer Prostaglandinwirkung beruhen.

Um diese These weiter zu prüfen, haben wir die morphologischen Veränderungen nach Gabe von Adrenalin und Prostaglandin miteinander verglichen.

Vergleich Prostaglandin – Adrenalin

Cynomolgusaffen wurden 4–5 Tage lang täglich mit 4 µg $PGF_{2\alpha}$ behandelt. Die Versuche sowie die physiologischen und ophthalmologischen Untersuchungen dieser Tiere erfolgte ebenfalls durch Prof. Kaufman im Institut für Ophthalmologie an der Universität Madison/Wisconsin/USA [9, 10].

Der IOP war nach Prostaglandin $F_{2\alpha}$ deutlich erniedrigt. Über die Sekretionsrate können wir keine Aussage machen, da diese nicht gemessen wurde. Morphologisch wies der Ziliarkörper der behandelten Tiere deutlich Zirkumferenzunterschiede auf. In durchschnittlich 40% der Zirkumferenz des Auges fand sich im vorderen Bereich der Ziliarfortsätze eine leichte Ödembildung und eine deutliche Erweiterung der Stromakapillaren. Die Epithelzellen erschienen leicht aktiviert, die Veränderungen waren aber nach 4tägiger Prostaglandinbehandlung insgesamt weit weniger ausgeprägt als nach 2–6monatiger Behandlung mit Adrenalin.

Auch wenn die Ergebnisse der beiden Versuchsserien nicht direkt vergleichbar sind, weisen die Ähnlichkeiten der morphologischen Veränderungen doch darauf hin, daß hier ähnliche Wirkungsmechanismen zugrunde liegen. Wenn jedoch beide Pharmaka, nämlich Adrenalin und Prostaglandin $F_{2\alpha}$ die Kammerwassersekretionsrate nicht senken, sondern eventuell sogar erhöhen, worauf beruht dann die drucksenkende Wirkung dieser Medikamente? Physiologische Untersuchungen verschiedener Arbeitsgruppen haben ergeben, daß die IOP-senkende Wirkung von $PGF_{2\alpha}$ auf einer Erhöhung des uveoskleralen Abflusses beruht [9, 10]. Tatsächlich fanden wir morphologisch im Ziliarkörper von $PGF_{2\alpha}$ behandelten Versuchstieren eine Verminderung des extrazellulären Materials im Ziliarkörper und eine Erweiterung der uveoskleralen Abflußwege. Wird durch Adrenalingabe sekundär eine Prostaglandinwirkung induziert, so könnte ein Teil der Adrenalinwirkung ebenfalls auf einer Erhöhung des uveoskleralen Abflusses beruhen. Ob Adrenalingabe darüberhinaus auch noch über Beeinflussung kontraktiler Elemente im Skleralsporn oder anderer Strukturen im Bereich der konventionellen Abflußwege wirkt, bedarf weiterer Untersuchungen.

Zusammenfassend weisen unsere morphologischen Befunde darauf hin, daß durch Timololbehandlung im Langzeitversuch bei Primaten sowohl die Ultrafiltration als auch die aktive Sekretionsleistung des Ziliarepithels vermindert wird. Ob dabei zunächst die aktive Pumpleistung des Epithels durch Blockade β-adrenerger Rezeptoren beeinflußt und die Durchblutung dann sekundär vermindert wird oder ob beide Systeme gleichzeitig betroffen sind, kann durch unsere Befunde zunächst noch nicht geklärt werden.

Auf der anderen Seite beruhen Adrenalin- und Prostaglandinwirkung nach unseren Untersuchungen nicht auf einer Sekretionsminderung, sondern auf einer Erhöhung des KaWa-Abflusses. In allen drei Versuchsserien waren Gefäßsystem und Epithel gleichsinnig verändert. Erweiterung der Gefäße war mit Aktivierung des Epithels, Verengung der Gefäße mit verminderter Aktivität verbunden, d.h. Epithel und angrenzende Stromakapillaren wirken im Langzeitversuch als funktionelle Einheit und beeinflussen sich offensichtlich gegenseitig.

Literatur

1. Yablonski ME, Zimmerman TJ, Waltman SR, Becker B (1978) A fluorophotometric study of the effect of topical timolol on aqueous humor dynamics. Exp Eye Res 27: 135–142
2. Coakes RL, Brubaker RF (1978) The mechanism of timolol in lowering intraocular pressure in the normal eye. Arch Ophthalmol 96: 2045–8
3. Kolker AE, Hetherington J Jr (1983) Becker-Shaffer's diagnosis and therapy of the glaucomas, 5th ed. CV Mosby, St. Louis, pp 84–106, 393–407
4. Sears ML (1966) The mechanism of action of adrenergic drugs in glaucoma. Invest Ophthalmol 5: 115–9
5. Townsend DJ, Brubaker RF (1980) Immediate effects of epinephrine on aqueous formation in the normal human eye as measured by fluorophotometry. Invest Ophthalmol Vis Sci 19: 256–66
6. Schenker HI, Yablonski ME, Podos SM, Linder L (1981) Fluorophotometric study of epinephrine and timolol in human subjects. Arch Ophthalmol 99: 1212–6
7. Lütjen-Drecoll E, Kaufman PL, Eichhorn M (1986) Long-term timolol and epinephrine in monkeys. I. Functional morphology of the ciliary processes. Trans Ophthalmol Soc UK 105: 180–195
8. Lütjen-Drecoll E, Kaufman P (1986) Long-term timolol and epinephrine in monkeys. II. Morphological alterations in trabecular meshwork and ciliary muscle. Trans Ophthalmol Soc UK 105: 105–107
9. Lütjen-Drecoll E, Tamm E (1989) The effects of ocular hypotensive doses of $PGF_{2\alpha}$-Isopropylester on anterior segment morphology. The ocular effects of Prostaglandin and other eicosanoids. Alan R. Liss, Inc, New York, pp 437–446
10. Lütjen-Drecoll E, Tamm E (1988) Morphological study of the anterior segment of cynomolgus monkey eyes following treatment with Prostaglandin $F_{2\alpha}$. Exp Eye Res 47: 761–769

Korrespondenzadresse
Professor Dr. med. E. Lütjen-Drecoll
Vorstand des Anatomischen Institutes, Lehrstuhl II, Universität Erlangen–Nürnberg, Krankenhausstraße 9, D-8520 Erlangen

Modulation of the Ciliary Process Vasculature by Vasoactive Substances

R. H. W. Funk

Abstract

Scanning electron microscopic (SEM) studies on the vasculature of the ciliary body in rabbit, monkey and man have shown that there are three different territories in the ciliary process vasculature characterized by separate afferent arterioles and efferent venules. Both the afferent and the efferent vascular segments are characterized ultrastructurally by a special medial layer with numerous nerve endings.

Using the newly developed methods of "functional resin casting" and intraocular microendoscopy in the albino rabbit it was found that the afferent arterioles react predominantly to vasocontrictory drugs such as α_1-adrenergetic agents, NPY (Neuropeptide Y) and Endothelin while the efferent venules contract exclusively after administration of ANF (Atrio Natriuretic Factor) or cholinergic agents. Doses of epinephrine above 50 ng/kg b. w. result in a complete stop of blood flow in the ciliary process vasculature, while NPY (1 ng/kg b. w.) leads to a blood flow reduction in the capillary bed of the main ciliary processes but not in the marginal venule. This marginal venule seems to be a thoroughfare channel from the ciliary process arterioles to the pars plana vessels. After CGRP (Calcitonin Gene Related Peptide) or Bradykinin as well as after paracentesis the most extensive vasodilation was found in the iridial ciliary processes. This was accompanied by a leakage of FITC (Fluorescein Iso Thio Cyanate) in this region whereas the major ciliary processes still retained the FITC underneath the ciliary epithelium.

Introduction

Till the last decade the action of vasoactive substances on the ciliary process vasculature was exclusively measured by indirect methods like measuring the temperature in the anterior chamber by thermocouples (Cole and Rumble, 1970) or counting the amount of radioactively labelled microspheres in preparations of the ciliary body or ciliary processes (Bill and Helsing, 1965). However, the latter method provided many insights into important functional features of the anterior eye vasculature (Bill 1974; O'Day et al., 1971; Alm et al., 1973a, b, c for review see Bill, 1985; Bill and Nilsson, 1982).

Gramer/Kampık (Hrsg.) Pharmakotherapıe am Auge
© Springer-Verlag Berlın Heıdelberg 1992

With the application of the new morphologic method of scanning electron microscopy of vascular resin casts to the eye vessels the astonishing complexity of the vascular architecture in the ciliary processes became visible. In the meantime the patterns of the ciliary process vessels have been investigated thoroughly in many mammalian species (Matsuo, 1973; Shimizu and Ujiie, 1978; Morrison and van Buskirk, 1983, 1984a, b, 1987a, b; Sharpnak et al., 1984; Funk and Rohen, 1985, 1987a, 1988a, 1990a). In human autoptic eyes, too, we could use this method for investigation of the ciliary process vessel architecture (Funk and Rohen, 1990b).

Results and Comments

Architecture of the Ciliary Process Vasculature in the Human and Rabbit Eye

A short comparison between the architecture of the ciliary process vessels in the rabbit and that in the human eye will show that despite some interspecies' variations there are many common principles. Thus, also the in vivo observations which we made in the rabbit eye (see below) possibly have a more common value.

In the rabbit and in the primate (cynomolgus monkey and man) as well as in all other mammalian species we have studied (rat, dog, cat, cow), the ciliary processes are supplied by three different vascular territories with discrete arterioles and venules (Figs. 1, 2).

In the rabbit the capillary net of the *first territory* is located in the iridial ciliary processes (Fig. 1) whereas in the human eye this territory is found in the anteriormost part of the major processes at the transition zone towards the iris root (Fig. 2).

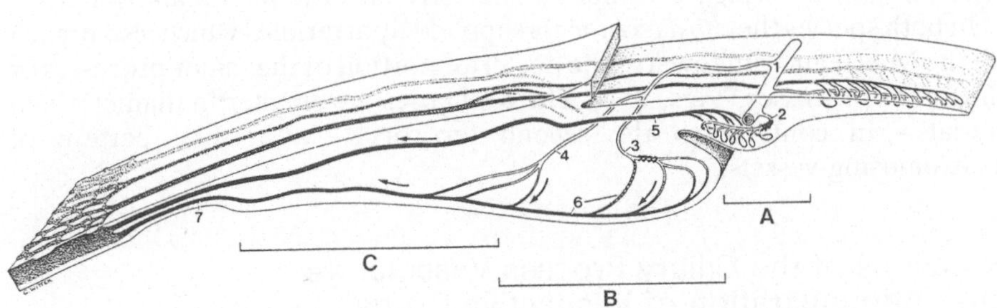

Fig. 1. Schematic drawing of the vascular architecture in the rabbit ciliary body. *A* = First vascular territory; *B* = second vascular territory; *C* = third vascular territory. *1* = major arterial circle of iris (MACI); *2* = terminal arteriole (afferent segment) of A (iridial ciliary processes); *3* = terminal arteriole (afferent segment) of B; *4* = arteriole of C; *5* = basal venule of A; *6* = marginal route; *7* = efferent venous segment of the marginal venule

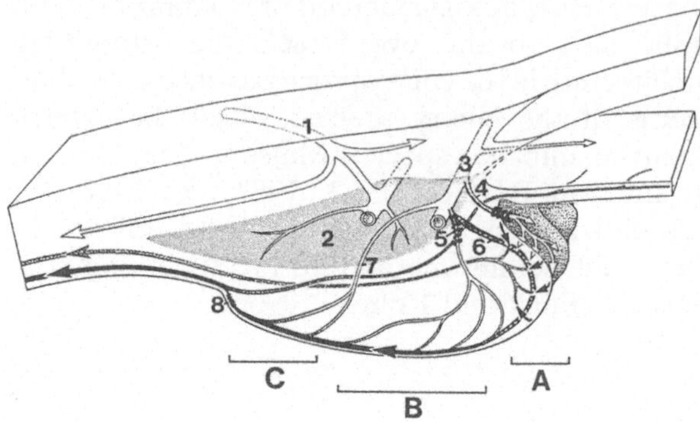

Fig. 2. Schematic drawing of the vascular architecture in the human ciliary body. *A* = First vascular territory; *B* = second vascular territory; *C* = third vascular territory. *1* = perforating branch of the anterior ciliary arteries (ACA); *2* ciliary muscle microvasculature; *3* = major arterial circle of iris (MACI); *4* = terminal arteriole (afferent segment) of A; *5* = terminal arteriole (afferent segment) of B; *6* arteriole leading to the marginal route; *7* arteriole of the third vascular territory; *8* = efferent venous segment of the marginal venule

In both species the *second territory* comprises the vasculature of the anterior portion of the major ciliary processes where the capillaries are relatively wide and tortuous. In the human eye this region is supplied by arterioles which lie anteriorly to the major arterial circle of iris (MACI) like those of the first territory (*anterior arterioles*, Fig. 2), whereas in the rabbit these arterioles are located posteriorly to the MACI and bend anteriorly in a long curve (Fig. 1).

There are arterioles which supply exclusively the capillary net of the second territory and others which bypass this capillary network and directly join the marginal venule situated at the inner edge of the major processes (marginal route, Figs. 1, 2). This marginal venule runs straight posteriorly towards the pars plana. At the posterior end of the ciliary processes it forms the *"efferent venous segment"*, which continues posteriorly into the pars plana-venule.

In both species the *third territory* is supplied by arterioles which also branch off the MACI and run towards the posterior portion of the major processes or the minor processes (Figs. 1, 2). The capillaries are smaller in diameter and reveal – in contrast to the second territory – a net-like pattern of anastomosing vessels.

Reactions of the Ciliary Process Vasculature after Administration of Vasoactive Drugs

Method of the Functional Resin Casting. By the *method of the functional resin casting* (low-viscous plastic injected under physiological pressure and temperature after drug administration) we could found that in the rabbit, cynomolgus monkey and in man the terminal arterioles, especially of the first and second vascular territory have a great potential to react with contractions or to a lesser degree with dilations (Funk and Rohen, 1987a, 1988a, 1990b). The ability to change the diameter superceeds all other vascular segments of the ciliary processes.

However, during plastic injection the reactions of the ciliary process vessels can not be controlled by direct in vivo observation like e.g. iris vessels (Funk, 1986). Furthermore, the resin casts only represent "punctually" the dynamic course of a drug response.

We therefore developed an endoscopic method in order to observe the ciliary process vasculature in vivo, at least in albino animals – the intraocular microendoscopy (Funk and Rohen, 1987b, 1989).

Intraocular Microendoscopy. An endoscope with an outer diameter of 1.9 mm held by a micromanipulator is introduced into the vitreous by a trephined hole through the sclera and the choroid 4 mm posterior to the limbus and placed tangentially to the lens near the ciliary processes (Fig. 3). During these and the later manipulations the intraocular pressure (IOP) was stabilized at a level of 15–20 mmHg by a needle connected to an open reservoir of salt solution which was inserted into the vitreous.

The ocular of the endoscope is attached to a light sensitive color camera and a video equipment by a magnifying system which shifts the focus nearer to the endoscope (up to 1 mm). Thus magnifications up to values of $\times 500$ can be achieved. At this magnification levels objects larger than 3–5 μm are visible, so that even single capillaries can be discerned.

The whole microvasculature of the ciliary processes and choroid can be observed. In addition, the blood flow pattern and velocity of the blood stream can be measured after bolus injections of Evans Blue into the common carotid artery. Furthermore, the blood-oxygenation can be estimated from the color of the vascular blood column, which varies from light-red to dark-blue.

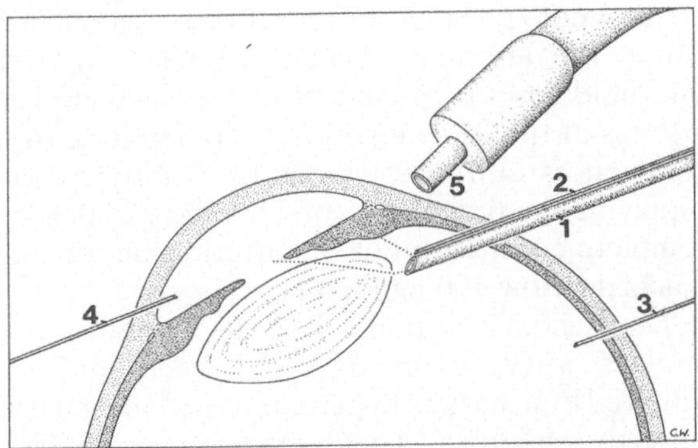

Fig. 3. Schematic drawing of the position of the tip of the endoscope (*1*) within the eye; *2* = tube for direct injections; *3* = canula to hydrostatic reservoir; *4* = canula for IOP-monitoring; *5* = tip of light-guide

The microendoscopy itself causes no apparent circulatory disturbance, at least within the first 60 minutes. In the iris, no miosis or hyperemia is found during an observation period of one hour. In addition, no changes of intraocular pressure (IOP) are seen if the hydrostatic reservoir is clamped *after* insertion, and the endoscope rests without movement. The vessel diameters seen with the endoscope correlated well with those which were found in the functional resin casts of the rabbit ciliary processes (Funk and Rohen, 1987a). Another proof of the usefullness of this method is that no leakage of fluorescein-isothiocyanat (FITC)-dextran was seen from the ciliary epithelium during microendoscopy carried out under undisturbed conditions (Funk and Rohen, 1989).

Generally, a very rapid flow of light red blood is visible within the capillaries and even in the venules – especially in the wide marginal venule situated at the inner edge of the major processes. After a bolus injection of Evans blue into the common carotid artery the dye always appeares earlier in the marginal venule of the major ciliary process than in the capillary network of the processes. This indicates the existence of a thoroughfare channel from the ciliary process arterioles via the marginal venule. In addition, this thorough-fare channel remains still open after doses of a given constrictory agent which at the same time leads to a complete stoppage of blood flow in the capillary system of the second territory.

Because of this phenomenon we can exclude in the second territory which is the main vascular territory (Fig. 1) effective *control segments* of the blood flow which are located proximally to the terminal arterioles. Otherwise the blood flow in the whole ciliary processes or at least in that second territory would cease after constrictory agents. In addition, observations of injected dye before and after drug administration lead to a in vivo localisation of this afferent vascular segment which was already presumed in the functional resin cast studies (see above).

Of all components of the ocular (vascular) innervation the adrenergic is the most extensively studied and adrenergic agents are commonly used in ophthalmology. Thus, we tested these agents at first and observed predomi-nantly the afferent vascular segments. Interestingly we found that the threshold doses for comparable responses are very different in the individual arteries of the three territories: epinephrine or phenylephrine given via the common carotid artery leads to a complete constriction of the arterioles supplying the first and second territory in dosages of 10 and 15 ng/kg b.w. A complete constriction of the arteriole supplying the third territory was not reached below 100 ng/kg b.w.

The ischemic response lasts 1–2 minutes after intracarotidal and 15–20 minutes after conjunctival or direct application. The constriction was followed by a marked hyperemic reaction which lasted 3 (intraarterially) or 50 (directly) minutes. The hyperemic response can be moderated by i.v. pretreatment with indomethacin.

The afferent vascular segments of the first and the second territory (the main vascular territory, Fig. 1) constrict after intracarotidal injection of epinephrine or phenylephrine in dosages of 1-1.5 ng/kg b.w. whereas the arterioles of the third territory are far less responsive. Similar reactions were obtained by topical application via a small tube fixed on the tip of the endoscope. Using clonidine, DL-isoproterenol and common adrenergic blockers (phenoxybenzamine, prazosine, yohimbine, timolol) it was found that the afferent segments are especially sensitive to α_1-adrenergic agents. Characteristically, the threshold for these reactions of the afferent segments was about 10 times lower than that for the remaining part of the arteriolar tree supplying the ciliary processes.

It is important to stress the biphasic mode of the above mentioned vascular reactions after adrenergic agents: by the method of radiactively labelled microspheres it was found that topical application of epinephrine leads to a reduction of *blood flow* in the anterior uvea of the *monkey* after 30–60 minutes (Alm, 1980). Three hours after topical application of epinephrine in *rabbits* (where the decrease in IOP is nearly maximal; see Langham and Kriegelstein 1976) the *blood flow* in the ciliary processes, measured with radioactively labelled microspheres, is greatly enhanced (Morgan et al. 1981). All these observations – short term reduction of blood flow and long term increase – correlate well with our direct in vivo observations. However, most studies dealing with blood flow or changes in IOP after adrenergic agonists begin the measurements not before 30 minutes after drug application – that means in the phase of *reactive* hyperemia of the ciliary process vasculature.

Among the numerous neuropeptides localized in peripheral ocular nerves (for review see Stone et al., 1987; Stone and Kuwayama, 1989) we tested Neuropeptid Y (NPY), Calcitonin Gene Related Peptide (CGRP) and Vasointestinal Peptide (VIP) because a rich innervation containing these neuropeptides is found in the anterior eye (Stone et al., 1987).

Neuropeptid Y-like nerve fibers closely parallel that of adrenergic nerves and mostly derive from the ipsilateral superior cervical ganglion (see Stone and Kuwayama, 1989).

After carotidal or direct application (via the tube attached to the endoscope) of NPY (0.1–0.5 ng/kg b.w.) it was found that the blood flow in the capillaries of the second territory was markedly reduced (Fig. 4a, b), again, in the marginal venule the blood flow was not affected substantially. It is noteworthy that NPY is very effective even at very low doses (compared to epinephrine) and the constriction phase lasts longer (5–10 minutes) than after epinephrine.

Calcitonin Gene Related Peptide (CGRP) and substance P (SP) are neuropeptides which are confined to sensory neurons of the anterior uvea (Terenghi et al., 1985). In the irritative response of the rabbit eye SP is involved in the miotic reaction (Stjernschantz et al., 1981) whereas the vascular effects are caused by CGRP (Oksala and Stjernschantz, 1988).

Direct application of CGRP via the tube attached to the endoscope (0.5 µg/kg b.w.) lead to *dilations* of the arterioles, capillaries and especially the venules in the first and second territory (venules: 130% of the initial

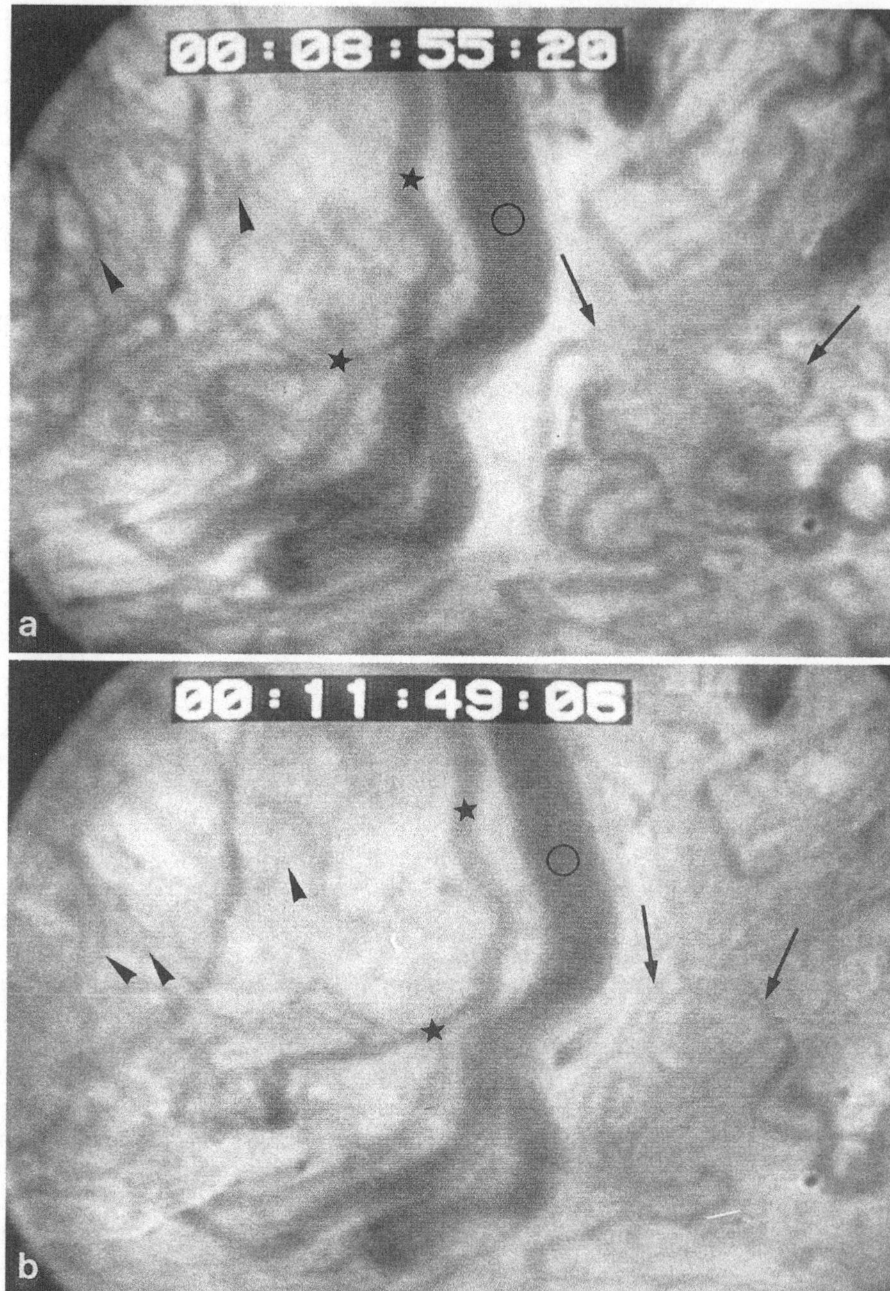

Fig. 4a,b. Microendoscopic monitor photographs before (**a**) and 1 minute after (**b**) intracarotidal injection of NPY (0.3 ng/kg b.w.). The terminal arterioles of the first (arrows) and second territory (arrowheads) are constricted so that the related capillary net is perfused not any longer whereas the diameters in the thoroughfare channel (asterisks) and in the marginal venules (circles) have only changed slightly

values about 3 min. after application). The same dosages injected into the anterior chamber caused exactly the same reactions.

Interestingly, a marked *constriction* of the whole arteriolar tree of the ciliary processes took place within one minute after carotidal application of CGRP (1–10 ng/kg b.w.). Possibly central reflectory mechanisms cause this phenomenon.

After intracarotidal administration of VIP (0.1–100 ng/kg b.w.) no substantial effect on the ciliary process vasculature was seen.

After paracentesis (IOP-reduction to 5 mmHg) a dilation of the capillaries and venules especially in the first territory (iridial ciliary processes) takes place within 2–5 minutes.

Using "*fluorescence-microendoscopy* with i.v. administrated FITC-dextran we found that an extravasation of FITC-dextran appears around the iridial ciliary processes. During the following 10–15 minutes, the fluorescence spreads out along the posterior surface of the iris, forming radial stripes which extend from the iridial ciliary processes as far as the pupilary margin. In the major ciliary processes the fluorescence was stopped underneath the ciliary epithelium.

These results indicate that a breakdown of the blood aqueous barrier must have occurred predominantly in the iridial ciliary processes, because in the untouched rabbit eye, FITC-dextran, in contrast to fluorescein-sodium does not pass through the blood aqueous barrier (Unger, 1979). In addition to the vascular reactions we have found electronmicroscopically a swelling of the whole region and an enlargement of the pigmented epithelium of the iridial ciliary processes forming wide protein-containing spaces (Funk, 1989).

The iridial ciliary processes (first territory) of the rabbit show similar reactions after paracentesis like the anterior-most portion of the primate ciliary processes where we have localized the first vascular territory (see above. Barthels et al. (1979) demonstrated swelling and breakdown of the blood aqueous barrier in this region of the rhesus monkey ciliary processes. For the cynomolgus monkey eye Okisaka (1976) pointed out the extreme sensivity of this region to paracentesis. Furthermore, in the cynomolgus monkey Ohnishi and Tanaka (1981) found changes in the tight junctions between the non-pigmented epithelial cells after paracentesis predominantly in this territory. This is discussed as a mechanism for the leakage of serum protein.

"Efferent Venous Segment"

The marginal venules of the ciliary processes continue posteriorly into the pars plana veins. At the transition zone between these two regions the morginal venule possesses a specific "efferent venous segment" (Figs. 1, 2) which appeared particularly sensitive to vasoactive drugs (Funk and Rohen, 1988b). By its localization distally to the capillary bed the efferent venous segment can influence the *intracapillary hydrostatic pressure* especially in the second territory, because e.g. a constriction of this segment leads to elevated intracapillary hydrostatic pressures. Here, some analogies exist to the renal glomerular vasculature and its reactions (see Steinhausen et al., 1983 and Marin-Grez et al., 1986).

The efferent venous segment was also analyzed by intraocular microendoscopy: three minutes after intracarotidal administration of atriopeptin (ANF) (15 ng/kg b.w.) this segment showed a marked vasoconstriction for 2–3 minutes (Fig. 5a, b), followed by a dilation of 30 minutes (120–130% of the initial diameters) whereas vessel segments distally and proximally remained unresponsive. Similar effects were obtained by topical application.

Nathanson (1987) recently found a long-term (72 hours) IOP-decrease after intravitreal injection of r-ANF 1–28 in the rabbit. Tsukahara et al. (1988) could also show an IOP-decrease after intravenous ANF in rabbits. Apart from other mechanisms these effects on IOP might be explained by e.g. a long-term dilation during the biphasic vascular response of the efferent vascular segment which we have found after ANF.

To sum up, our microendoscopical observations of the rabbit ciliary process vasculature revealed very differentiated reactions after vasoactive stimuli which were specific for defined vascular segments. Especially the afferent (arteriolar) segments of the first and second territory and the efferent venous

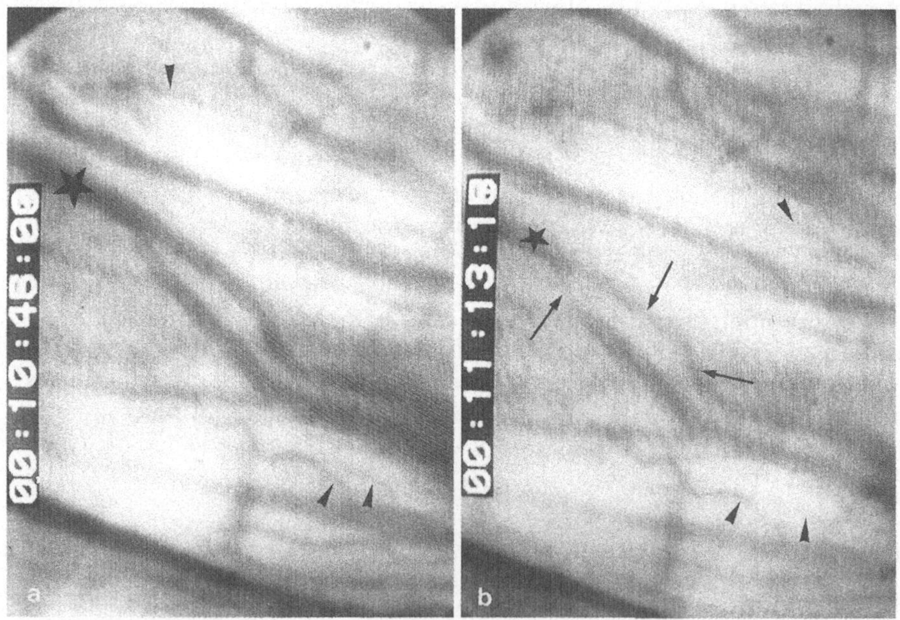

Fig. 5a,b. Microendoscopic monitor photographs before (**a**) and 2 minutes (**b**) after intracarotidal injection of ANF (Atriopeptin III, 15 ng/kg b.w.). asterisks = marginal venules; arrowheads = ciliary muscle capillaries. Localized constrictions (arrows in b) were found at the efferent venous segment whereas the segments located proximally or distally are affected only slightly. The short constrictory phase was followed by a long-lasting dilatory phase

segment seemed to be the most important control segments of the related microvasculature. The reactivity of the *afferent segments* possibly serves for a constant *blood flow* through the ciliary processes despite changes of the systemic arterial blood pressure and may also prevent a breakdown of the blood aqueous barrier in the first vascular territory under conditions of high arterial pressure (cf. Beausang-Linder, 1982). On the other hand the *intracapillary hydrostatic pressure* may be influenced by the *efferent segment*. Thus, besides the ciliary epithelium the ciliary process vasculature, too, seems to play an active role in the process of aqueous humor production.

References

Alm A (1980) The effect of topical 1-epinephrine on regional ocular blood flow in monkeys. Invest Ophthalmol 19: 487

Alm A, Bill A, Young FA (1973a) The effects of pilocarpine and neostigmine on the blood flow through the anterior uvea in monkeys. A study with radioactively labelled microspheres. Exp Eye Res 15: 31

Alm A, Bill A (1973b) The effect of stimulation of the sympathetic chain on retinal oxygen tension and uveal, retinal and cerebral blood flow in cats. Acta Physiol Scand 88: 84–94

Alm A, Bill A (1973c) Ocular and optic nerve blood flow at normal and increased intraocular pressures in monkeys (Macaca irus): a study with radioactively labeled microspheres including flow determinations in brain and some other tissues. Exp Eye Res 15: 15

Barthels SP, Pederson JE, Gaasterland DE, Armaly MF (1979) Sites of breakdown of the blood aqueous barrier after paracentesis of the rhesus monkey eye. Invest Ophthalmol 18: 1050–1060

Beausang-Linder M (1982) Effects of sympathetic stimulation on cerebral and ocular blood flow. Acta Physiol Scand 144: 217–224

Bill A (1974) Effects of acetazolamide and carotid occlusion on the ocular blood flow in unanesthetized rabbits. Invest Ophthalmol 13: 954–958

Bill A (1985) Some aspects of the ocular circulation. Invest Ophthalmol 4: 410–424

Bill A, Helsing K (1965) Production and drainage of aqueous humor in the cynomolgus monkey (Macaca irus). Invest Ophthalmol 4: 920

Bill A, Nilsson S (1982) The blood supply of the eye and its regulation. In: Lütjen-Drecoll E (ed) Basic aspects of glaucoma research. Schattauer, Stuttgart New York, pp 39–48

Cole DF, Rumble R (1970) Effects of catecholamines on circulation in the rabbit iris. Exp Eye Res 9: 219–232

Funk R (1986) Studies on the functional morphology of rat ocular vessels with SEM. Acta Anatomica 125: 252–257

Funk R (1989) Functional morphology of rabbit iridial ciliary processes. Ophthalmic Res 21: 249–260

Funk R, Rohen JW (1987a) SEM-studies on the functional morphology of the rabbit ciliary process vasculature. Exp Eye Res 45: 579

Funk R, Rohen JW (1987b) Intraocular microendoscopy of the ciliary process vasculature in albino rabbits; Effects of vasoactive agents. Exp Eye Res 45: 597

Funk R, Rohen JW (1988a) SEM-studies of the functional morphology of the ciliary process vasculature in the cynomolgus monkey; reactions after application of epinephrine. Exp Eye Res 47: 653

Funk R, Rohen JW (1988b) Reactions of efferent venous segments in the ciliary process vasculature of albino rabbits. Exp Eye Res 46: 95–104

Funk R, Rohen JW (1989) Microendoscopy of the anterior segment vasculature in the rabbit eye. Ophthalmic Res 21: 8–17

Funk R, Rohen JW (1990a) Functional morphology of the vasculature in anterior eye segment. Monograph in: Basic aspects of glaucoma research II. Schattauer, Stuttgart

Funk R, Rohen JW (1990b) Scanning electron microscopic study on the vasculature of the human anterior eye segment especially with respect to the ciliary processes. Exp Eye Res 51: 651

Langham ME, Kriegelstein GK (1976) The biphasic intraocular pressure response of rabbits to epinephrine. Invest Ophthalmol 15: 119–127

Marin-Grez M, Fleming JT, Steinhausen M (1986) Atrial natriuretic peptide causes pre-glomerular vasodilatation and post-glomerular vasoconstriction in rat kidney. Nature (London) 324: 473–476

Matsuo N (1973) Scanning electron microscopic studies on the corrosion casts of the blood vessels of the ciliary body. Acta Soc Ophthal Jap 77 (8): 928–935

Morgan TR, Green K, Bowman K (1981) Effects of adrenergic agonists upon regional ocular blood flow in normal and ganglionectomized rabbits. Exp Eye Res 32: 691

Morrison JC, Van Buskirk EM (1983) Anterior collateral circulation in the primate eye. Ophthalmology 90: 707

Morrison JC, Van Buskirk EM (1984a) Ciliary process microvasculature. Am J Ophthalmol 97: 372–384

Morrison JC, Van Buskirk EM (1984b) Sequential microdissection and scanning electron microscopy of ciliary microvascular castings. Scanning Electron Microscopy II. 857–865

Morrison JC, DeFrank MP, Van Buskirk EM (1987a) Regional microvascular anatomy of the rabbit ciliary body. Invest Ophthalmol 28: 1314–1324

Morrison JC, DeFrank MP, Van Buskirk EM (1987b) Comparative microvascular anatomy of mammalian ciliary processes. Invest Ophthalmol 28: 1325–1340

Nathanson JA (1987) Atriopeptin-activated guanylate cyclase in the anterior segment. Identification localization, and effects of atriopeptins on IOP. Invest Ophthalmol 28: 1357–1364

O'Day DM, Fish MB, Aronson SB, Pollycove M, Coon A (1971) Ocular blood flow measurements by nuclide labelled microspheres. Arch Ophthalmol 86: 205

Ohnishi Y, Tanaka M (1981) Effects of pilocarpine and paracentesis on occluding junctions between the nonpigmented ciliary epithelial cells. Exp Eye Res 32: 635–47

Okisaka S (1976) Effects of paracentesis on the blood-aqueous barrier: a light and electron microscopic study on cynomolgus monkey. Invest Ophthalmol 15: 824

Oksala O, Stjernschantz J (1988) Effects of calcitonin gene-related peptide in the eye. Invest Ophthalmol 29: 1006–1011

Sharpnack DD, Wyman M, Anderson BG, Anderson WD (1984) Vascular pathways of the anterior segment of the canine eye. Am J Vet Res 45, 7: 1287–1294

Shimizu K, Ujie K (1978) Structure of ocular vessels. Igaku-Shoin, Tokyo, pp 1–7, 92–107

Steinhausen M, Snoli H, Parekh N, Baker R, Johnson PC (1983) Hydronephrosis: a new method to visualize vas afferens, efferens and glomerular network. Kidney Intern 23: 794–806

Stone RA, Kuwayama Y (1989) The nervous system and intraocular pressure. In: Ritch R, Shields MB, Krupin T (eds) The glaucomas. Mosby, New York, p 257

Stone RA, Kuwayama Y, Laties AM (1987) Regulatory peptides in the eye. Experientia 43: 791

Therenghi G, Polak JM, Ghatei MA, Mulderry PK, Butler JM, Unger WG, Bloom SR (1985) Distribution and origin of calcitonin gene-related peptide (CGRP) immunoreactivity in the sensory innervation of the mammalian eye. J comp Neurol 233: 506–516

Tsukahara S, Sasaki T, Yamabayashi S, Furuta M, Ushiyama M, Yamamoto T (1988) Effect of alpha-human atrial natriuretic peptides on intraocular pressure in normal albino rabbits. Ophthalmologia, Basel 197: 104–109

Unger WG (1979) Changes in the anterior uveal vessels and epithelium in the inflamed rabbit eye. 10th Europ. Conf. Microcirculation, Cagliari (1978), Bibliotheca anat. 18: 278

Corresponding Address

Professor Dr. med. R. H. W. Funk

Anatomisches Institut der Universität Erlangen–Nürnberg, Krankenhausstr. 9, D-8520 Erlangen

Apraclonidine Hydrochloride Therapy for Glaucoma Laser Surgery

Y. Kitazawa, K. Sugiyama, T. Taniguchi, and T. Inoue

Introduction

Several different kinds of lasers are widely employed for the treatment of glaucomas. They comprise iridotomy, trabeculoplasty, goniophotocoagulation, sclerostomy ab interno or externo. Except for sclerostomy, all the procedures share the potentially serious complication, that is the acute elevation of intraocular pressure (IOP) which occurs immediately after the treatment.

In an attempt to circumvent this ominous complication, various attempts had been made unsuccessfully until the advent of apraclonidine hydrochloride, an adrenergic alpha-2 agonist [1–3]. In the present contribution we like to share with you what we have learned in our clinical studies which were done to evaluate the ability of apraclonidine to suppress the acute IOP spike and to shed some lights on the mechanism(s) of its action.

Q-Switched Nd:YAG Laser Iridotomy

Acute IOP elevation following laser iridotomy occurs regardless of whether an argon or Q-switched Nd:YAG laser is used [4–7]. We carried out a prospective study in primary angle-closure glaucoma patients to evaluate the effect of topical apraclonidine on the IOP response to Q-switched Nd:YAG laser iridotomy.

We included 24 consecutive patients (29 eyes) with chronic angle-closure glaucoma who underwent Q-switched Nd:YAG laser iridotomy. In all patients 0.5% apraclonidine ophthalmic solution was instilled every 30 minutes during the 2 hours prior to and immeditely after Nd:YAG laser iridotomy, which was done using a TOPAZ (LASAG, Thus, Switzerland) and an iridotomy lens (CGT, LASAG).

From the clinical records of 117 chronic primary angle-closure glaucoma eyes in which neither topical or systemic drugs were used to prevent the acute IOP elevation, we chose 29 eyes as controls by matching the factors reported to influence the IOP response to laser iridotomy [6–8].

IOP Rise: The mean preoperative IOP was 13.2 ± 3.8 mmHg in the apraclonidine-treated eyes and 13.8 ± 3.9 mmHg in the controls. The change

Gramer/Kampik (Hrsg.) Pharmakotherapie am Auge
© Springer-Verlag Berlin Heidelberg 1992

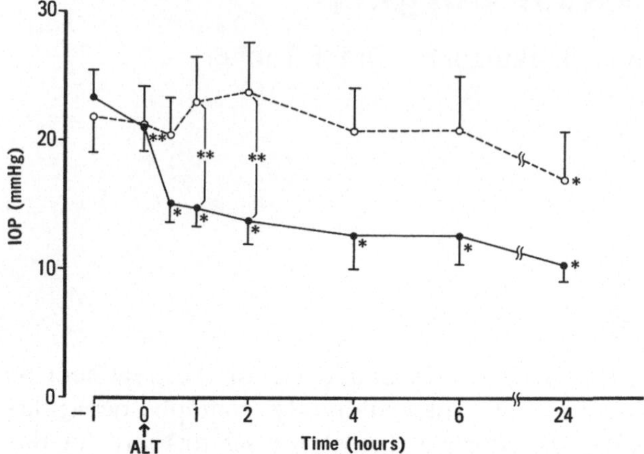

Fig. 1. Intraocular pressure following Q-switched Nd:YAG laser iridotomy. At time 0, iridotomy was performed immeditely after tonometry. The dotted line indicates eyes not treated with apraclonidine ophthalmic solution. The solid line represents the eyes treated with 0.5% apraclonidine. Each circle indicates the mean, and vertical bars denote the standard error of the mean (SEM). The difference in IOP between the apraclonidine treated and the control eyes was significantly different at each measured time for 24 hours postoperatively (P < 0.05, Wilcoxon rank sum test). (From [3] with permission of Ophthalmic Surgery)

in the average IOP over time is illustrated in Fig. 1. The difference in the IOP rise was statistically highly significant (p < 0.01, Wilcoxon rank sum test). The mean difference in IOP prelaser and postlaser maximal value was 1.4 ± 2.8 mmHg in the apraclonidine-treated eyes, while it was 6.4 ± 5.8 mmHg in the untreated controls. IOP rise greater than 19 mmHg was noted in 5 of the untreated eyes (7.2%) and in only one eye (3.4%) in the apraclonidine-treated eyes.

Other Complications: Immediately following the procedure, the anterior chamber was filled with the dispersed pigment and tissue debris in all cases, irrespective of apraclonidine treatment. Bleeding from the iridotomy site was seen in 4 eyes (13.8%) in the apraclonidine-treated group and in 12 (41.4%) of the control eyes. The difference was statistically significant (P < 0.05, X^2 test).

Argon Laser Trabeculoplasty (ALT)

We enrolled 19 primary open-angle glaucoma or capsular glaucoma patients who were decided to receive ALT. The indications for ALT were the uncontrollable IOP with the maximum tolerable medication. The patients were randomly assigned to either topical 1% apraclonidine or placebo treatment. Thus, 19 eyes were allocated to the apraclonidine treatment and 10 eyes to the placebo. Fifty microliter of either apraclonidine or placebo was

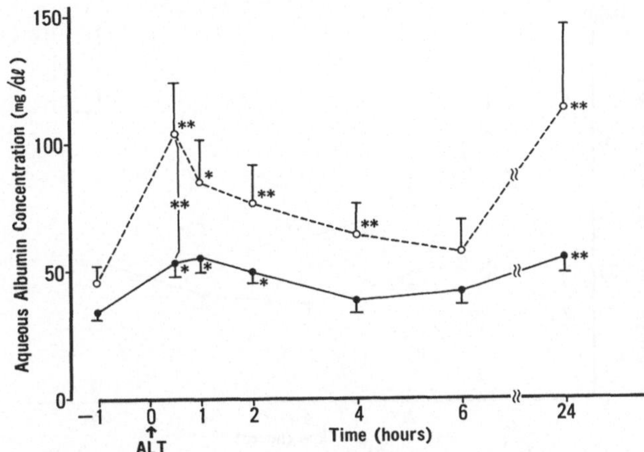

Fig. 2. Intraocular pressure following argon laser trabeculoplasty (ALT). At time −1 and 0, 50 μl of 1% apraclonidine was instilled. ALT was done immediately after tonometry. The dotted line indicates eye treated with placebo. The solid line represents the eyes treated with apraclonidine. Each circle indicates the mean, and vertical bars denote the standard error of the mean (SEM). *P < 0.01; **P < 0.05. (From [3], Wilcoxon rank sum test for the intergroup comparison and Wilcoxon signed rank test for the intragroup comparison)

instilled one hour prior to and immediately after ALT. Equally spaced 50 burns of continuous blue-green argon laser beam were applied to the trabecular pigment band over half the circumference of the chamber angle.

The IOP and the aqueous flare intensity were determined at the designated time points for 24 hours after ALT. The IOP was measured with a Goldmann applanation tonometer and the flare intensity was determined with a Flare-Cell Meter (FC-1000, Kowa, Japan) [9]. The flare intensity was converted to albumin concentration using the conversion table.

The IOP change is illustrated in Fig. 2. The significant IOP rise was observed in the placebo-treated eyes. In contrast, the apraclonidine-treated eyes showed a singificant IOP decrease. The findings are in good agreement with the previous reports in that apraclonidine significantly reduces the IOP spike immediately after ALT [1–3].

Moreover, IOP rise equal to or greater than 5 mmHg exceeding the pre-ALT value was seen in 9 (64%) among the 14 placebo-treated eyes, while it was noted in only one eye (8%) in the apraclonidine-treated eye. The difference is statistically significant (P < 0.01, Fisher, exact probability test). The maximum IOP change after ALT expressed as the maximum post-ALT minus the pre-ALT value was 6.6 ± 5.5 mmHg in the placebo group. While it was − 4.6 ± 4.0 mmHg indicating that on the average the peak, post-ALT IOP was lower than the pre-ALT baseline in the apraclonidine treated group.

The flare intensity converted into the albumin content was more conspicuously elevated in the placebo-treated eyes as compared with the apraclon-

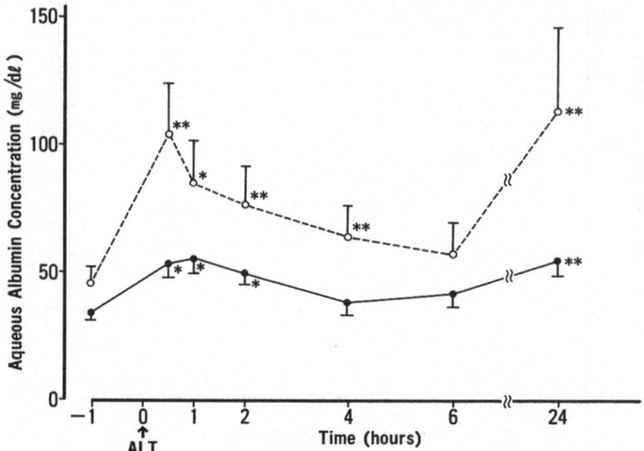

Fig. 3. Aqueous flare following ALT in the same groups of patients as illustrated in Fig. 2. The solid line represents the eyes treated with apraclonidine. Each circle indicates the mean, and vertical bars denote the standard error of the mean (SEM). *P < 0.01; **P < 0.05. (From [3], Wilcoxon rank sum test for the intergroup comparison and Wilcoxon signed rank test for the intragroup comparison)

idine treated. At one hour after ALT, the flare intensity was significantly higher in the placebo as compared with the apraclonidine group. Besides, the duration of the increase was shorter in the apraclonidine treated eyes (Fig. 3). The extent of IOP rise was found to be directly proportional to the increase in aqueous flare in the placebo-treated eyes.

Discussion

The exact mechanism of the acute IOP rise after laser surgery remains unknown. The striking inhibitory effect of apraclonidine on the acute IOP rise seems to indicate that clarifying the mechanism of action of this compound on the IOP response to laser surgery will presumably help identifying the factors responsible for the IOP spike. The results of our studies strongly suggest the following two possibilities: first, apraclonidine prevents the breakdown of the blood-aqueous barrier, which has been documented to follow laser-induced trauma to the intraocular structures. Second, the ocular hypotensive effect of apraclonidine plays a significant role in suppressing the acute IOP rise.

It has been demonstrated that the aqueous protein concentration elevates concurrently with IOP rise after laser application to the iris [10, 11] in animals. Our study also confirmed the increase in aqueous protein concentration in men following ALT, which was suppressed by apraclonidine. The results of these studies support the notion that apraclonidine acts to minimize the breakdown of the integrity of the blood-aqueous barrier, thereby preventing the IOP from elevating in response to laser application to iris or trabecular meshwork [12].

Apraclonidine reduces IOP by reducing aqueous formation in normal human subjects [13] and glaucoma patients. Hence, it is possible that the suppression of the postlaser IOP rise is at least in part attributable to the hypotensive effect of this compound.

Thus, it may be concluded that apraclonidine suppresses the acute postlaser IOP spike by preserving the integrity of the blood-aqueous barrier and by inhibiting the aqueous formation.

References

1. Schrems W, van Drop HP, Mechler W, Krieglstein GK (1983) The time course of laser-induced disruption of the blood aqueous barrier in the rabbit. Graefe's Arch Clin Exp Ophthalmol 221: 65
2. Gailitis R, Peyman GA, Pulido J, Mitchell MD, Weinreb RM (1986) Prostaglandin release following Nd:YAG iridotomy in rabbits. Ophthalmic Surg 17: 467
3. Kitazawa Y, Taniguchi T, Sugiyama K (1989) Use of apraclonidine reduces acute intraocular pressure rise following Q-switched Nd:YAG laser iridotomy. Ophthalmic Surg 20: 49
4. Robin AL, Pollack IP (1984) A comparison of neodymium: YAG and argon laser iridotomies. Ophthalmology 91: 1011
5. Moster MR, Schwartz LW, Spaeth GL, Wilson RP, McAllister A, Poryzees EM (1986) Laser iridotomy: A controlled study comparing argon and neodymium YAG. Ophthalmology 93: 20
6. Taniguchi T, Rho SH, Gotoh Y, Kitazawa Y (1987) Intraocular pressure rise following Q-switched neodymium: YAG laser iridotomy. Ophthalmic Laser Therapy 2: 99
7. Shirato S, Yumita A, Yamamoto T, Kitazawa Y (1987) Q-switched Nd:YAG laser iridotomy vs argon laser iridotomy. New Trends Ophthalmol 2: 314
8. Tuulonen A (1984) Effect of topical indomethacin on acute pressure rise in laser trabeculoplasty. Proc VIIth Cong Eur Soc Ophthalmol, pp 592–593
9. Sawa M, Tsurumaki Y, Tsuru T, et al (1988) New quantitative method to determine protein concentration and cell number in aqueous in vivo. Jpn J Ophthalmol 32: 132–142
10. Weinreb RN, Weaver D, Mitchell MD (1985) Prostanoids in rabbit aqueous humor: Effect of laser photocoagulation of the iris. Invest Ophthalmol Vis Sci 26: 1087
11. Schrems W, van Drop HP, Wendel M, Krieglstein GK (1984) The effect of yag laser iridotomy in the blood aqueous barrier in the rabbit. Graefes Arch Clin Exp Ophthalmol 221: 179
12. Sugiyama K, Kitazawa Y, Kawai K (1990) Apraclonidine effects on ocular responses to YAG laser irradiation to the rabbit iris. Invest Ophthalmol Vis Sci 31: 708
13. Gharazagozloo NZ, Relf SJ, Brubaker RF (1988) Aqueous flow is reduced by the alpha-adrenergic agonist, apraclonidine hydrochloride (ALO 2145). Ophthalmology 95: 1217

Corresponding Address
Professor Y. Kitazawa, M.D.
Chairman, Department of Ophthalmology, Gifu University School of Medicine, Tsukasa – Machi 40, Gifu, 500 Japan

Medical Management of Cycloplegic-Induced Intraocular Pressure Spikes

R.A. Hill, D.S. Minckler, M. Lee, D.K. Heuer, G. Baerveldt, and J.F. Martone

Abstract

Tropicamide is routinely used for diagnostic mydriasis in many glaucoma clinics. This agent is the most effective available in the United States for short duration dilation of the pupil for visual field examination, stereoscopic disc examination, photography, and peripheral retinal examination. Previously published reports indicate that clinically significant intraocular pressure (IOP) spikes (≥ 6 mmHg) occur in approximately 2% of normal, 23% of chronic open angle glaucoma (COAG) eyes, and in 30–50% of COAG eyes on miotic therapy following the use of cycloplegics. This report includes preliminary data on a randomized, prospective, double masked study investigating the efficacy of Apraclonidine prophylaxis to prevent cycloplegic-induced IOP spikes in glaucoma patients and provides guidelines for management of this complication.

Introduction

A clinically significant (≥ 6 mmHg) pressure elevation has been detected after pharmacologic pupillary dilation in 2% of normal eyes, 23% of eyes with open angle glaucoma, and as many as 33% to 50% of patients on miotic therapy [1–4]. Among glaucoma patients using miotics, intraocular pressure (IOP) spikes can sometimes reach the heights of pressures seen clinically in acute angle closure glaucoma even though the angles of these eyes are open. High IOP spikes can be dangerous in an eye with a badly damaged optic nerve and may be difficult to manage if the patient is already on maximum medical therapy. Apraclonidine hydrochloride may be a useful alternative to oral or intravenous hyperosmotic therapy in such patients.

Apraclonidine is an alpha-adrenergic agonist that has been approved by the Federal Drug Administration in the United States to prevent IOP spikes following laser procedures including capsulotomies, trabeculoplasties, and iridectomies [5–8]. This drug may produce an intense anterior segment vasoconstriction and is thought to lower intraocular pressure by reduction of aqueous formation. The onset of action is within one hour and becomes maximal in terms of reduction of IOP three-five hours after topical

Gramer/Kampik (Hrsg.) Pharmakotherapie am Auge
© Springer-Verlag Berlin Heidelberg 1992

application of a single drop of 1% solution. Apraclonidine has been proven safe in normal volunteers who used it continuously for a period of four weeks [9]. Anecdotal uses of this agent in emergent situations in our own clinics have suggested its potential benefit in patients at risk for post-cycloplegic IOP spikes. This report summarizes a larger study reported elsewhere and describes the effects of Apraclonidine prophylaxis on the incidence and severity of post-cycloplegic IOP spikes in glaucoma patients [9].

Materials and Methods

Approval of the study protocol and informed consent form were obtained from the Los Angeles County-University of Southern California's Human Studies Institutional Review Board Committee. Patients with open angle glaucoma, who were to undergo pharmacologic pupillary dilation for diagnostic purposes were offered participation in the study. Patients were entered in the study provided that they:

1) did not have systemic hypertension;
2) were not on monoamine oxydase inhibitors;
3) were not pregnant;
4) were not less than 18 years old;
5) were willing and able to give informed consent;
6) had not undergone glaucoma filtering surgery or penetrating keratoplasty;
7) had not undergone Argon laser trabeculoplasty; and
8) had no history or findings consistent with angle closure glaucoma.

Patients accepted into the study were divided into those using miotics and those not using miotics before being randomly assigned to receiving Apraclonidine or placebo prior to dilation with tropicamide (1%) and phenylephrin (2.5%). Patients were designated as being in one of four groups. Group 1 consisted of patients with open angle glaucoma not on miotic therapy who received a placebo (artificial tear solution) prior to dilation. Group 2 consisted of open angle glaucoma patients without miotic therapy who received Apraclonidine prior to dilation. Group 3 consisted of open angle glaucoma patients using miotic therapy who received a placebo (artificial tear solution) prior to dilation. Group 4 included open angle glaucoma patients with miotic therapy who received Apraclonidine prior to dilation. Statistically significant results were obtained in both nonmiotic and miotic groups between eyes showing elevation of intraocular pressure after placebo vs. those showing elevation of intraocular pressure after Apraclonidine (Tables 1 and 2).

Goldmann applanation tensions as described in the Glaucoma Laser Trial [11] were then taken by qualified ophthalmic technicians prior to dilation. Follow-up intraocular pressures were taken approximately one hour after dilation agent instillation by the treating physician using the same technique.

Table 1. Open angle glaucoma without miotic therapy

	Group 1 Placebo	Group 2 Apraclonidine	Total
Patients	13	16	29
Eyes	26	32	58
Eyes with > IOP	10	2	12
($\geq$ 6 mmHg)	(p = 0.003; Chi-square)		

Table 2. Open angle glaucoma with miotic therapy

	Group 3 Placebo	Group 4 Apraclonidine	Total
Patients	15	18	33
Eyes	25	33	58
Eyes with > IOP	9	3	12
($\geq$ 6 mmHg)	(p = 0.012; Chi square)		

Zeiss gonioscopy was performed by an ophthalmologist before and after dilation. Patients with occludable angles (Shaffer grade 2 or narrower) were excluded. The patients were pretreated with the placebo or Apraclonidine ten minutes prior to instillation of both the dilating agent (tropicamide 1%) and phenylephrine (2.5%). Treatment with phenylephrine has been shown to have little effect on intraocular pressure elevation after mydriasis [4] and was included only to mask the effects (vasoconstriction or dilation) of Apraclonidine. Intraocular pressure was checked one to two hours after pupillary dilation and Zeiss gonioscopy was repeated in all patients. If a clinically significant (greater than $\geq$ 6 mmHg) or hazardous intraocular pressure spike occurred, appropriate additional therapy was given usually consisting of a hyperosmotic agent.

Results

In eight cases only one eye was included in the study from each patient. Seven of these eyes were fellow eyes in the miotic group not receiving miotic therapy. One additional patient in this group had undergone unilateral filtration surgery. Among the four groups, Group one (nonmiotic; placebo) recorded the highest intraocular pressure spikes (21 and 27 mmHg), with four patients having intraocular pressure rises over 10 mmHg. In group two (nonmiotic; Apraclonidine) only one patient had a pressure rise over 10 mmHg (12 mmHg). Within the miotic therapy groups, only group three (miotic; placebo) had patients (5) with pressure elevations above 10 mmHg.

Discussion

Apraclonidine is widely used as prophylaxis against IOP spikes following laser procedures. Its short duration of action and low incidence of side effects appear to make it an ideal drug for prophylaxis against cycloplegic-induced pressure spikes. Its ocular effects are primarily limited to transient upper lid elevation (1.3%), conjunctival blanching (0.4%), mydriasis (0.4%) and transient burning or foreign body sensation [8]. Apraclonidine may also be a useful agent in the acute treatment of nauseated patients with primary or secondary angle closure. Other possible uses of this agent include treatment of transient IOP elevation after cataract surgery, panretinal photocoagulation and retinal surgery. Within the nonmiotic placebo group, the incidence of IOP elevations (38%) was slightly higher than results previously reported [1, 2]. The miotic control group (36%) was within previously reported parameters [3, 4]. Fellow eyes generally had similar elevations of IOP, although the exact amount of pressure elevation was variable.

These preliminary results clearly show a clinically important difference between placebo and treatment groups in terms of the risk of IOP elevation following pharmacologic pupillary dilation with a cycloplegic agent. If IOP elevation did occur in eyes receiving Apraclonidine prophylaxis, the spike was generally not as great as the IOP spike in the placebo group. Finally, in only three patients (5%), did IOP rise to potentially problematic levels during these initial studies.

We recommend as a clinical routine, that patients with severely compromised optic nerves have their IOP measured before and after pupillary dilation with tropicamide or similar agents. Assuming there are no contraindications, Apraclonidine is a rational prophylactic therapy to prevent or decrease the risk of high IOP elevation following mydriasis in patients with known risk or advanced glaucomatous optic nerve injury.

Acknowledgments. The Apraclonidine used in this study was donated by Alcon Surgical. Secretarial support and editorial assistance was provided by Teresa Gonzales and Melissa C. Hill.

Literature

1. Harris LS (1968) Cycloplegic-induced intraocular pressure elevations: A study of normal and open-angle glaucomatous eyes. Arch Ophthalmol 79: 242–246,
2. Galin MA (1961) The mydriasis provocative test. Arch Ophthalmol 66: 87–89
3. Harris LS, Galin MA (1969) Cycloplegic provocative testing: Effect of miotic therapy. Arch Ophthalmol 81: 544–547
4. Schimek RA, Lieberman WJ (1961) The influence of cyclogyl and neosynephrine on tonographic studies of miotic control in open-angle glaucoma. Am J Ophthalmol 51: 781–784
5. Weinreb RN, Ruderman J, Juster R, Zweig K (1983) Immediate intraocular pressure response to argon laser trabeculoplasty. Am J Ophthalmol 95: 279–286

6. Hoskins HD, Hetherington J, Minckler DS, Lieberman MF, Shaffer RN (1983) Complications of laser trabeculoplasty. Ophthalmology 90: 796–799
7. Robin AL, Pollack IP, House B, Enger C (1987) Effects of ALO 2145 on intraocular pressure following argon laser trabeculoplasty. Arch Ophthalmol 105: 646–650
8. Robin AL, Pollack IP, deFaller JM (1987) Effects of topical ALO 2145 (p-aminoclonidine hydrochloride) on the acute intraocular pressure rise after argon laser iridotomy. Arch Ophthalmol 105: 1208–1211
9. Hill RA, Minckler DS, Lee M, Heuer DK, Baerveldt G, Martone JF (1991) Apraclonidine therapy to prevent cycloplegic-induced IOP spikes, a chlinical study. Ophthalmology 98: 1083–1086
10. Abrams DA, Robin AL, Pollack IP, deFaller JM, DeSantis L (1987) The safety and efficacy of topical 1% ALO 2145 (p-aminoclonidine hydrochloride) in normal volunteers. Arch Ophthalmol 105: 1205–1207
11. Glaucoma Laser Trial Research Group. Handbook. Springfield, Virginia: National Technical Information Service; 1985. Accession No. PB 86-101039, March

Corresponding Address

Professor D. S. Minckler, M.D.
Director, University of Southern California School of Medicine, Department of Ophthalmology, Glaucoma Services, Estelle Doheny Eye Institute, 1355 San Pablo Street, Ste. 406E, Los Angeles, CA 90033/USA

Zur Logik der medikamentösen Kombinationstherapie beim Glaukom

M. Diestelhorst und G. K. Krieglstein

Die lokale Verträglichkeit und die Lebensqualität spielen eine wichtige Rolle bei der Therapie des chronisch erkrankten Glaukompatienten.

Oft führt mangelnde Compliance zum Versagen und Abbruch der Therapie. Die Compliance wird durch die Vielzahl von Applikationen verschiedener Präparate negativ beeinflußt. Doch mehr als 35 % der Glaukompatienten benötigen bei einem Ausgangsdruckniveau von > 32mmHg zwei oder mehr Antiglaukomatosa, um eine Konstanz von Papille und Gesichtsfeld zu erzielen.

Eine ausreichende intraokulare Druckregulierung ist notwendig, da die Inzidenz der Gesichtsfeldausfälle und Papillenschädigung mit steigendem intraokularen Druck zunimmt. Papillenveränderungen sind bei hohem intraokularen Druckniveau in kürzeren Zeitabständen zu beobachten. Diese in Tiermodellen gezeigte Druckschädigung der Papille ist als ein gesicherter Pathomechanismus – neben anderen – bei Glaukom allgemein anerkannt.

Die Möglichkeiten der Kombinationstherapie werden durch mehrere miteinander verknüpfte Faktoren beeinflußt:

- Wirkung und Nebenwirkung der kombinierten Antiglaukomatosa,
- Glaukomform,
- Alter und Tätigkeit des Patienten,
- bestehende Unverträglichkeitsreaktionen,
- bestehende systemische und lokale Therapie,
- Ausgangsniveau von intraokularem Druck – intraokularer Druck ohne Therapie,
- Zustand von Papille und Gesichtsfeld,
- Begleiterkrankungen des Patienten.

Die drei Hauptsäulen der Glaukomtherapie sind die Parasympathomimetika, Sympatholytika und die Karboanhydrasehemmer.

Ihre Angriffspunkte zur Drucksenkung sind:
1. Verbesserung der Abflußleichtigkeit (Parasympathomimetika),
2. Einschränkung der Kammerwasser-Sekretion
    - Rezeptorblockade (Sympatholytika)
    - Enzymhemmung (Karboanhydrasehemmstoffe).

Gramer/Kampik (Hrsg.) Pharmakotherapie am Auge
© Springer-Verlag Berlin Heidelberg 1992

Hinzugekommen sind die Adrenergika in Form des Epinephrins und dessen „Prodrug". Sie verbessern die Fazilität und den uveoskleralen Abfluß über die Veränderung des Gefäßtonus.

Ziel des behandelnden Ophthalmologen ist es, die geeignete Kombination dieser Pharmakagruppen bezüglich der jeweiligen Glaukomform und Patienten herauszufinden, um Gesichtsfeld und Papille über Jahre konstant zu erhalten. Dabei sind die oben genannten Faktoren – insbesondere eine gute Compliance – zu berücksichtigen. Eine Glaukom-Maximaltherapie (Miotikum 4mal, Betarezeptorenblocker 2mal, Epinephrin 2mal, Karboanhydrasehemmer 3mal ½ Tablette) ist mit einem geregelten Berufsleben nur schwer in Einklang zu bringen.

Der Vorteil fixer Kombinationspräparate liegt auf der Hand: der Patient benötigt weniger Fläschchen, hat keinen komplizierten Applikationsplan einzuhalten, die Therapie kann nicht verwechselt werden, die Compliance steigt, es werden weniger Konservierungsstoffe appliziert, der Patient kann mit seiner Erkrankung besser leben.

Die Kombination von Antiglaukomatosa sollte wenn möglich eine fazilitätsverbessernde Substanz beinhalten. Pilokarpin, Aceclidin oder Carbachol haben hier den größten meßbaren Effekt gezeigt. Irreversible Cholinesterasehemmer, wie das DFP-Fluostigmin oder Ecothiophat, werden heute nur noch in Ausnahmefällen angewandt. Allergien, Iriszysten, Ziliarkörperspasmen, Schmerzen, Schwindel, Übelkeit waren einige der Gründe für die limitierte Ordination.

Die Kombination von Pilokarpin mit Betablockern ist in Deutschland seit einigen Jahren eingeführt. Sie erfüllt die Regel, wonach keine Pharmaka gleicher Wirkung kombiniert werden sollten. Die Betarezeptorenblockade drosselt die Kammerwassersekretionsrate um bis zu 40 % und unterstützt dadurch zusätzlich die durch Pilokarpinapplikation verbesserte Abflußleichtigkeit im Bereich des Trabekelmaschenwerkes. Eine dritte Leitschiene der Kombinationstherapie wird durch die Applikation geringer Konzentrationen erreicht. Es hat sich gezeigt, daß eine Erhöhung der Konzentration eines Wirkstoffes nur bedingt zu einer verbesserten intraokularen Drucksenkung führt. Die verschiedenen Untersuchungen bezüglich der Drucksenkung gleicher Betarezeptorenblocker unterschiedlicher Konzentration haben hierüber Aufschluß gegeben.

Werden Parasympathomimetika mit Adrenalinpräparaten kombiniert, so ist insbesondere auf die adrenalinbedingte Mydriasis zu achten. Sie ist bei älteren Patienten mit Cataracta incipiens oft hilfreich, kann bei engerem Kammerwinkel jedoch den akuten Glaukomanfall begünstigen. Da die Halbwertszeit von Adrenergika länger ist als diejenige von Pilokarpin, ist hier bei nachlassender Pilokarpinwirkung ein negativer Effekt nicht auszuschliessen.

Die Kombination wird derzeit in Deutschland von zwei Herstellern angeboten und kann bei weitem Kammerwinkel sinnvoll eingesetzt werden. Eine weitere Kombinationsmöglichkeit besteht für Betarezeptorenblocker und Epinephrin-Augentropfen. Hier wirken Kammerwassersekretionshemmung und die Verbesserung des uveoskleralen Abflusses zusammen drucksenkend. Zusätzlich zu den bekannten Nebenwirkungen der Betarezeptorenblocker (Asthma, Emphysembronchitis, AV-Block II. u. III. Grades) muß hier auf eine Verstärkung der Mydriasis bei dieser Kombination hingewiesen werden. Beide Pharmakagruppen „unterstützen" sich bezüglich des mydriatischen Effektes bei alpha-1-Stimulation des M. dilatator pupillae. Ein weiter Kammerwinkel ist also Voraussetzung Nummer 1 für diese Kombination, falls kein Miotikum zusätzlich appliziert wird.

Karboanhydrasehemmstoffe sind als Kombination mit allen genannten Antiglaukomatosa denkbar und möglich. Aus der systemischen Enzymhemmung resultiert eine etwa 50 %ige Reduktion der Kammerwassersekretion. Dieser maximale therapeutische Effekt auf den intraokularen Druck durch ein einzelnes Pharmakon konnte durch die Applikation lokaler Karboanhydrasehemmstoffe bisher nicht erreicht werden.

Die sich derzeitig in der zweiten klinischen Phase befindlichen lokalen Karboanhydrasehemmstoffe haben auch in Kombination mit lokalen Betarezeptorenblockern eine additive Wirkung beider drucksenkender Mechanismen bestätigen können. Enzymhemmung und Rezeptorenblockade ergänzen sich also auch bei lokaler gleichzeitiger Applikation.

Eine zusätzliche fixe Therapiemöglichkeit besteht seit Anfang der 80er Jahre in der Kombination von Adrenergika mit Guanethidin. Guanethidin verändert sowohl die Speicherfähigkeit für die adrenerge Überträgersubstanz als auch die Membraneigenschaften der postganglionären sympathischen Nervenendstrecke (periphere, chemische Sympathektomie). Die so behandelten Gewebsstrukturen werden für adrenerge Substanzen empfindlicher. Die mit Adrenalin verbundenen Nebenwirkungen (Blutdruckanstieg, Pulsanstieg, Gefäßverengung, Schmerzen) sind reduziert. Beide Präparate sind in geringster Konzentration kombiniert. Die mydriatische Wirkung des Epinephrins kann jedoch auch bei dieser Kombination bei engem Kammerwinkel zum Glaukomanfall führen.

Wird eine Kombinationstherapie mehrerer Antiglaukomatosa erforderlich, sollte vor Therapiebeginn die Medikamentenanamnese bei den Patienten wiederholt werden. Ein mit Betarezeptorenblockern systemisch behandelter Hypertoniker bedarf nicht der zusätzlichen Betarezeptorenblockade am Auge. Andererseits wird ein latenter Hypertonus durch lokale Adrenalintherapie negativ beeinflußt. Die nasolacrimale Resorption lokal applizierter wäßriger Augentropfen unter Umgehung des „first pass"-Effektes zeichnet für die systemischen Nebenwirkungen verschiedener Augentropfen verantwortlich.

Der Vorteil der Therapie mehrerer Einzelpräparate beruht auf der Möglichkeit des selektiven Dosierungsschemas und des selektiven Abbruchs eines Pharmakons, z.B. bei möglicher Allergisierung oder auftretenden Nebenwirkungen. Dennoch scheint unter Berücksichtigung aller Aspekte die fixe Kombinationstherapie für viele Glaukompatienten eine sinnvolle, die Compliance verbessernde Alternative. Sie vereinfacht das Therapieverständnis für die Patienten und verbessert zusätzlich ihre Lebensqualität.

Welche neuen Kombinationspräparate erscheinen möglich? Die Einführung der lokalen Karboanhydrasehemmer läßt eine Kombination mit Miotika (Fazilitätsverbesserung) oder mit Betarezeptorenblockern (Kammerwassersekretionsminderung) sinnvoll erscheinen.

Die ebenfalls noch in der klinischen Erprobung befindlichen Prostaglandine F2-alpha könnten z.B. mit Betarezeptorenblockern kombiniert werden. Eine Verbindung mit Miotika ist dagegen jedoch unwahrscheinlich, da die Ziliarkörperkontraktion den uveoskleralen Abfluß signifikant hemmt.

Literatur beim Verfasser

Korrespondenzadresse
Dr. med. M. Diestelhorst
Universitätsaugenklinik Köln, Joseph-Stelzmann-Str. 9, D-5000 Köln 41

Beta-Blockers and Ocular Bloodflow

W. Soudijn

The pharmacological effect of a beta-blocker on a local tissue e.g. the non-pigmented epithelium of the ciliary processes, the trabecular meshwork or the various ocular vascular beds, depends on a combination of several factors.

One of these factors is the concentration of the drug in a specific receptor-compartment which depends on the ability of the compound to cross a number of barriers in order to reach the receptors.

Other factors are the kind and number of different receptor types and subtypes present in the receptor compartment.

And last but not least there is the pharmacological profile of the betablocker itself.

The affinity of a beta-blocker for a beta-adrenergic receptor is a measure for its beta-blocking potency. Beta-1-selective beta-blockers like betaxolol have a higher affinity for beta-1-adrenoceptors than for beta-2-adrenoceptors while for non-selective beta-blockers like timolol the affinity is about the same for both receptor subtypes.

Fairly recently the existence of a third beta-adrenoceptor subtype was discovered. Because of some similarity in properties with the beta-2-adrenoceptor is called a beta-2-like- or a beta-3-adrenoceptor. Some beta-blockers like (−)pindolol or (±)alprenolol and probably several others stimulate instead of block this receptor at concentrations far above those necessary to block beta-1 and beta-2 receptors.

These beta-blockers are called by Kaumann, non conventional partial agonists [1].

Beta-3-receptors are found in heart tissue and in bloodvessels in coexistence with beta-2-receptors and having a similar effect on stimulation. This might also be the case in the non-pigmented epithelium of the ciliary processes, the epithelium of the trabecular meshwork and in retinal blood vessels were the existence of beta-2-receptors unambiguously has been demonstrated.

It is generally accepted that beta-blockers topically administered reduce the intra-ocular pressure by reducing the inflow of aqueous humor. Although it is tempting to assume that the mechanism of action is by blocking the beta-2-receptors of the non-pigmented epithelium of the ciliary processes, there are some serious objections to be made.

Gramer/Kampik (Hrsg.) Pharmakotherapie am Auge
© Springer-Verlag Berlin Heidelberg 1992

First of all there is no correlation between the potency of a beta-blocker to block beta-2-receptors in other tissues and its IOP lowering potency. The R(+) isomers of beta-blockers having generally a very low affinity for beta-2-receptors are still able to reduce the intraocular pressure. Secondly not all beta-blockers despite high concentrations in the aqueous humor effectively lower IOP.

However, there is a possibility that the beta-2-receptors in the epithelial membranes of the ciliary processes are at least partly beta-2-like receptors differing from the classical beta-2-receptors in other tissues of the body. Some evidence was recently presented by Nathanson [2].

Isoprenaline, a non-selective beta-agonist stimulates adenylate cyclase to produce c-AMP from ATP in heart tissue via beta-1-receptors and in the isolated ciliary process epithelium via beta-2-receptors.

This effect is blocked by beta-blockers (Table 1).

The optical isomer S(−) timolol used in ophtalmology as an IOP lowering agent does not discriminate between the beta-1 and beta-2 receptors as the potency ratio is about 1 in this biochemical test system.

However rather unexpectedly the S(−) isomer of betaxol does not, and its enantiomer R(+) hardly discriminates between the two receptor types, while in other tissues the discrimination ratio varies between 100 and 250. The R(+) isomer of timolol in this test discriminates rather well between beta-1 and beta-2 receptors and is clearly a beta-2-selective antagonist. These data may explain why R(+) timolol as well as the clinically used S(−) timolol lowers the IOP as both are equipotent on beta-2-receptors of the ciliary processes epithelium.

On the other hand the data on betaxolol show that at least part of the receptor population of the ciliary processes epithelium consists of beta-2-like receptors which may play a role in the IOP lowering mechanism of beta-blockers whether they are beta-1-selective or not.

Also in cultured human trabecular meshwork cells the beta-2-adrenoceptor population may consist at least in part of beta-2-like receptors as can be inferred from data given by Polansky [3].

From this data (Table 2) it appears that the affinity of betaxolol for the beta-2-receptors in this tissue ($K_d = 40–60$ nM) is about 4 times higher than in

Table 1. Isoprenaline (beta-agonist) stimulated adenylate cyclase in heart (beta-1) and ciliary process (beta-2) blocked by beta-blockers. (From [2])

	K_i Micro M		
	Heart	Ciliary process	Ratio
S-Timolol	0.0064	0.0055	1.2
R-Timolol	0.28	0.0045	62
S-Betaxolol	0.17	0.15	1.1
R-Betaxolol	90.0	29.0	3.1

Table 2. Beta-2-adrenoceptors. (From [3])

Beta-2-adrenoceptors in:

Human trabecular meshwork

	K_d	nM
Timolol	0.5	
Betaxolol	40–60	

Other beta-2 rich tissues

Timolol	0.5
Betaxolol	150–220

in other classical beta-2-receptor rich tissues (K_d = 150–200 nM). The non-selective beta-blocker timolol does not discriminate between the beta-2-receptors in the trabecular meshwork and beta-2-receptors in other tissues.

The affinity of timolol for the trabecular meshwork beta-2-receptors appears to be 100 times higher than the affinity of betaxolol for these adrenoceptors.

There is another factor that should be kept in mind.

After topical administration the beta-blocker concentration in the aqueous humor for several hours is 100–1000 times higher than needed for blocking either beta-1 or beta-2-receptors in other tissues.

This should prompt us to take a closer look at the capabilities of beta-blockers to bind to other than beta-adrenoceptors.

This is easily done by in vitro receptor binding studies, either by determining the dissociation constant K_d for certain receptor which is a measure for the affinity of the compound for this receptor (see Table 3) or by determining the IC_{50} or the inhibition constant K_i often expressed as pK_i of the beta-blocker for a certain non-beta-adrenergic receptor (see Table 3).

Table 3. In vitro receptor binding studies

K_d = dissociation constant = measure of the affinity of a compound for its receptor

   K_d large = low affinity
   K_d small = high affinity

IC_{50} = concentration of a compound necessary to displace 50 % of a radioligand from its receptor

$$K_i = \text{inhibition constant} = \frac{IC_{50}}{1 + \dfrac{L}{K_d}}$$

where L = concentration radioligand
K_d = diss. constant radioligand

pK_i = negative logarithm of K_i
pK_i = 9 K_i = 10^{-9} molar = 1 nanomolar
pK_i = 6 K_i = 10^{-6} molar = 1 micromolar

A low value of K_i or a higher value for pK_i denotes a high affinity for the receptor under investigation.

In this way we investigated betaxolol and timolol for their affinities for 28 different receptors (Fig. 1). We did not discriminate between beta-1- and beta-2-affinity because this is already well known from the literature on the non-selective timolol and the beta-1-selective betaxolol. Besides our interest was to know whether both drugs had affinities for other receptors and in how far they differ in their affinities for these receptors.

From the results it appears that both drugs have a low affinity ($pK_i < 5$ $K_i > 10.000$ nanoM) for the majority of the receptors tested.

Betaxolol however has a significant affinity for the serotonin 5-HT-1A receptor ($pK_i = 6.84$; $K_i = 145$ nM) and a neglible affinity for all the other serotonin receptor subtypes while timolol has a 10 fold less affinity for the 5-HT-1A receptor and a low ($pK_i = 5.3$) but clear cut affinity for the 5-HT-1C receptor (Fig. 2).

Interestingly betaxolol also has affinity for the verapamil binding site ($pK_i = 6.3$, $K_i = 480$ nM).

Verapamil is a calcium entry blocker on the potential dependent calcium channels of the smooth muscle of arterial vascular beds.

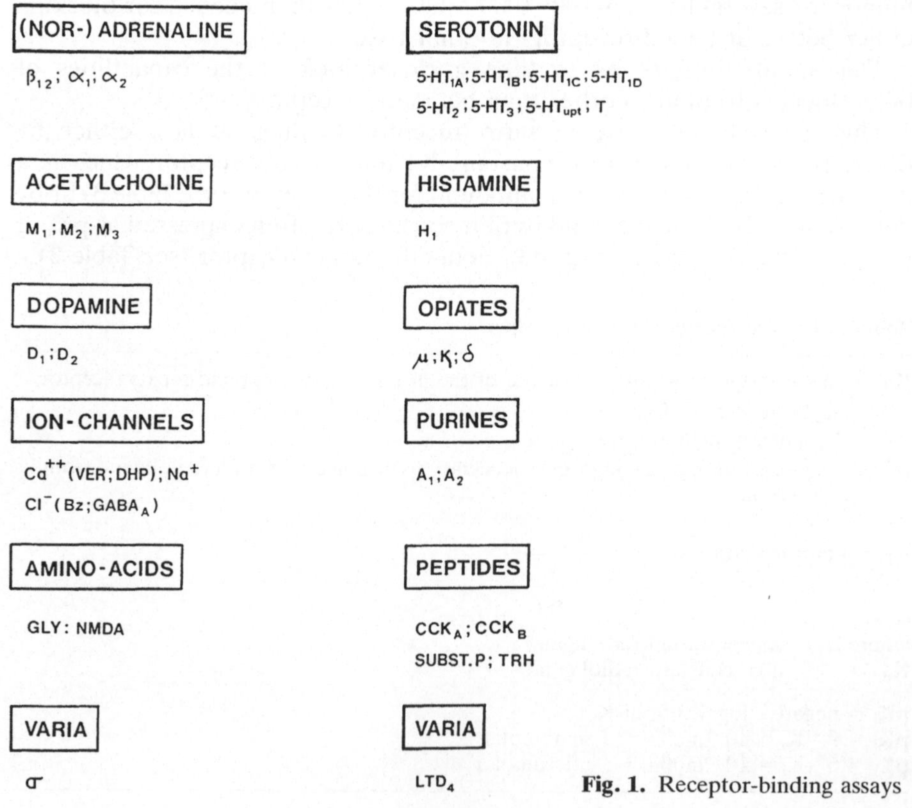

Fig. 1. Receptor-binding assays

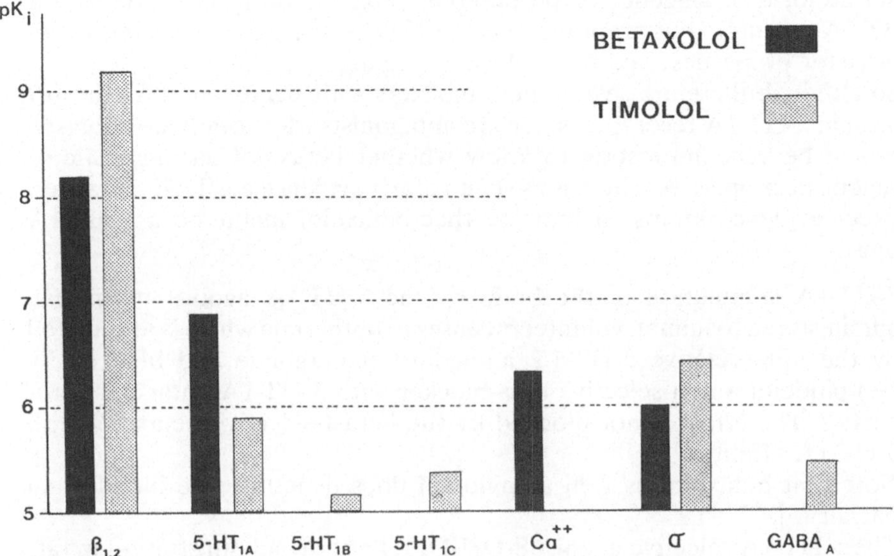

Fig. 2

The effect of verapamil on the coronary vascular system is vasodilatation. The affinity of betaxolol for the verapamil binding site on the calcium channel, if it is expressed as a verapamil like activity, could be of advantage for the interaction of the drug with arteries in the ocular vascular bed. The interaction of timolol with the verapamil binding site is negligible ($pK_a < 5$).

Timolol has some affinity for the Gaba-A-receptor ($pK_i = 5.27$) were betaxolol has none, and affinity for the central sigma receptor ($pK_i = 6.41$, $K_i = 390$ nM) where the affinity of betaxolol for this receptor is two times lower ($pK_i = 6.0$, $K_i = 1000$ nM). These affinities have probably nothing to do with the IOP lowering effect of the drugs neither with a possible effect on the ocular vascular beds.

From the differences in binding profile of betaxolol and timolol it can surmised that there might be differences in the effect of these drugs on local vascular beds.

Excepting the well-known difference in selectivity and affinity for beta-adrenoceptors, the most striking difference is the relatively high affinity of betaxolol for the serotonin 5-HT-1A receptor compared to timolol and the moderate affinity for the calcium channel blocking binding site of verapamil which is lacking in timolol.

Recently it was demonstrated by Verbeuren et al. [4] that reno-vasodilation by the beta-blocker tertatolol was most probably caused by stimulation of 5-HT-1A receptors in the reno-vascular bed and partly dependent on the presence of vasal endothelium.

Tertatolol is a congener of propranolol (Fig. 3). Both have affinity for 5-HT-1A receptors but propranolol is a 5-HT-1A antagonist with renovaso-constrictor properties, and tertatolol is an agonist.

So although there are several beta-blockers with significant affinities for serotonin 5-HT-1A receptors, some are antagonists while other are agonists. It would be very interesting to know whether betaxolol has agonistic or antagonistic properties. There is as yet no direct evidence available, however, indirect evidence seems to indicate that betaxolol might be a 5-HT-1A agonist.

- 5-HT-1A stimulation in the brain by the 5-HT-1A agonist ipsapirone administered to human volunteers causes hypothermia which is attenuated by the non-selective 5-HT-1/2 antagonist metergoline and blocked by (−)-pindolol a non-selective beta-blocker with 5-HT-1A antagonist properties. The effect is not blocked by the beta-1-selective betaxolol with 5-HT-1A affinity.
  Note that betaxolol as well as pindolol does penetrate the blood-brain barrier [5].
- The 5-HT-1A selective agonist 8-OH-DPAT after iv administration in rats increases plasma adrenalin levels and induces hyperglycaemia. (−)-pindolol diminishes the rise in adrenalin levels and blocks the hyperglycemic effect.
  Betaxolol does not block the effects of 8-OH-DPAT neither does the beta-2-antagonist ICI 118.551 [6].

BETAXOLOL
β₁- SELECTIVE
5-HT₁ₐ AGONIST
TIMOLOL
NON-SELECTIVE
5-HT₁ₐ (AGO/ANTA?)
PROPRANOLOL
NON-SELECTIVE
5-HT₁ₐ ANTAGONIST
TERTATOLOL
NON-SELECTIVE
5-HT₁ₐ AGONIST

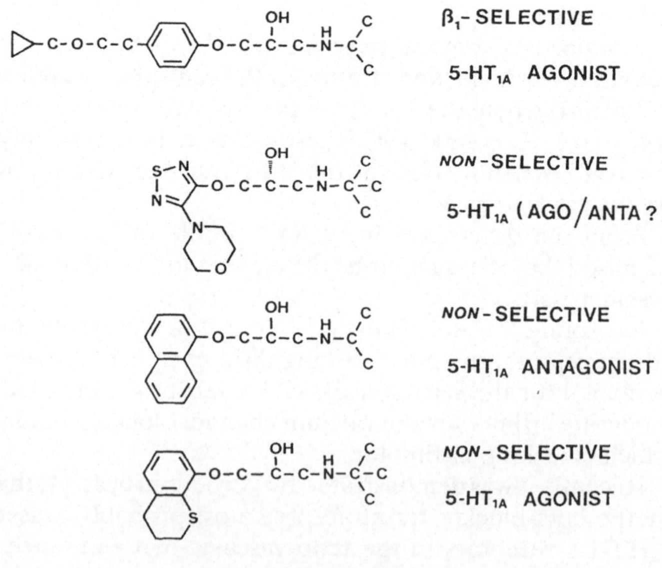

Fig. 3. Beta-blockers

These experiments show that betaxolol is probably not a 5-HT-1A antagonist but direct evidence is needed to show that betaxolol can act in vivo as a 5-HT-1A agonist in local vascular beds.

Little is known about 5-HT-receptors and their subtypes in ocular beds and in-depth research in this area could be very useful.

The effect of topically administered beta-blockers on the ocular vasculature depends on the concentration of the beta-blockers in this particular receptor compartment and the population of relevant receptors present in the compartment.

For instance it is assumed that in the uveal vascular bed there are only alpha-adrenergic receptors present, which on stimulation result in vasoconstriction, while in the ciliary processes and choroid cholinergic or peptidergic (VIP) nerves are active (Table 4). These receptors do not interact with beta-blockers commonly used in lowering the IOP.

However in the retinal vessels, although they are not innervated in the intra-ocular part of the retinal vascular bed, alpha-1, alpha-2 and beta-1 and beta-2-receptors are shown to be present (Table 5) by G. Ferrari Dileo et al. [7].

The exact function and localisation of these receptors is not known yet. If they are localized on the smooth muscle of arteries and arterioles, stimulation

Table 4. Ocular vascular beds

Innervation
Uveal: adrenergic only alpha receptors stimulation → vasocontraction also cholinergic in
          ciliary processes and choroïd (peptidergic, VIP)
Retinal: intraocular no innervation

Autoregulation
Uveal: Iris and ciliary body partly
Retinal: Autoregulated

Precapillary sphincters are absent in choroïdal and retinal beds

---

Table 5. Bovine retinal vessels. (From [7])

Adrenergic receptors:
Present; alpha-1 and 2, beta-1 and 2
Localisation unkown

If on smooth muscle:
Stimulation alpha → contraction
            beta → relaxation

If on endothelium:
Stimulation alpha-2 → relaxation

Angiotensin II receptors:
Stimulation → contraction

---

of the alpha-receptors leads to contraction of the vessels. However if the alpha-2-receptors are localized in the endothelium membranes, stimulation leads to vasodilation of the retinal vessels (Table 5). Whatever the case may be, beta-blockers having no affinity whatsoever for alpha-receptors cannot interfere directly with the mechanism of action of the alpha-receptors in the retinal vascular system.

However, if on the contrary non-selective beta-blockers like for instance timolol block the beta-2-receptors on the smooth muscle of retinal arteries, the result could be a vasoconstriction of the intra-ocular retinal arteries. This was indeed shown to be the case by X.D. Martin and P.A. Rabineau [8] who demonstrated that topical administration of 0.5 % timolol in one eye twice daily for one week to human volunteers decreased the diameter of retinal arteries by 4 % in the treated eye, compared to the untreated, controlateral eye. This indicates that neither a blood-pressure lowering effect nor transportation of timolol by the circulation to the untreated eye can account for this effect.

According to Poiseulle's law this reduction in arterial diameter should lead to a reduction in retinal arterial bloodflow of about 17 %.

If the reduction is due to arterial beta-2-receptor blocking, this is not to be expected for beta-1-selective blockers like betaxolol.

It is questionable whether timolol can reach receptors on the luminal side of the vascular endothelium by way of the vitreous because of the blood-retinal barrier localized on this endothelium.

(Timolol is too hydrophilic to pass the blood-brain barrier while more lipophil beta-blockers like e.g. betaxolol, pindolol and propranolol can.) Interaction with the endothelial receptors by timolol transported by the systemic circulation is of course possible but that does not explain the difference between the vessels in the treated and untreated eye.

It should be interesting to test betaxolol under similar conditions as in the timolol experiment in order to conclude whether the difference in the pharmacological profile of both drugs could lead to different effects on the retinal vascular bed.

It is clear that beta-blockers used in ophthalmology may have quite different pharmacological profiles and thus may have different effects on the ocular vascular beds. More clinical pharmacology with different beta-blockers is needed to gain more insight in the relationship between IOP-lowering beta-blockers and ocular vascular blood flow.

References

1. Kaumann AJ (1989) Trends in Pharmacol Sci 10: 316
2. Nathanson JA (1988) Pharmacol Exp Ther 245: 94
3. Polansky JR (1990) Int Ophthalmology Clinics 30: 219
4. Verbeuren TJ et al. (1990) Eur J Pharmacol 183: 666. (Abstracts IUPHAR symposium Amsterdam 1990.) See also: J Pharmacol Exp Ther 246: 628 (1988). Am J Hypertension (Suppl) Vol 2 Part 2, 219S (1989). Here is demonstrated that the renovasodilating effect

is not blocked by adrenergic, dopaminergic, cholinergic, histaminergic, or opioïd antagonists.

5. Lesch KP et al. (1990) Eur J Clin Pharmacol 39: 17
6. Chaouloff F et al (1990) NS Arch Pharmacol 341: 381
7. Ferrari Dileo G (1988) Invest Ophthal Vis Sci 29: 695, 28: 1741, 1747 (1987)
8. Martin XD, Rabineau PA (1987) Graefe's Arch Clin Exp Ophthalmol 227: 526

Corresponding Address
Professor W. Soudijn, Ph.D.
Gorlaeus Laboratories, Leiden University, P.O. Box 9502 N-2300 RA Leiden, Niederlande

Neue Kombinationspräparate mit nur zwei Applikationen täglich als Bestandteil einer medikamentösen Drei- oder Vierkomponententherapie des Glaukoms

E. Gramer

Zusammenfassung

Drei neue Kombinationspräparate werden vorgeschlagen:

1. Die fixe Kombination aus Carbachol und Betaxolol.
2. Die fixe Kombination aus Carbachol und DPE.
3. Die fixe Kombination aus DPE und Betaxolol.

1. Carbachol ist ein direktes Parasympathomimetikum mit gleichzeitiger Cholinesterasehemmung und weist aufgrund dieser Doppelwirkung in wäßriger Lösung in einer Konzentration von 3 % eine längere Wirkungsdauer (ca. 12 Stunden) als Pilocarpin-Augentropfen 2 % (ca. 4 Stunden) auf und zeigt eine höhere Augeninnendrucksenkung als Pilocarpin-Augentropfen 2 % (IOD-Senkung von Carbachol 3 % entspricht Pilocarpin 8 %).
2. Bei unter gleichzeitiger Betablockergabe reduzierter Kammerwasserproduktion ergibt sich eine geänderte Pharmakokinetik und höhere Bioverfügbarkeit des Carbachols und damit eine höhere und längere augeninnendrucksenkende Wirkung als bei freier Kombination der Medikamente.
3. Die Suspensionstechnologie ist auf den Betablocker und auf Carbachol anwendbar, was zu einer besseren Penetration und langsameren Wirkstoffabgabe führt, so daß bei gleicher Wirkungsstärke und gleicher Wirkungsdauer die Konzentration des Betablockers (von 0.5 % auf 0,28 %) und von Carbachol (von 3 % auf weniger als 3 %) im Kombinationspräparat reduziert werden kann. Dies führt zu einer besseren lokalen und systemischen Verträglichkeit unter Wegfall des Bolus-Charakters der Medikamente und zu einer konstanten Miosis.

Diese 3 Gründe erlauben für das neue Kombinationspräparat aus Carbachol und Betaxolol (Suspension oder Lösung) mit höherer Wahrscheinlichkeit die Reduzierung der Applikationshäufigkeit auf 2× täglich bei konstanter Augeninnendrucksenkung und konstanter Miosis als bei einem Pilocarpin-Kombinationspräparat. Die nur noch 2× tägliche Applikation des Kombinationspräparats führt neben einer Verbesserung der Compliance auch zu einer Verminderung der Konservierungsmittelbelastung, einer geringeren

Gramer/Kampik (Hrsg.) Pharmakotherapie am Auge
© Springer-Verlag Berlin Heidelberg 1992

Gefahr der Ausbildung einer Subsensitivität und Allergisierung und einer besseren Anpassung des Therapieschemas an den Tagesablauf des Patienten. Das vorgeschlagene Carbachol-Betaxolol-Kombinationspräparat wie auch das vorgeschlagene Carbachol-DPE-Kombinationspräparat weist daher gegenüber Pilocarpin-Betablocker-Kombinationspräparaten oder Pilocarpin-DPE-Kombinationspräparaten, die wegen der kurzen Wirkungsdauer des Pilocarpins 4× täglich appliziert werden sollten, deutliche Vorzüge auf. Durch den Beta-1-selektiven Betablocker als Betablockerkomponente im Carbachol-Betaxolol-Kombinationspräparat ergibt sich eine bessere Kombinierbarkeit mit DPE (Drei-Komponenten-Therapie) oder mit DPE-Guanethidin-Kombinationspräparaten (Vier-Komponenten-Therapie). Um eine selektive Umstellung von Teilkomponenten unter Beibehaltung der Vorzüge des Kombinationspräparats mit 2× täglicher Applikation zu gewährleisten, sind folgende Kombinationspräparate wünschenswert: Carbachol-Betaxolol-Kombination; Carbachol-DPE-Kombination; DPE-Betaxolol-Kombination, die alle nur noch 2× täglich appliziert werden müssen. Die vorgeschlagenen 3 neuen Kombinationspräparate können die Stufenleiter der medikamentösen Kombinationstherapie verlängern und sind in anbetracht der steigenden Lebenserwartung der Bevölkerung eine medizinische und ethische Notwendigkeit.

Medikamentöse Kombinationstherapie bei Glaukom

Die medikamentöse Therapie des Glaukoms wird üblicherweise mit einer Monotherapie begonnen. Bei nicht ausreichender Drucksenkung kann dann auf eine Monotherapie mit anderer Substanzklasse ausgewichen werden oder bei nachgewiesener Wirksamkeit dieser Monosubstanz, die erforderlichenfalls durch Auslaßversuch gesichert sein muß, kann es, abhängig von der Höhe des angestrebten Augeninnendruckniveaus individuell auch sinnvoll sein, auf die Kombination mit einer zusätzlichen Monosubstanz mit anderer Wirkungsweise auszuweichen. Erweist sich die Kombination aus 2 Substanzen in der Tagesdruckkurve dann als ausreichend drucksenkend, sollten die beiden Präparate – wenn möglich – aus Compliance-Gründen durch ein Kombinationspräparat mit fixer Kombination dieser beiden Wirksubstanzen ersetzt werden. Läßt sich mit einem solchen Kombinationspräparat dann das angestrebte therapeutische Augeninnendruckniveau dennoch nicht dauerhaft erreichen, so kann, wenn eine operative Therapie primär nicht infrage kommt, zu diesem Kombinationspräparat eine zusätzliche Medikation appliziert werden. Es entstehen so Dreier- oder gar Viererkombinationen von Medikamenten. Solche bisher relativ wenig wissenschaftlich untersuchten, aber dennoch gebräuchlichen Mehrfachkombinationen müssen als Ultima ratio bei anders nicht therapierbarem Glaukom angesehen werden. Die praktische Anwendbarkeit muß unter dem Aspekt der additiven Wirkung und unter dem Gesichtspunkt der Compliance [34] sorgfältig geprüft werden.

So zeigen z.B. Untersuchungen von Kass et al. (1978) zur Compliance, daß bei verordneter 4× täglicher Pilocarpinanwendung im Mittel nur 2,5 Tropfen pro Tag vom Patienten appliziert werden, wobei am Tag des Arztbesuchs (Kass et al. 1983) Applikationen selten vergessen werden. Untersuchungen von Davidson et al. (1983) zeigen, daß die Mittagsapplikation am häufigsten vergessen wird. Zur Compliance bei langdauernder Glaukomtherapie sei auf die Übersicht von Noack [34] mit weiterführenden Literaturangaben verwiesen. Complianceverbessernd wirken Pharmaka mit geringen Nebenwirkungen sowie ein einfaches Therapieschema (2 × tägl.). Ein Therapieschema kann nicht nur durch neue Wirksubstanzen verbessert werden, sondern es kann auch versucht werden, bekannte Substanzen statt bisher in freier Kombination in fixer Kombination anzuwenden, wobei die Kombination von Medikamenten mit langer Wirkdauer (z.B. Carbachol-Betablocker-Kombinationspräparte) und andere galenische Wege (z.B. Suspensionstechnologie) die pharmakokinetischen Eigenschaften des Kombinationspräparates dahingehend verändern können, daß es stärker und länger augeninnendrucksenkend wirkt als die freie Kombination der Einzelsubstanzen und somit mit nur noch 2× täglicher Applikation eine konstante Augeninnendrucksenkung erzielbar ist.

Die Logik eines solchen Therapiekonzepts und die zu erwartenden Verbesserungen gegenüber der freien Kombination von Medikamenten aufzuzeigen, ist das Ziel dieser Arbeit.

Die Kombination folgender Substanzen, einzeln oder als Kombinationspräparat, sind bisher in ihrer Wirkung gesichert: Betablocker und Pilocarpin [2, 37] oder Dipivalyl-Epinephrin (DPE) und Pilocarpin [27] oder Adrenalin bzw. DPE und Guanethidin [18, 19, 21, 38, 52]. Kontrovers diskutiert wird die Kombination aus einem Betablocker mit einem Sympathomimetikum [3, 23, 31, 40, 41, 44, 49, 51, 54], wie im folgenden noch dargestellt wird.

Vor-/Nachteile fixer Medikamenten-Kombinationen

Ein Vorteil der Kombinationspräparate liegt in der besseren Compliance. Ein besonders für ältere Patienten oft kompliziertes Behandlungsschema aus mehreren Medikamenten läßt sich durch Reduzierung der Zahl der Medikamentenfläschchen und damit Reduzierung der Zahl der Applikationen über die Anwendung eines Kombinationspräparates wesentlich vereinfachen. Durch Reduzierung der Applikationshäufigkeit auf 2× täglich – wenn möglich – läßt sich ferner das Therapieschema besser an den spezifischen Tagesablauf des Patienten anpassen. Eine erhebliche Verbesserung der Lebensqualität des Patienten kann die Folge sein. Die Zusammenfassung von 2 Medikamenten in einem Kombinationspräparat hat ferner den Vorteil, daß weniger Konservierungsstoffe als bei Anwendung von 2 Tropfenfläschchen angewandt werden und somit weniger epithelschädigende Nebenwirkungen entstehen. Die fixe Kombination von Medikamenten hat, wie verschiedene Untersuchungen zeigen, möglicherweise auch eine längere

Wirkungsdauer und/oder eine höhere Drucksenkung zur Folge als Kombination der Einzelsubstanzen [2, 46].

Der Wirkungsmechanismus der Kombinationspräparate scheint nicht immer nur die Summe der Einzelmechanismen der Monopräparate zu sein, sondern die verlängerte augeninnendrucksenkende Wirkung des Kombinationspräparates läßt auch eine Änderung der Pharmakokinetik und/oder eine andere Interaktion der Medikamente im Auge vermuten.
Nachteilig bei Kombinationspräparaten ist jedoch, daß keine selektive Dosierung der Einzelsubstanzen mehr möglich ist und auch kein selektiver Abbruch der Therapie bei Nebenwirkungen besteht.

Voraussetzung für ein sinnvolles Kombinationspräparat ist, daß

1. keine Substanzen mit gleichem Wirkungsmechanismus und gleichem Angriffsort enthalten sind,
2. mindestens eine der Substanzen über eine Verbesserung der Abflußleichtigkeit wirkt und
3. die Einzelsubstanzen additive drucksenkende Wirkung aufweisen.

Behandlungszielgruppe für Kombinationspräparate sind Patienten mit schwer einstellbarem Glaukom mit hohen intraokularen Druckwerten, Glaukom mit einem großen Glaukomvorschaden an Papille und Gesichtsfeld [14] oder Glaukome, bei denen das gewünschte therapeutische Augeninnendruckniveau anders nicht erreichbar ist [15]. Kombinationspräparate können dann individuell eine Alternative oder eine Ergänzung zum operativen Vorgehen darstellen.

Bisher verfügbare Kombinationspräparate und ihre Kombinierbarkeit

In Deutschland stehen uns, im Gegensatz z.B. zu anderen Ländern, eine Reihe von Kombinationspräparaten mit fixer Kombination von Medikamenten zur Verfügung (Tabelle 1, oben).

Kombinationspräparate aus einem Miotikum mit einem Betablocker oder aus einem Miotikum mit Adrenalin: So gibt es die fixe Kombination aus folgenden Augentropfen als Lösung: Pilocarpin 2 % und Metipranolol 0,1 % (Normoglaucon) oder Pilocarpin 1 % und Dipivalyl-Epinephrin (DPE) 0,1 % (Thiloadren) oder Pilocarpin 2 % und Epinephrin 2 % (Piladren). Das Kombinationspräparat, das die DPE-Komponente, also das Adrenalin Prodrug enthält, hat wegen der geringeren Nebenwirkungen des Prodrugs Vorteile [22, 27] (vergl. Tab. 1, oben).

Weitere Kombinationspräparate bestehen aus: *einem indirekten Sympatholytikum und einem direkten Sympathomimetikum:* So gibt es die fixe Kombination aus Guanethidin 0,5 % und DPE 0,1 % (Thilodigon 0,5 %)

Tabelle 1. Bisher erhältliche und wünschenswerte neue Kombinationspräparate zur Vereinfachung des Therapieschemas der medikamentösen Glaukomtherpaie

Vorhandene Kombinationspräparte:

Direktes Parasympathomimetikum/Direktes Sympatholytikum
Pilocarpin 2% und Metipranolol 0,1% (Normoglaucon®)

Direktes Parasympathomimetikum/Direktes Sympathomimetikum
Pilocarpin 1% und Dipivalylepinephrin 0,1% (Thiloadren®)
Pilocarpin 2% und Epinephrin 2% (Piladren®)

Indirektes Sympatholytikum/Direktes Sympathomimetikum
Guanethidin 0,5% und Dipivalylepinephrin 0,1% (Thilodigon® 0,5%)
Guanethidin 1% und Adrenalin 0,2% (Suprexon®)
Guanethidin 3% und Adrenalin 0,5% (Suprexon®-forte)

Direktes Parasympathomimetikum/reversibler Cholinesterasehemmer
Pilocarpin 2% und Neostigmin 1% (Syncarpin®)
Pilocarpin 2% und Physostigmin 0,25% (Isopto-Pilomin®)
Pilocarpin 2% und Physostigmin 0,5% (Pilo-Eserin®)

Wünschenswerte fixe Kombination mit 2 × täglicher Applikation

Direktes Parasympathomimetikum mit gleichzeitiger Cholinesterasehemmung/Direktes Sympatholytikum
Carbachol S (z.B. 3%) und Betaxolol S 0,28% (NN)
Carbachol 3%-Lösung und Betaxolol-0,5%-Lösung) (NN)

Direktes Parasympathomimetikum mit gleichzeitiger Cholinesterasehemmung/Direktes Sympathomimetikum
Carbachol S (z.B. 3%) u. DPE (Dipivalylepinephrin 0,1%) (Suspension) (NN)
Carbachol-3%-Lösung und DPE (Dipivalylepinephrin 0,1%) (Lösung) (NN)

Direktes Sympathomimetikum/Direktes Sympatholytikum
Dipivalylepinephrin 0,1% und z.B. Betaxolol-S-0,28% (Suspension) (NN)
DPE (Dipivalylepinephrin 0,1%) und z.B. Betaxolol 0,5% (Lösung) (NN)

oder Guanethidin 1% und Adrenalin 0,2% (Suprexon) oder Guanethidin 3% und Adrenalin 0,5% (Suprexon forte). Das Kombinationspräparat mit dem DPE läßt wiederum Vorteile durch Reduzierung der Adrenalinnebenwirkungen erwarten [39] (vergl. Tab. 1, Mitte).

Andere Kombinationspräparate bestehen aus *einem direkten Parasympathomimetikum und einem reversiblen Cholinesterasehemmer:* So gibt es die fixe Kombination aus Pilocarpin 2% und Neostigmin 1% (Syncarpin) oder Pilocarpin 2% und Physostigmin 0,25% (Isopto-Pilomin) oder Pilocarpin-AT 2% und Physostigmin 0,5% (Pilo-Eserin) (vergl. Tab. 1, Mitte). Da Acetylcholin und Pilocarpin am gleichen Rezeptor wirken, wird zwischen diesen Komponenten eher ein kompetitiver als ein additiver Effekt angenommen [17, 45]. Eine verlängerte Wirkungsdauer ist jedoch gegeben. So beträgt die Wirkungsdauer von Pilocarpin 2% ca. 4 Stunden und von Neostigmin 1% ca. 8–12Stunden [11]. Die Kombinierbarkeit von DPE mit Cholinesterasehemmern wird kontrovers diskutiert. Dies betrifft z.B. die

Kombinationsfähigkeit von Neostigmin 1 %, enthalten im Syncarpin oder von Physostigmin 0,25 %, enthalten im Isopto-Pilomin mit DPE oder DPE-Kombinationspräparaten.

Untersuchungen von Abramovsky und Mindel [1] zeigen, daß im Tierversuch Cholinesterasehemmer möglicherweise unspezifisch die adrenalinfreisetzende Esterase mithemmen können und so die Umwandlung des DPE in Adrenalin hemmen können. Beim Menschen wurde jedoch über einen additiven Effekt berichtet [36].

Bei der Kombination anderer Medikamente mit Adrenalinpräparaten oder DPE ist generell zu berücksichtigen, daß die Adrenalinwirkung ihr Maximum nach 4 Stunden hat und die Wirkung 12 und mehr Stunden anhalten kann. Bei Anwendung von Adrenalin oder eines Adrenalin-Kombinationspräparats ist dies hinsichtlich der Pupillenerweiterung mitzuberücksichtigen. Die fixe Kombination mit einem längerwirkenden Miotikum, z.B. Carbachol 3 %, kann daher individuell sinnvoll sein (vgl. Tabelle 1, unten, Tabelle 2b und Tabelle 4).

Vier-Komponenten-Therapie durch Kombination von zwei Kombinationspräparaten mit nur zwei Applikationen täglich: Carbachol/Betablocker und DPE/Guanethidin

Aus Compliance-Gründen sollte die Vielfach-Medikation, insbesondere für den älteren Patienten möglichst nicht aus mehr als 2 Medikamentenfläschchen bestehen (Tabelle 2a). Kombinationspräparate sind also bei diesem Therapieschema unverzichtbar. Eines der beiden Kombinationspräparate kann z.B. aus der fixen Kombination eines Betarezeptorenblockers und einem Miotikum, also in der Kombination von Betablocker und Pilocarpin oder Betablocker und Carbachol bestehen (vgl. Tabelle 2a, links). Der Betarezeptorenblocker reduziert die Kammerwassersekretion während das Miotikum eine Verbesserung der Abflußleichtigkeit bewirkt. Bisher ist nur ein Pilocarpin-Betablocker-Kombinationspräparat in Deutschland im Handel (vergl. Tabelle 1, oben), ein anderes ist in der Entwicklung [2].

Wünschenswert wäre zusätzlich ein weiteres Kombinationspräparat aus einem Betablocker in fixer Kombination mit Carbachol 3 % (vergl. Tabelle 1, unten, Tabelle 2a), was gegenüber der bisherigen fixen Pilocarpin-Betablokker-Kombination in der Vier-Komponenten-Therapie viele Vorzüge hätte, wie im folgenden noch ausführlich dargestellt wird. Von einem Kombinationspräparat aus einem Beta-1 selektiven Betablocker (Betaxolol) und Carbachol 3 % (besonders in Suspension), kombiniert mit dem Kombinationspräparat aus DPE und Guanethidin (vgl. Tabelle 2a, rechts), ist ein besonders hoher augeninnendrucksenkender Effekt zu erwarten. Unsere Untersuchungen zeigen (vgl. Abb. 1), daß bereits die Kombination der Monosubstanzen Carbachol 3 % und Betablocker 0,5 % zusammen mit dem Kombinationspräparat aus DPE und Guanethidin eine sehr hohe Augenin-

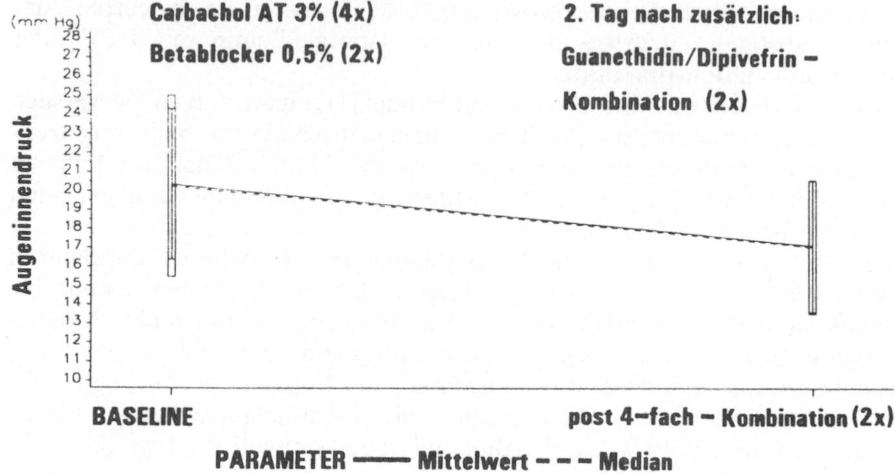

Abb. 1. Mittlere Änderung des Augeninnendrucks (Mittelwert, Median) bei 10 Patienten mit Glaucoma chronicum simplex. Durch die freie Kombination von Carbachol-AT-Lösung 3 % 4× tägl. und Betablocker 0,5 % 2× tägl. war, ausgehend von hohen Augeninnendruckwerten, eine Drucksenkung auf im Mittel 20,5 mmHg (Baseline) möglich. Durch zusätzliche Therapie mit dem Kombinationspräparat aus Guanethidin/DPE konnte am 2. Tag im Mittel eine zusätzliche Augeninnendrucksenkung auf 17 mmHg im Rahmen einer Vier-Komponenten-Therapie erzielt werden

Tabelle 2a. Wirkungsweise der Vier-Komponenten-Therapie bestehend aus einem neuen Kombinationspräparat aus einem direkten Sympatholytikum und einem direkten Parasympathomimetikum mit gleichzeitiger Cholinesterasehemmung (Carbachol/Betaxol-Kombinationspräparat) als Bestandteil einer Vier-Komponenten-Therapie aus zwei Kombinationspräparaten (Kombinationspräparat I und II mit nur 2 Applikationen täglich)

Kombinationspräparat I
- Direktes Sympatholytikum
  Beta-Rezeptorenblocker

- Direktes Parasympatho-
  mimetikum mit gleichzeitiger
  Cholinesteraseemmung
  Carbachol

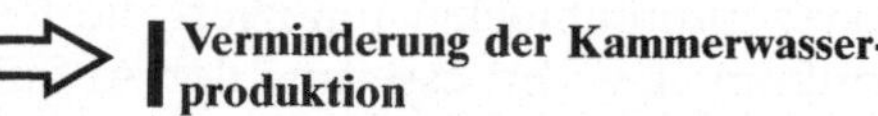 **Verminderung der Kammerwasserproduktion**

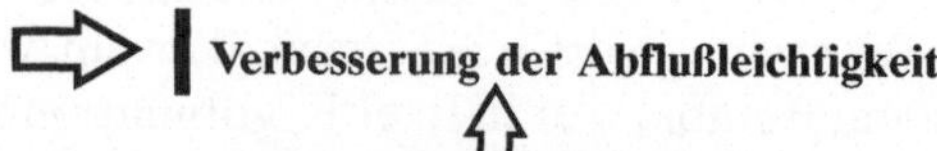 **Verbesserung der Abflußleichtigkeit**

Kombinationspräparat II
- Direktes Sympathomimetikum
  Dipivalylepinephrin (DPE) 0,1 %

- Indirektes Sympatholytikum
  Guanethidin

Guanethidin: Sensibilisierung der adrenergen Rezeptoren infolge pharmakologischer Sympathektomie

Tabelle 2b. Vorgeschlagenes neues Kombinationspräparat aus einem direkten Parasympathomimetikum mit gleichzeitiger Cholinesterasehemmung und einem direkten Sympathomimetikum (Carbachol-DPE-Kombinationspräparat). Durch Überwiegen der Miotikawirkung könnte sich in dieser fixen Kombination auch eine Erweiterung des DPE-Anwendungsbereiches beim Glaucoma chronicum simplex mit engem Kammerwinkel ergeben. Durch die fixe Kombination der Medikamente ist im Gegensatz zur freien Kombination der Monosubstanzen ausgeschlossen, daß der Patient durch fehlerhafte Anwendung nur DPE appliziert und so einen Glaukomanfall auslöst (Applikation 2× täglich). Dargestellt ist das vorgeschlagene Carbachol-DPE-Kombinationspräparat in Kombination mit einem Betablocker (Drei-Komponenten-Therapie)

● Direktes Sympatholytikum
  Beta-Rezeptorenblocker   ⇨ | **Verminderung der Kammerwasserproduktion**

Kombinationspräparat
● Direktes Parasympathomimetikum mit
  gleichzeitiger Cholinesterasehemmung
  Carbachol   ⇨ | **Verbesserung der Abflußleichtigkeit**

● Direktes Sympathomimetikum
  Dipivalylepinephrin (DPE) 0,1 %   ⇨ |

Tabelle 2c. Vorgeschlagenes neues Kombinationspräparat aus einem direkten Sympatholytikum und einem direkten Sympathomimetikum (DPE-Betaxolol-Kombinationspräparat) wobei experimentelle Untersuchungen eine bessere Kompatibilität mit einem Beta-1-selektiven Betablocker vermuten lassen. Ein besonderer Einsatzbereich dieses Kombinationspräparats könnte beim Neovaskularisationsglaukom liegen (Applikation 2× täglich). Dargestellt ist das vorgeschlagene Betaxolol-DPE-Kombinationspräparat in Kombination mit Carbachol (Drei-Komponenten-Therapie)

Kombinationspräparat
● Direktes Sympatholytikum
  Beta-Rezeptorenblocker   ⇨ | **Verminderung der Kammerwasserproduktion**

● Direktes Sympathomimetikum
  Dipivalylepinephrin (DPE) 0,1 %   ⇨ | **Verbesserung der Abflußleichtigkeit**

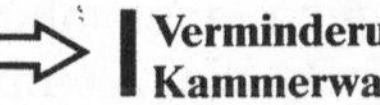

● Direktes Parasympathomimetikum mit gleichzeitiger Cholinesterasehemmung
  Carbachol

nendrucksenkung ergeben. Bei fixer Kombination von Carbachol 3 % und Betaxolol 0,28 %-Suspension ist eine noch ausgeprägtere Drucksenkung bei der Vier-Komponenten-Therapie zu erwarten, als bei freier Kombination der Präparate, wie im folgenden dargelegt wird. Da ein Carbachol-Kombinationspräparat jedoch derzeit noch nicht zur Verfügung steht, wird aus Compliance-Gründen häufig auf die Kombination aus dem bisher verfügbaren fixen Pilocarpin-Betablocker-Kombinationspräparat (Normoglaucon-AT 4× tägl.) und der verfügbaren fixen Kombination aus Guanethidin und DPE (Thilodigon 0,5 % 2× tägl.) ausgewichen. Pilocarpin-Betablocker-Kombinationspräparate haben jedoch den Nachteil, daß sie bei hohen Augeninnendruckwerten meist 4× täglich appliziert werden müssen, wegen der relativ kurzen Wirkungsdauer der Pilocarpinkomponente. Tabelle 2a zeigt die Wirkungsweise der Einzelkomponenten bei der Vier-Komponenten-Therapie. Der Betablocker wirkt über eine Verminderung der Kammerwasserproduktion, während das direkte Parasympathikomimetikum (Carbachol bzw. Pilocarpin), wie auch das direkte Sympathomimetikum (DPE), unterstützt durch Guanethidin, zu einer Verbesserung der Abflußleichtigkeit führt. Guanethidin führt durch pharmakologische Sympathektomie zu einer Sensibilisierung der adrenergen Rezeptoren und – wahrscheinlich auch durch eine zahlenmäßige Vermehrung der adrenergen Rezeptoren – zu einer erheblichen Wirkungsverstärkung des Adrenalinprodrugs DPE [38].

Das im Vergleich zum Adrenalin besser lipidlösliche Prodrug wird erst durch Esterasen in der Hornhaut aktiviert, so daß erst dann nach Aktivierung das freie Adrenalin das Kammerwasser erreicht. DPE wird nicht wie Adrenalin in 1–2 %iger Konzentration angewandt, sondern hat in 0,1 %iger Konzentration bereits dieselbe augeninnendrucksenkende Wirkung bei geringeren lokalen und systemischen Nebenwirkungen. Das vorgeschlagene neue Kombinationspräparat in fixer Kombination aus Betaxolol und Carbachol in Suspensions-Technologie als Betaxolol-S-Carbachol-S-Kombinationspräparat oder in wäßriger Lösung als Betaxolol-Lösung-Carbachol-Lösung-Kombinationspräparat, ist hinsichtlich seiner Beta-1-selektiven Betablocker-Komponente mit DPE oder DPE-Kombinationspräparaten ohne Wirkungsverlust der DPE-Komponente kompatibel. Adrenalin wirkt im wesentlichen über eine Verbesserung der Abflußleichtigkeit (vgl. Tabelle 2a). Bekannte Mechanismen einer medikamentösen Augeninnendrucksenkung können sich so durch die Kombination der 2 Kombinationspräparate addieren, wobei 3 der 4 Komponenten im wesentlichen über eine Verbesserung der Abflußleichtigkeit und die Betablocker-Komponente über eine Verminderung der Kammerwasserproduktion wirkt (vgl. Tabelle 2a). Welches

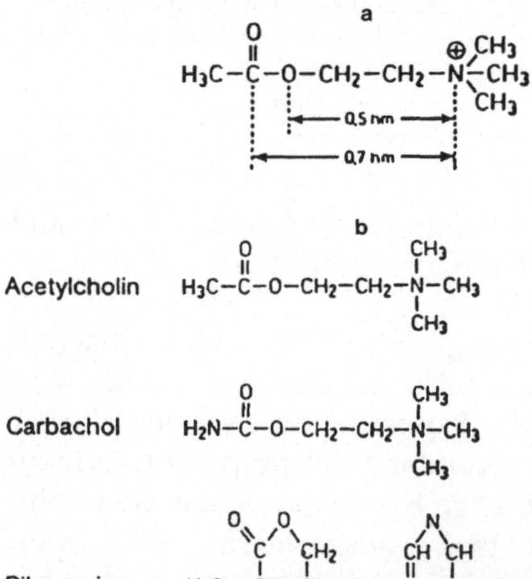

Abb. 2a, b. Chemische Struktur von Acetylcholin, Carbachol und Pilocarpin. Die Abstände der reaktionsfähigen Zentren (a) sind verantwortlich für die Wirkung der Parasympathomimetika. Carbachol, ein synthetisches Cholinderivat, unterscheidet sich vom Acetylcholin nur dadurch, daß die Acetylgruppe durch eine Carbamyl-Gruppe ersetzt ist. Daraus entsteht eine Doppelwirkung: Carbachol wirkt erstens als direktes Parasympathomimetikum und zweitens durch die Carbamyl-Gruppe als Cholinesterasehemmer. Daraus erklärt sich die lange Wirkungsdauer. Diese Doppelwirkung gibt dieser Substanz im Rahmen eines Kombinationspräparats mit nur 2× tägl. Anwendung Vorteile gegenüber anderen Miotika

Miotikum und welcher Betablocker für ein Kombinationspräparat im Rahmen der Vier-Komponenten-Therapie besser geeignet ist, sowie die Logik der Interaktion der 4 Teilkomponenten, vor allem des Betablockers mit Carbachol und mit DPE, soll im folgenden dargestellt werden.

Welches Miotikum ist theoretisch für ein Miotikum-Betablocker-Kombinationspräparat oder für ein DPE-Betablocker-Kombinationspräparat besser geeignet: Pilocarpin oder Carbachol?

Pilocarpin. Pilocarpin ist ein Alkaloid und somit eine schwache organische Base [30]. Es ist kein Ester wie das Carbachol und hat im Gegensatz zu den Cholin-Derivaten keinen quartären Stickstoff (vgl. Abb. 2 b). Die therapeutische Wirkung einer 2 prozentigen Pilocarpin-Lösung tritt nach 45 Minuten ein und kann 4 Stunden anhalten, jedoch nicht länger [3]. Angewandt wird das Hydrochlorid in 0,25 prozentiger bis 4 prozentiger Lösung, das Borat in 0,5 prozentiger bis 2 prozentiger Lösung. Ferner gibt es Anwendungen als ölige Lösung, als Salbe oder Gel zur Erhöhung der Wirkungsdauer. Eine Kombination des Betablockers mit Pilocarpin 2 % Augentropfen erfordert in anbetracht der im Vergleich zu Carbachol kürzeren Wirkungsdauer von Pilocarpin 2 % von ca. 4 Stunden, bisher ein relativ hohes Dosierungsschema mit 4 Applikationen täglich. Bei 4 Applikationen täglich besteht eine größere Gefahr der Allergisierung und durch die Daueranwendung von Pilocarpin auch eine höhere Gefahr der Ausbildung einer Subsensitivität [30] gegenüber Pilocarpin als bei 2× täglicher Applikation des Betablocker-Carbachol-Präparates. Die lokalen Nebenwirkungen, wie akkommodative Myopisierung oder Ziliarspasmen sind konzentrationsabhängig bei Pilocarpin und bei Carbachol möglich.

Carbachol. Eine Kombination von Carbachol mit Betablockern, also die Anwendung eines stärkeren Miotikums hat Vorteile wegen der deutlich erhöhten Wirkungsdauer. Carbachol kann chemisch als Carbamoylester des Cholins angesehen werden und ist durch die Cholinesterase weniger leicht hydrolysierbar als Acetylcholin und damit länger wirksam [3]. Aufgrund der dem Acetylcholin ähnlichen molekularen Struktur wirkt es auf den Rezeptor, wie in Abbildung 2 dargestellt. Bereits die 1,5 % Carbachol-Lösung führt bei Einmalapplikation, wie Abb. 3 zeigt, zu einer über 12 Stunden nahezu konstanten Miosis, wobei die pupillenverengende Wirkung über mehr als 48 Stunden sichtbar ist. Die Dauer der Pupillenverengung ist dabei nicht gleichzusetzen mit der Dauer der Augeninnendrucksenkung, die konzentrationsabhängig ist und nach Untersuchungen von Findall und Drance [12] nur bei Carbachol 3 %-Lösung länger als 8 Stunden anhält (Abb. 4). Bei Carbachol 3 %-Lösung (oder einer unter Suspensionstechnologie bei gleicher Bioverfügbarkeit entsprechend verringerten Konzentration) ist so bei 2× täglicher Applikation mit einer nahezu konstanten Miosis zu rechnen. Es ist denkbar, daß dadurch nach einer gewissen Gewöhnungsphase – vergleich-

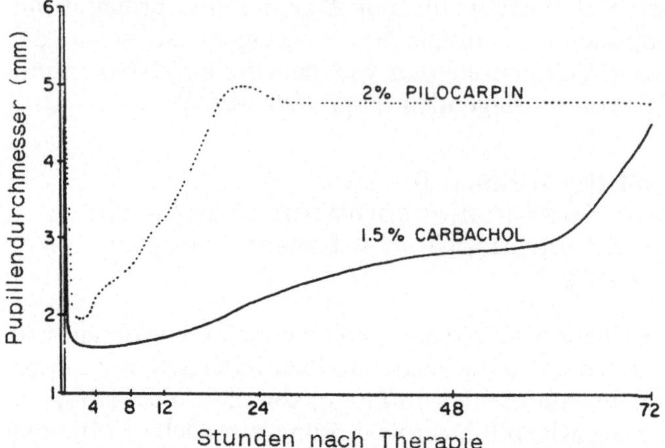

Abb. 3. Mittleres Ausmaß und Dauer der medikamentösen Miosis bei 10 gesunden Erwachsenen nach einer Einzelapplikation von Pilocarpin 2 % und Carbachol-AT 1,5 %. (Nach [37])

bar dem Medikamententräger-System Ocusert – die bei Pilocarpin-Augentropfen bestehenden Miosisschwankungen und die akkommodativen Schwankungen dadurch weitgehend reduziert werden und so dieser visusbeeinträchtigende Nebeneffekt zumindest reduziert ist. Dies würde bei Langzeitanwendung zu einer besseren subjektiven Verträglichkeit mit entsprechend verbesserter Compliance führen. Neben die direkte parasympathische Wirkung tritt bei Carbachol auch eine leichte Hemmung der Cholinesterase, d.h. es verzögert zusätzlich den Abbau von Acetylcholin, wie im folgenden noch dargestellt wird. Im Falle einer Pilocarpin-Allergie läßt sich Carbachol als Austauschmittel einsetzen. Nachteilig ist, daß beim Carbachol wegen seiner hydrophilen Eigenschaften, also seiner schlechten Fettlöslichkeit, das Penetrationsvermögen durch die Cornea herabgesetzt ist.

Erst durch die Verwendung des Konservierungsmittels Benzalkoniumchlorid als oberflächenwirksames Agens (sog. wetting agent) ergibt sich eine resorbierbare Lösung. Durch den Zusatz von Methylcellulose als visköse Trägersubstanz wird eine gewisse Depotwirkung erreicht. Wird Carbachol 3 % zusammen mit Betaxolol 0,28 %-Suspension als fixe Kombination hergestellt, ist eine zusätzliche Verbesserung des Penetrationsvermögens und damit eine höhere Bioverfügbarkeit, auch für Carbachol zu erwarten, da Carbachol an die Suspension gebunden wird, wenn auch in etwas geringerem Ausmaß als bei Betaxolol. Es handelt sich bei der neuen Suspensions-Technologie um eine neuartige Trägersubstanz aus Poly-(Styrol-Divinylbenzol) Sulphonsäure (Amberlite IRP-69) und Carbomer 934 P (56), die dazu führt, daß das Pharmakon aus der Suspension langsam und kontinuierlich abgegeben wird, im Gegensatz zur mehr bolusartigen Wirkung der Lösung. Diese Suspensions-Technologie erlaubte die Konzentration von Betaxolol-Lösung 0,5 % auf Betaxolol-Suspension 0,28 % zu senken, bei identischer

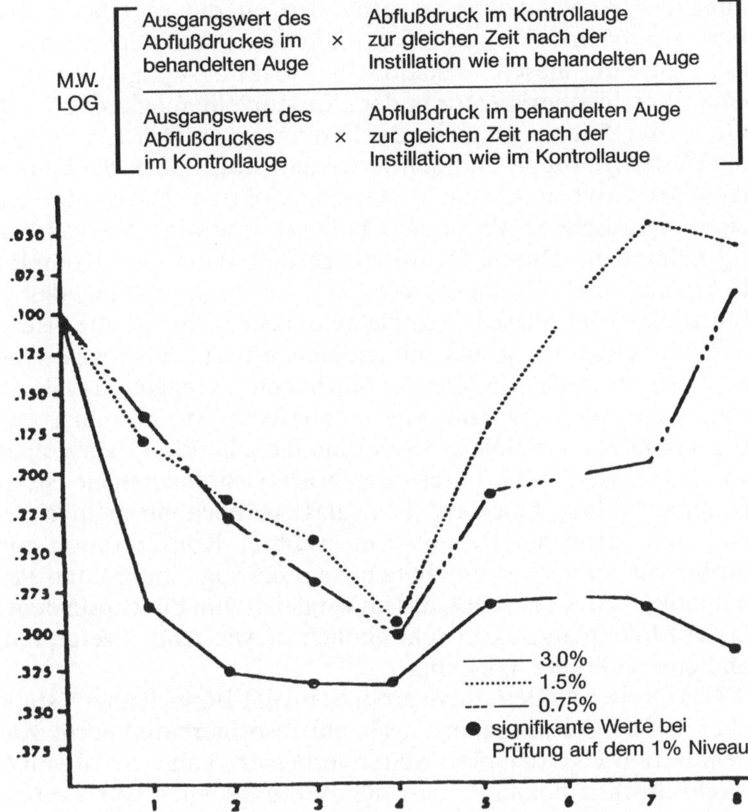

Abb. 4. Konzentrationsabhängige mittlere Wirkung von Carbachol-AT 3 %, 1,5 %, 0,75 % auf den Abflußdruck (IOD −10 mmHg) bei 24 Augen mit erhöhtem Augeninnendruck nach Einmalapplikation in ein Auge. Ein Anstieg im logarithmischem Verhältnis (Kurvenabfall) zeigt eine durch das Präparat bewirkte Senkung des Augeninnendrucks an. Carbachol erreicht die maximale Augeninnendrucksenkung danach im Mittel nach 4 Stunden, wobei die Wirkung konzentrationsabhängig ist und nur Carbachol 3 % länger als 8 Stunden wirkt. (Nach [12])

augeninnendrucksenkender Wirkung, was neben der langsameren Abgabe der Wirksubstanz auch insgesamt durch die Reduzierung der Konzentration für Betaxolol und Carbachol geringere lokale und systemische Nebenwirkungen sowohl für den Betablocker als auch für das Carbachol erwarten läßt bei längerer Wirkungsdauer der fixen Kombination im Vergleich zu den Einzelsubstanzen. Carbachol hat als quartäres Amin gegenüber anderen Miotika den Vorteil, daß es systemisch schlecht resorbiert wird, was die Gefahren zentraler und systemischer Wirkungen reduziert [17]. Mit einer 0,75–1,5 prozentigen Carbachol-Lösung stellt sich ein Maximum der Pupillenverengung nach ca. 4 Stunden ein.

Kurz zum Wirkungsmechanismus des Carbachols: Die spezifische Wirkung des Acetylcholins ist gebunden an die räumliche Zuordnung der Estergruppe und der quartenären Stickstoffbase von 0,7 μm (vgl. Abb. 2 a) [8]. Stoffe mit diesen Abständen der reaktionsfähigen Zentren können mit dem Acetylcholinrezeptor in der Effektorzelle reagieren, der dann mit zwei dieser drei Zentren reagiert. Die Estergruppe teilt sich dabei nochmals auf in die Carbonylgruppe und den Estersauerstoff. Auch die Cholinesterase hat diese spezifischen Abstände reagibler Zentren. Durch eine anionische und eine esteratische Stelle an der Cholinesterase wird Acetylcholin komplexartig gebunden. Durch Hydrolyse zerfällt dann der Komplex in Cholin, Essigsäure und Cholinesterase, was zur Inaktivierung des Acetylcholins führt. Der auf dieses Acetylcholinmuster eingestellte Rezeptor in der Effektorzelle vermag auch mit anderen Stoffen, deren wirksame Zentren die gleichen Abstände wie Acetylcholin haben, zu reagieren (vgl. Abb. 2 b). Eine cholinerge Wirkung tritt ein, wenn diese Stoffe selbst eine erregende Eigenschaft haben. Diese Stoffe sind die „direkten Parasympathikomimetika". Wird die Cholinesterase durch acetylcholinähnliche Stoffe durch eine Komplexbildung blockiert, kann das Acetylcholin nicht abgebaut werden und steht dann am Rezeptor in erhöhter Konzentration zur Verfügung. Stoffe, die diese Wirkung haben, sind die sog. „indirekten Parasymathikomimetika" (8). Carbachol, das im Vergleich zum Pilocarpin dem Acetylcholin in der Molekularstruktur sehr ähnlich ist, wie Abb. 2 zeigt, hat eine direkte und eine indirkete Wirkung.

Das Derivat N-Demethylcarbol ist im pH-Bereich über 7 stabil und liegt zu über 10 % in undissoziierter, als gut resorbierbarer Form vor [3], was die Penetrationseigenschaften weiter verbessern kann. So ist von Carbachol als Monosubstanz bekannt, daß die Wirkungsdauer von Carbachol 3 % der Wirkungsdauer von Pilocarpin-Augensalbe 2 % mit einer Wirkungsdauer von 8–12 Stunden entspricht [9, 12, 43]. Im Ausmaß der Augeninnensenkung entsprechen Carbachol-Augentropfen 3 % nach Untersuchungen von Richardson (43) der Wirkung von Pilocarpin-Augentropfen 8 % [11] (Tabelle 3). In seiner miotischen und augeninnendrucksenkenden Wirkung und in der Wirkungsdauer ist Carbachol somit dem Pilocarpin überlegen [12]. Abbildung 5 zeigt die deutlich erhöhte augeninnendrucksenkende Wirkung von Carbachol 1,5 % (3× täglich) im Vergleich zu Pilocarpin-AT 2 % (4× täglich). Die sich daraus ergebende höhere Drucksenkung und längere Wirkungsdauer wird mit höherer Wahrscheinlichkeit als bei Anwendung von Pilocarpin 2 % eine Reduzierung des Dosierungsschemas auf 2× täglich bei

Tabelle 3. Vergleich der augeninnendrucksenkenden Wirkung von Pilocarpin, Carbachol und Aceclidin nach Untersuchungen von Richardson. (Nach [11])

Pilocarpin	Carbachol	Aceclidin
1 %	0,75 %	
2 %	1,50 %	2 %
4 %	2,25 %	
8 %	3,00 %	

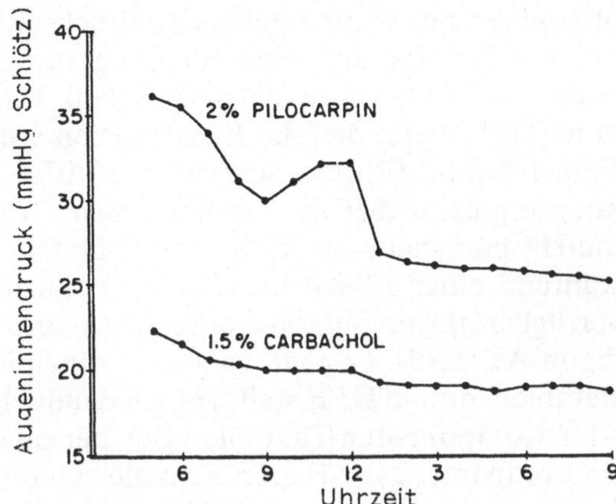

Abb. 5. Mittlere Tagesdruckkurven bei 34 Augen mit Glaucoma chronicum simplex, behandelt mit Pilocarpin-AT 2% (4× tägl.) und mit 1,5% Carbachol-Lösung (3× tägl.). (Nach [39])

Anwendung von Carbachol 3% erlauben. Die nur 2× tägliche Applikation hat neben den genannten Vorteilen (geringere Gefahr der Allergisierung und Subsensitivität) eine weitere Verbesserung der Compliance zur Folge. Das im Vergleich zum Pilocarpin etwas in Vergessenheit geratene Carbachol hat durch seine hohe augeninnendrucksenkende Wirkung und seine lange Wirkungsdauer infolge seiner Doppelwirkung als direktes Parasympathiko-mimetikum und als Cholinesterasehemmer Eigenschaften, die es für die Verwendung als Miotikum bei 2× täglicher Anwendung in einem Kombinationspräparat mit Betaxolol S oder Betaxolol-Lösung oder anderen Substanzen mit 2× täglicher Anwendung, z.B. DPE, empfehlen.

Carbachol 1931 von Kreitmeier synthetisch hergestellt und 1933 durch Velhagen erstmals in der Ophthalmologie angewandt, zeigte wegen seiner hydrophilen Eigenschaften eine schlechte Hornhautpenetration, die erst durch Swan und O'Brien durch Zusatz von Benzalkoniumchlorid als oberflächenaktives Agenz sowie durch Zusatz von Methylcellulose, das zu einer Erhöhung der Hornhautkontaktzeit führte, verbessert werden konnte [9]. Die Anwendung der Suspensions-Technologie auf Carbachol und auf das Carbachol-Betaxolol-Kombinationspräparat im besonderen wird die Bioverfügbarkeit von Carbachol im Auge trotz nur noch 2× täglicher Applikation weiter erhöhen.

Ist für ein Carbachol-Betablocker-Kombinationspräparat oder für ein DPE-Betablocker-Kombinationspräparat jeder Betablocker gleich gut geeignet?

a) Betaxolol-DPE-Wechselwirkung bei Drei- oder Vier-Komponenten-Therapie

Timolol und Carbachol haben eine gesicherte additive augeninnendrucksenkende Wirkung [35], wobei bei Timolol im Gegensatz zu Betaxolol bei gleichzeitiger Gabe von Adrenalin eine Reduktion des drucksenkenden Effektes von Adrenalin um 25% erfolgt [31]. Thomas et al. [49] berichten über einen nur vorübergehenden drucksenkenden Effekt bei der Kombination von Timolol- und Adrenalin-Augentropfen mit vollständigem Verlust des additiven Effekts nach einigen Wochen. Eine prospektive Studie von Parrow et al. [11] zeigte, daß die Kombination von DPE mit einem unspezifischen Beta-1-Beta-2-Blocker auch eine additive augeninnendrucksenkende Wirkung ergibt, wobei die Addition von DPE zu einer IOD-Senkung von 2 mmHg und mehr bei 50 % und 3 mmHg und mehr bei 19 % der Augen während einer 12-Wochen-Therapie führte. Eine Kombination der bisher verfügbaren Kombinationspräparate Normoglaucon-AT 4× tägl. und Thilodigon-AT 0,5 % 2× tägl. ist somit prinzipiell möglich. Die Interaktion von Betablocker und DPE stellt jedoch dennoch einen kritischen Punkt in dieser Vier-Komponenten-Therapie oder bei einem DPE-Betablocker-Kombinationspräparat dar. Experimentelle Untersuchungen von Robinson and Kaufmann [44] zeigen, daß die Abflußverbesserung von Adrenalin im Tierversuch durch unspezifische Betablocker zwar nicht aufgehoben, aber doch reduziert werden kann, wobei Betaxolol, ein Beta-1-spezifischer Blocker [44] diese Wirkung überraschenderweise nicht zeigte. Betaxolol weist ferner weniger pulmonale und kardiale Nebenwirkungen auf [4–7, 10, 47, 48, 55]. Betaxolol wirkt gut augeninnnendrucksenkend, wobei im Vergleich zu Levobunolol oder Timolol über eine schwächere Drucksenkung berichtet wird [33, 53]. Gut kombinierbar ist Betaxolol mit Adrenalin [3]. Denkbar ist, daß der abflußverbessernde Effekt des Adrenalin über Beta-2-Rezeptoren erfolgt und so der die Adrenalinwirkung blockierende Effekt des Beta-1-selektiven Betaxolols geringer ist als bei Beta-1-Beta-2-Blockern. Hinsichtlich der allgemeinen Wirkungen und Nebenwirkungen der verschiedenen Betablocker sei auf eine eigene frühere Übersichtsarbeit verwiesen [13]. Bei der Drei-Komponenten-Therapie des Carbachol-Betablocker-Kombinationspräparates mit DPE oder bei der Vier-Komponenten-Therapie mit dem Kombinationspräparat aus DPE und Guanethidin wäre somit in anbetracht der DPE-Komponente und ihrer besseren Kompatibilität mit einem Beta-1-spezifischen Blocker eine fixe Kombination aus Betaxolol S oder Betaxolol-Lösung mit Carbachol von Vorteil.

Eine optimale Vier-Komponenten-Therapie könnte somit in der Kombination von 2 Kombinations-Präparaten, der fixen Kombination aus Carbachol 3 % und Betaxolol S bzw. Betaxolol-Lösung bei 2× täglicher Applikation und der fixen Kombination aus DPE und Guanethidin bestehen, das morgens zusätzlich 1 × appliziert wird. Der Patient muß also nur noch morgens und abends seine Medikamente anwenden, mit insgesamt nur noch 3 Tropfenapplikationen pro Tag. Unter Verwendung des selektiven Beta-1-Blockers bei Kombination von DPE mit dem Carbachol-Betaxolol-Kombinationspräparat bleibt die Abflußverbesserung durch Adrenalin uneingeschränkt erhalten. Diese bessere Kompatibilität von Betaxolol und DPE [44] und die in fixer Kombination längere Wirkungsdauer des Carbachol-Betaxolol-Kombinationspräparats im Vergleich zur freien Kombination läßt eine weitere Verbesserung der Augeninnendrucksenkung, die dann auch im Rahmen einer Vier-Komponenten-Therapie möglich ist, bei nur 2 Anwendungen täglich erwarten (vergl. Tabelle 2a).

b) Suspensionstechnologie

Bei der neuen Carbachol-Betaxolol-Suspension hat Betaxolol S eine längere Verweildauer auf der Hornhaut und wird dadurch besser resorbiert, so daß die Betablockerkonzentration auf 0,28 % bei gleicher Augeninnendrucksenkung reduziert werden konnte [56]. Wird Betaxolol-Suspension mit Carbachol als fixe Kombination verabreicht, so wird auch Carbachol an den Trägermechanismus der Suspension gebunden und somit auch die Resorption des schwer lipidlöslichen Carbachol durch die Suspensionstechnologie verbessert. Betaxolol selbst hat eine hohe Lipophilie, was wiederum in fixer Kombination mit Carbachol die Penetration für Carbachol erhöhen könnte. Bei der Carbachol-Monosubstanz verbesserte bereits die bisher verwendete visköse Trägersubstanz Methylzellulose als sog. „wetting agent" neben dem Konservierungsmittel Benzalkoniumchlorid, das diesen positiven Nebeneffekt beim Carbachol hat, die Aufnahme des Wirkstoffs ins Auge. Eine höhere Bioverfügbarkeit mit noch längerer Wirkungsdauer des Carbachol 3 % ist daher zusammen mit der Betaxolol-Suspension einmal durch die höhere Penetration und längere Verweildauer auf der Hornhaut als auch durch die geringere intraokulare „turnover"-Rate des Carbachol bei unter Betaxolol reduzierter Kammerwassersekretion möglich. Carbachol 3 % als Monosubstanz entspricht einer Wirkungsdauer von Pilocarpin-AS 2 % und einer drucksenkenden Wirkung von Pilocarpin-AT 8 % [9, 12, 43]. Die längere Wirkungsdauer von Carbachol, die im Kombinationspräparat, insbesondere mit der Betaxolol 0,28 % Suspension noch höher ist, macht eine konstante Augeninnendurcksenkung bei konstanter Pupillenweite auch bei nur zweimaliger Applikation des Kombinationspräparats wahrscheinlich. Die langdauernde konstante Miosis durch Carbachol läßt eine gute subjektive Verträglichkeit, ohne die bei Pilocarpin üblichen Visusschwankungen erwarten. Die langdauernde Miosis des Carbachol sowie die hohe und langdauernde Augeninnendrucksenkung läßt auch eine fixe Kombination mit DPE sinnvoll erscheinen (vergl. Tabelle 1).

Welche Bedeutung hat die 4. Komponente, das Guanethidin?

Guanethidin, das selbst drucksenkend wirkt, führt zusätzlich infolge pharmakologischer Sympathektomie zur Sensibilisierung der adrenergen Rezeptoren [18, 19] und damit zur Wirkungsverstärkung des DPE, das zusammen mit dem selektiven Beta-1-Blocker uneingeschränkt wirkt (vergl. Tabelle 2a). Möglicherweise erlaubt dies dann die Reduzierung der Applikationshäufigkeit des 2. Kombinationspräparates aus DPE und Guanethidin auf 1 × morgens bei der Vier-Komponenten-Therapie oder auf DPE 1 × morgens bei der Drei-Komponenten-Therapie.

Bei einer Einmalapplikation sollte Adrenalin morgens angewandt werden, da Adrenalin die im Schlaf physiologischerweise herabgesetzte Kammerwasserproduktion erhöhen kann [41]. Das Prodrug DPE ist bekanntlich besser lipidlöslich als Adrenalin, so daß mit 0,1 prozentiger Konzentration die gleiche augeninnendrucksenkende Wirkung erreicht wird wie mit Adrenalin-AT 1 % bei geringerer lokaler und systemischer Nebenwirkung [28, 29]. Betaxolol erlaubt die Nutzung der vollen Adrenalinwirkung. Denkbar ist, daß auch das neue Apraclonidin [20, 24], das geringere blutdrucksenkende Nebenwirkungen als Clonidin hat [25] oder Clonidin, additiv eingesetzt werden kann. Deren additive Wirkung zur fixen Carbachol-Betaxolol-Kombination eröffnet weitere Perspektiven einer Kombinationstherapie, ebenso die Kombination der fixen Carbachol-Betaxolol-Kombination mit lokalen Carboanhydrasehemmern [42].

Überraschend hohe Augeninnendrucksenkung

Bei schwer einstellbarem Glaucoma chronicum simplex konnte nach eigenen Untersuchungen bereits durch Kombination der Monopräparate von Carbachol-AT 3 % 4× tägl. und Betablocker 0,5 % 2× tägl. eine mittlere Drucksenkung (Baseline) von 20,5 mmHg im Mittel erreicht werden (vergl. Abb. 1). Durch zusätzliche Gabe des Kombinationspräparates aus DPE/Guanethidin war eine zusätzliche Augeninnendrucksenkung im Mittel von 4 mmHg am 2. Tag nach zusätzlicher Therapie zu erzielen (vgl. Abb. 1). Die überraschend hohe augeninnendrucksenkende Wirkung der Vier-Komponenten-Therapie insgesamt macht ferner zusätzliche Mechanismen wahrscheinlich, welche die Anwesenheit dieser Komponenten erfordern. Die Kombination der 4 Komponenten zeigt eine additive Augeninnendrucksenkung. Durch die Suspensionstechnologie, welche die Penetration des Betablockers und auch des Carbachols verbessert, wird sich, wie für den Betablocker belegt [56], auch die Konzentration des Carbachols um ein noch nicht bekanntes Ausmaß reduzieren lassen, auf eine Dosis, die bei zweimaliger Applikation eine weitgehend konstante Miosis und konstante Augeninnendrucksenkung erlaubt. Die Bereitstellung einer Carbachol-Betaxolol-Suspension und/oder einer Carbachol-Betaxolol-Lösung, die als Bestandteil einer Vier-Komponenten-Therapie einsetzbar ist, erscheint daher sinnvoll. Tabelle 4 faßt die Vorteile der Carbachol-Betablocker-Kombination gegenüber der freien Kombination und gegenüber Pilocarpin-Betablocker-Kombinationspräparaten zusammen (Tabelle 4). Tabelle 5 zeigt die Konservierungsmittel bei vorhandenen Glaukomtherapeutica auf (Tabelle 5a–c), die bei der Kombination von Medikamenten mit berücksichtigt werden sollten, um bei den Medikamenten ein einheitliches Konservierungsmittel zu

Tabelle 4. Kombinationspräparate mit Carbachol und Betablocker, Carbachol und DPE, DPE und Betablocker (Vor- und Nachteile)

1. Carbachol als direktes Parasympathikomimetikum mit gleichzeitiger Cholinesterasehemmung hat eine längere Wirkungsdauer und höhere Augeninnendrucksenkung als z.B. Pilocarpin und damit eine prinzipiell höhere Wahrscheinlichkeit zur Reduzierung der Applikationshäufigkeit auf 2 × täglich bei konstanter Augeninnendrucksenkung.

2. In Kombination mit z.B. einem Betablocker ergibt sich durch eine Verminderung der Kammerwasserproduktion eine geänderte Pharmakokinetik und damit eine längere Bioverfügbarkeit des Carbachols mit höherer Wahrscheinlichkeit einer konstanten Augeninnendrucksenkung bei nur noch 2 × täglicher Applikation.

3. Die Suspensionstechnologie, die auf den Betablocker und auf Carbachol anwendbar ist, ergibt im Kombinationspräparat für beide Substanzen eine bessere Penetration und langsamere Wirkstoffabgabe (Bolus-Charakter der Medikamente entfällt) und damit eine höhere Bioverfügbarkeit mit höherer Wahrscheinlichkeit der konstanten Augeninnendrucksenkung bei nur 2 × täglicher Applikation bei gleichzeitig bestehender Möglichkeit der Reduzierung der Konzentration des Betablockers (von 0,5 % auf 0,28 %) und von Carbachol (von 3 % auf weniger als 3 %) ohne Einschränkung der Wirkungsdauer und Wirkungsstärke.

4. Die Zweimal-Applikation und die bei Anwendung der Suspensionstechnologie geringere Konzentration der Wirkstoffe führt zu geringeren lokalen und systemischen Nebenwirkungen und damit zu einer Verbesserung der Compliance.

5. Die langdauernde pupillenverengende Wirkung von Carbachol ergibt eine nahezu konstante Miosis zwischen den Einzelapplikationen bei 2 × täglicher Applikation.

6. Die 2 × tägliche Applikation führt zu einer Reduzierung der Konservierungsmittelbelastung und damit geringerer Gefahr der Allergisierung und geringerer Gefahr der Ausbildung einer Subsensitivität.

7. Carbachol wäre auch einsetzbar in fixer Kombination mit DPE, wobei durch Überwiegen der Miotikawirkung DPE im Kombinationspräparat auch bei Glaucoma chronicum simplex mit engem Kammerwinkel mit hoher Wahrscheinlichkeit einsetzbar ist und sich so zwei abflußverbessernde Medikamente in einem Kombinationspräparat mit erweitertem Einsatzbereich ergänzen.

8. Die fixe Kombination aus DPE und einem Betablocker (Beta-1-selektiver Betablocker ist hier theoretisch von Vorteil) wäre ein zusätzliches Kombinationspräparat, das insbesondere beim Neovaskularisationsglaukom mit 2 × täglicher Applikation einsetzbar wäre. Diese zusätzlichen Kombinationspräparate (vgl. Tab. 1, unten) würden z.B. bei Auftreten von Nebenwirkungen eine selektive Umstellung von Teilkomponenten erlauben unter Beibehaltung der prinzipiellen Vorteile eines Kombinationspräparats.

9. Kombinationspräparate generell führen durch Reduzierung der Zahl der Medikamentenfläschchen zu einem einfacheren Therapieschema und einer besseren Anpassung des Therapieschemas an den Tagesablauf des Patienten durch Reduzierung der Applikationshäufigkeit (von z.B. Carbachol 3 × täglich und Betablocker 2 × täglich auf 2 × tägliche Applikation des Kombinationspräparats) zur Verbesserung der Compliance. Durch Wegfall des gegenseitigen Auswascheffekts bei Einzelapplikation und durch Änderung der Pharmakokinetik lassen Kombinationspräparate im allgemeinen eine höhere Wirkungsdauer und stärkere Drucksenkung als die freie Kombination der Einzelsubstanzen erwarten.

10. Carbachol hat wie andere starke Miotika den Nachteil der Myopisierung und des möglichen Auftretens eines Akkommodationsspasmus, so daß ein carbacholhaltiges Kombinationspräparat von jungen Patienten im allgemeinen nicht vertragen wird, insbesondere wenn keine Eingewöhnung durch Vorbehandlung mit z.B. Pilocarpin-Präparaten erfolgte.
Carbachol kann auch bei Allergisierung auf Pilocarpin als Ersatzpräparat verwendet werden. Der *Indikationsbereich* der Kombinationspräparate liegt jedoch in anbetracht der mit zunehmendem Alter größeren Häufigkeit des Glaukoms und schwereren Einstellbarkeit des Glaukoms mit Monopräparaten häufig bei Patienten mit höherem Alter oder bei hyperopen Patienten mit engem Kammerwinkel, bei denen Miotika besser toleriert werden. Die vorgeschlagenen drei neuen Kombinationspräparate können die „Stufenleiter" der medikamentösen Therapie verlängern, wozu in anbetracht der steigenden Lebenserwartung der Bevölkerung eine ethische Notwendigkeit besteht.

wählen. Nach Vorliegen der neuen Kombinationspräparate sind prospektive Studien zur Höhe der Augeninnendrucksenkung bei nur 2× täglicher Applikation, z. B. mit dem Carbachol-Betaxolol-Kombinationspräparat erforderlich [16]. Da die Compliance [34] so wichtig ist wie die Wirksamkeit des Medikaments, liegt in dem einfachen Therapieschema mit nur 2× täglicher Anwendung des im Vergleich zu Pilocarpinpräparten stärker und länger drucksenkenden Carbachol-Präparates ein wesentlicher Vorteil gegenüber bisherigen freien Medikamentenkombinationen. Die Logik der Interaktion der 3 Wirkstoffe Carbachol, Betaxolol und DPE, das erforderlichenfalls als DPE-Guanethidin-Kombinationspräparat verabreicht werden kann, läßt die vorgeschlagenen 3 neuen Kombinationspräparate sinnvoll erscheinen. Diese sind dann compliancegerecht einzeln, als Drei- oder Vierkomponententherapie einsetzbar.

Medikamente und ihre Konservierungsmittel in der Glaukomtherapie (Tab. 5a—c)

Tabelle 5a. Konservierungsmittel in Betablockern und Betablocker-Kombinationspräparaten

Handelsname	Substanzen	Konservierungsmittel
Arteoptic 1 %, 2 %	Carteolol-HCl	Benzalkoniumchlorid
Betamann 0,1 %, 0,3 %, 0,6 %	Metipranolol-HCl	Benzalkoniumchlorid
Betamann-EDO 0,3 %	Metipranolol-HCl	keine
Betoptima	Betaxolol-HCl	Benzalkoniumchlorid
Chibro-Timoptol 0,1 %, 0,25 %, 0,5 %	Timololhydrogenmaleat	Benzalkoniumchlorid
Dispatim 0,1 %, 0,25 %, 0,5 %	Timololhydrogenmaleat	Benzalkoniumchlorid
Durapindol 0,5 %, 1,0 %	Pindolol	Benzalkoniumchlorid
Glauconex 0,25 %, 0,5 %	Befunolol-HCl	Benzalkoniumchlorid
Glauco-Visken	Pindolol	Benzalkoniumchlorid
Ophtorenin 0,05 %, 0,1 %, 0,25 %, 0,5 %	Bupranolol	keine
Pindoptan 0,5 %, 1,0 %	Pindolol	Benzalkoniumchlorid
Thimohexal 0,1 %, 0,25 %, 0,5 %	Timololhydrogenmaleat	Benzalkoniumchlorid
Timosine (0,5 %)	Timololhydrogenmaleat	keine
Timosine mite (0,25 %)		keine
VistaganLiquifilm 0,5 %	Levobunolol-HCl	Benzalkoniumchlorid, Edetinsäure, Dinatriumsalz, Polyvinylalkohol
Kombinationspräparat Normoglaucon	Pilocarpin-HCl Metipranolol	Benzalkoniumchlorid

Tabelle 5b. Konservierungsmittel in Sympathikomimetika und Sympathikomimetika-Kombinationspräparten

Handelsname	Substanzen	Konservierungsmittel
d Epifrin 0,1 %	Dipivefrin-HCI	Benzalkoniumchlorid, Natriumdisulfit, Edetinsäure, Dinatriumsalz
Epiglaufrin 1 %, 2 %	Epinephrin	Edetinsäure, Dinatriumsalz, Benzalkoniumchlorid, Natriumdisulfit
Glaucothil 0,1 %	Dipivefrin-HCI	Benzalkoniumchlorid, Natriumdisulfit, Edetinsäure, Dinatriumsalz
Isoglaucon 1/8 %, 1/4 %, 1/2 %	Clonidin-HCI	Benzalkoniumchlorid
Links-Glaukosan	Epinephrinhydrogentartrat Adrenalon-HCI	Methyl-4-Hydroxybenzoat
Kombinationspräparate Glaucadrin	Aceclidin-HCI, Epinephrin	Benzalkoniumchlorid Natriumdisulfit
Piladren 1 %, 2 %, 4 %	Pilocarpin, Epinephrin	8-Chinolinsulfat, Edetinsäure, Dinatriumsalz, Borsäurelösung
Suprexon/Suprexon forte	Guanethidinsulfat Epinephrin	Benzalkoniumchlorid
Thiloadren	Dipivefrin-HCI Pilocarpin-HCI	Thiomersal, Natriumdisulfit, Edetinsäure, Dinatriumsalz
Thilodigon 0,5 %	Guanethidinsulfat Dipivefrin-HCI	Benzalkoniumchlorid, Edetinsäure, Dinatriumsalz

Das *DPE-Betaxolol-Kombinationspräparat* ist nur bei Glaukomen mit weitem Kammerwinkel anwendbar. Beim hämorrhagischen Glaukom z.B. erscheint seine nur 2× tägliche Anwendung besonders sinnvoll. Im Rahmen einer Dreikomponententherapie ist es mit allen Miotika, z.B. mit Ocusert oder Aceclidin bei jungen myopen Patienten oder bei Pigmentglaukom einsetzbar (vergl. Abb. 2c).

Das *Carbachol-DPE-Kombinationspräparat* ist durch die langdauernde, überwiegende Miosis der Carbacholkomponente mit hoher Wahrscheinlichkeit auch bei Glaukomen mit engem Kammerwinkel einsetzbar bei einer 2× täglichen Applikation. In fixer Kombination ergäbe sich damit eine Erweiterung des Indikationsbereiches für DPE, ohne daß eine periphere Iridektomie zur Anfallsprophylaxe ausgeführt werden müßte. Das bisherige Pilocarpin-DPE-Kombinationspräparat (Thiloadren) muß wegen der im Vergleich zum DPE kürzeren Wirkungsdauer der Pilocarpinkomponente 3 oder 4× täglich appliziert werden und ist nur bei Glaukomen mit weitem Kammerwinkel einsetzbar.

Im Rahmen einer Dreikomponententherapie ist das Carbachol-DPE-kom-

Tabelle 5c. Konservierungsmittel in Parasympathikomimetika und Parasympathikomimetika – Kombinationspräparaten

Handelsname	Substanzen	Konservierungsmittel
Borocarpin 0,5 %, 1 %, 2 %	Pilocarpinborat Naphazolin-HCI	Chlorobutanol
Borocarpin-N 0,5 %, 1 %, 2 %	Pilocarpinborat Pilocarpin-HCI Naphazolin-HCI	Chlorobutanol
Carbamann 1 %, 2 %, 3 %	Carbachol	Benzalkoniumchlorid
Chibro-Pilocarpin 1 %, 2 %	Pilocarpinnitrat	Benzododeciniumbramid
Glaucotat	Aceclidin-HCI	Benzalkoniumchlorid
Isopto-Carbachol 0,75 %, 1,5 %, 2,25 %, 3 %	Carbachol	Benzalkoniumchlorid
Isopto-Pilocarpin 0,5 %, 1 %, 2 %, 3 %, 4 %	Pilocarpin-HCI	Benzalkoniumchlorid
Miopos-POS schwach AS	Pilocarpinnitrat	
Pilocarpin 3 %	Pilocarpin-HCI	Benzalkoniumchlorid
Pilocarpol 1 %, 2 %	Pilocarpin	Cetalkoniumchlorid
Pilogel	Pilocarpin-HCI	Benzalkoniumchlorid
Pilomann 0,5 %, 1 %, 2 %, 3 %	Pilocarpin-HCI	Cetrimoniumchlorid
Pilomann-Öl 2 %	Pilocarpin	Chlorobutanol
Pilopos 0,5 %, 1 %, 2 %, 3 %	Pilocarpinnitrat	Benzalkoniumchlorid
Spersacarpin AS 1 %, 2 %, 3 %	Pilocarpin-HCI	Benzalkoniumchlorid
Thilo-Carpin 0,5 %, 1 %, 2 %	Pilocarpinborat	Thiamersal
Vistacarpin N 0,5 %, 1 %, 2 %, 3 %	Pilocarpin-HCI	Benzalkoniumchlorid
Indirekte Parasympathikomimetika Phospholinjodid	Ecothiopatiodid	Chlorobutanol
Kombinationspräparate Glaucadrin	Aceclidin-HCI Epinephrin	Benzalkoniumchlorid
Isopto-Pilomin	Pilocarpin-HCI Physostigminsalicylat	Chlorobutanol
Miopos-POS – stark AS	Pilocarpinitrat Physostigminsalicylat	
Normoglaucon	Pilocarpin-HCI Metipranolol-HCI	Benzalkoniumchlorid
Piladren 1 %, 2 %, 4 %	Pilocarpin Epinephrin	8-Chinololinsulfat, Editin- säure, Dinatriumsalz, Borsäurelösung
Pilo/Eserin (ölig)	Pilocarpin Physostiamin	Chlorobutanol
Pilo-Eserin Dispersa AT und AS	Pilocarpin-HCI Physostigminsalicylat	Dofamiumchlorid
Piloserin/Piloserin forte	Pilocarpin-HCI Physostigminsulfat	Benzalkoniumchlorid
Syncarpin-AT	Pilocarpinborat Neostigminbramid Naphazolin-HCI	Chlorobutanol
Syncarpin AS	siehe oben	Cetalkoniumchlorid
Thiloadren	Dipivefrin-HCI Pilocarpin-HCI	Thiamersal, Natrium- disulfit Editinsäure, Dinatriumsalz

binationspräparat z. B. mit Clonidin oder mit Betablockern kombinierbar, was dann die selektive Wahl der Betablockerkonzentration oder die Anwendung konservierungsmittelfreier Betablocker erlaubt (vergl. Abb. 2c).

Das *Carbachol-Betaxolol-Kombinationspräparat* ist auch bei Glaukomen mit engem Kammerwinkel anwendbar bei nur 2× täglicher Applikation. Im Rahmen einer Dreikomponententherapie ist es z. B. mit DPE oder als Vierkomponententherapie mit dem DPE/Guanethidin-Kombinationspräparat kombinierbar bei nur 2 Applikationen täglich (vergl. Tabelle 2a).

Sollte sich selbst mit einer Vier-Komponenten-Therapie keine ausreichende Drucksenkung ergeben, so ist ohne Zeitverzögerung und unter Verzicht auf die Argon-Laser-Therapie des Trabekelmaschenwerks die Ausführung einer filtrierenden Operation unumgänglich.

Die vorgeschlagenen drei neuen Kombinationspräparate können die „Stufenleiter" einer auch unter Compliance-Gesichtspunkten vertretbaren medikamentösen Glaukomtherapie verlängern und verbessern und sind in anbetracht der steigenden Lebenserwartung der Bevölkerung eine medizinische und ethische Notwendigkeit.

Literatur

1. Abramovsky I, Mindel JS (1979) Dipivefrin and echothiophate: contraindications to combined use. Arch Ophthal 97: 1937–1940
2. Airaksinen PJ, Valkonen R, Stenborg T, et al (1987) A double-masked study of timolol and pilocarpine. Am J Ophthal 104: 587–590
3. Allen RC, Epstein DL (1986) Additive effect of betaxolol and epinephrine in primary open angle glaucoma. Arch Ophthal 104: 1178–1184
4. Atkins JM, Pugh BR Jr, Timewell RM (1985) Cardiovascular effects of topical beta-blockers during exercise. Am J Ophthal 99: 173
5. Berry DP Jr, Van Buskirk EM, Shields MB (1984) Betaxolol and timolol. A comparison of efficacy and side effects. Arch Ophthal 102: 42
6. Brooks AMV, Gillies WE, West RH (1987) Betaxolol eye drops as a safe medication to lower intraocular pressure. Aust NZ J Ophthal 15: 125–129
7. Van Buskirk EM, Weinreb RN, Berry DP, Lustgarten JS, Podos SM, Berry MM (1986) Betaxolol in patients with glaucoma and asthma. Am J Ophthal 101:531
8. Dolder R, Skinner FS (Hrsg) (1983) Ophthalmika – Pharamkologie, Biopharmazie und Galenik der Augenarzneimittel. Wissenschaftliche Verlagsgesellschaft mbH, Stuttgart, S 110
9. Drance SM (1970) Use of cholinergic agents in the management of chronic simple glaucoma. In: Transactions of the New Orleans Academy of Ophthalmology, 18th meeting, Symposium on ocular pharmacology and therapeutics. Mosby, St. Louis, p 113
10. Dunn TL, Gerber MJ, Shen AS, Fernandez E, Iseman MD, Cherniak RM (1986) The effect of topical ophthalmic installation of timolol and betaxolol on lung function in asthmatic subjects. Am Rev Respir Dis 133: 264
11. Fechner PU, Teichmann KD (1982) Medikamentöse Augentherapie. Bücherei des Augenarztes 67. Enke, Stuttgart
12. Flindall RJ, Drance SM (1966) Dose response of intra-ocular pressure to carbaminoyl-choline chloride. Canad J Ophthal 1: 292
13. Gramer E (1987) Zur Betablocker-Therapie des Glaukoms. Biomedizinische Forschungsgesellschaft der Österreichischen Akademie der Wissenschaften, Grosdanoff P, Kaindl F, Kraupp O, Lehnert T, Lichtlen P, Schuster J, Siegenthaler W (Hrsg) de Gruyter, Berlin New York, S 319–338

14. Gramer E, Althaus G (1988) Zur Progredienz des glaukomatösen Gesichtsfeldschadens. Eine klinische Studie mit Programm Delta des Octopus-Perimeters 201 zum Einfluß des Vorschadens auf die Gesichtsfeldverschlechterung beim Glaucoma chronicum simplex. Fortschr Ophthal 85: 620–625
15. Gramer E, Althaus G (1990) Bedeutung des erhöhten Augeninnendrucks für den Gesichtsfeldschaden. Eine klinische Studie. Klin Mbl Augenheilk 197: 218–224
16. Gramer E (1992) Zur Beurteilung des Therapieeffektes bei Glaukom. In: G. K. Krieglstein (Hrsg.) Glaukom, Verlag ad manum medici, München, S. 39–64
17. Havener WH (1970) Ocular pharmacology. 2. Aufl. Mosby, St. Louis
18. Heilmann K (1983) Das Verhalten des intraokularen Drucks während einer Langzeitbehandlung mit der Kombination Guanethidin-Adrenalin. Klin Mbl Augenheilkd 183: 17–21
19. Hitchings RA, Glover D (1982) Adrenaline 1 % combined with guanethidine 1 % versus adrenaline 1 %: a randomised prosepective double-blind cross-over study. Brit Ophthal 66: 247–249
20. Hill RA, Minckler DS, Lee M, Heuer DK, Baerveldt G, Martone JF Medical management of cycloplegic-induced intraocular pressure spikes. In: Gramer E, Kampik A (1992) (Hrsg), Pharmakotherapie am Auge, Springer-Verlag Heidelberg; pp 116–120
21. Hoyng Ph FJ, Dake Cl (1979) The combination of guanethidine 3 % and adrenaline 0.5 % in 1 eyedrop (GA) in glaucoma treatment. Brit Ophthal 63: 56–62
22. Kass MA, et al (1979) Dipivefrin and Epinephrine treatment of elevated intraocular pressure. A comparative Study. Arch Ophthal Vol 97: 1865–1866
23. Kass MA (1983) Eficacy of combining timolol with other antiglaucoma medications. Surv. Ophthal. (Suppl.) 28: 274–279
24. Kitazawa Y, Sugiyama K, Taniguchi T, Inoue T (1992) Apraclonidine hydrochloride therapy for glaucoma laser surgery. In: Gramer E, Kampik A (Hrsg), Pharmakotherapie am Auge, Springer-Verlag Heidelberg; pp 111–115
25. Krieglstein GK, Gramer E (1978) The response of ophthalmic arteriel pressure to topically applied clonidine. A. v. Graefe's Arch Clin Exp Ophthalmol 207: 1–5
26. Krieglstein GK (1979) Response of the intraocular pressure to various ß-blocking agents. In: GK Krieglstein, W Leydhecker (Hrsg) Glaucoma Update, 179–186 Springer-Verlag, Berlin–Heidelberg–New York
27. Krieglstein GK, Leydhecker W (1979) Die augendrucksenkende Wirkung von Pilocarpin und Adrenalin-Dipivalat bei Glaucoma chronicum simplex: Eine kontrollierte klinische Studie. Klin Mbl Augenheilkd 175: 86–90
28. Krieglstein GK, Gramer E (1983) Allgemeine Nebenwirkungen augenärztlicher Medikamente. Intern. Praxis 23: 755–760
29. Krieglstein GK 1984 The uses and side effects of adrenergic drugs in the management of intraocular pressure. In: SM Drance, A Neufeld (Hrsg) Applied pharmacology in the medical treatment of glaucomas, 255–276, Grune & Stratton New York
30. Kreiglstein GK (1990) Perspektiven der cholinergen Glaukomtherapie. In. E Gramer (Hrsg) Glaukom – Diagnostik und Therapie, 146–148, Ferdinand-Enke-Verlag Stuttgart
31. Langham ME, Kitazawa Y, Hart RW (1971) Adrenergic responses in the human eye. J Pharmacol Exp Ther 179: 47
32. Lesar TS (1987) Comparison of ophthalmic betablocking agents. Clin. Pharm. 6: 451
33. Long DA, Johns GE, Mullen RS, et al (1988) Levobunolol and betaxolol – a double-masked controlled comparison of efficacy and safety in patients with elevated intraocular pressure. Ophthalmology 95: 735–741
34. Noack E (1991) Patienten-Compliance bei langdauernder Glaukomtherapie. Z Prakt Augenheilk 12: 223–228
35. Merkle W (1981) Timolol in Kombination mit anderen Antiglaucomatosa. Klin Mbl Augenheilkd 178: 50–54

36. Mindel JS, Yablonski ME, Tavitian HO, et al (1981) Dipivefrin and echothiophate. Efficacy of combined use in human beings. Arch Ophthal 99: 1583–1586
37. Ober M, Scharrer A (1986) Erfahrungen über Wirksamkeit und Verträglichkeit von Guanethidin/Dipivefrin-AT bei der Behandlung des erhöhten Augeninnendrucks. Klin Mbl Augenheilkd 188: 64–66
38. Ober M, Scharrer A, Dausch D (1987) Guanethidin/Dipivefrin und Pilocarpin bei der Behandlung des erhöhten intraokularen Drucks. Klin Mbl Augenheilkd 190: 103–104
39. O'Brien CS, Swan KC (1942) Carbaminoylcholine chloride in the treatment of glaucoma simplex. Arch Ophthalmol 27: 253
40. Parrow KA et al (1989) Is it worthwhile to add Dipivefrin HCL 01, % to topical β_1-, β_2-blocker therapy? Ophthalmology, Vol. 96, Nr. 9, 1338–1341
41. Pfeiffer N, Grehn F (1988) Augendrucksenkung durch Kombination von Timolol mit Adrenergika. Fortschr Ophthal 85: 456–458
42. Pfeiffer N, Greve E, Béchetoille A, Lippa E, Jaquet-Müller F, Gerling J. Grehn F (1990) Additive Wirkung von Timolol und dem lokalen Carboanhydrasehemmer MK-417. Vortrag bei der DOG Baden-Baden
43. Richardson KT (1973) Cellular response to drugs affecting aqueos dynamics. Arch Ophthal 89: 65–84
44. Robinson JC, Kaufmann PL (1990) Effects and interactions of epinephrine, norepinephrine, timolol, and betaxolol on outflow facility in the cynomolgus monkey. Am J Ophthal 109: 189–194
45. Sears ML (1984) Pharmacology of the eye. Springer-Verlag Berlin–Heidelberg-New York-Tokyo
46. Scharrer A, Ober M (1986) Metipranolol 0,1 % und Pilocarpin 2 % als fixe Kombination im Vergleich zu den Monosubstanzen in der Behandlung des Glaukoms. Klin Mbl Augenheilkd 189: 450–455
47. Schoene RB, Abuan T, Ward RL, Beasley CH (1984) Effects of topical betaxolol, timolol, and placebo on pulmonary function in asthmatic bronchitis. Am J Ophthal 97: 86
48. Stewart RH, Kimbrough RL, Ward RL (1986) Betaxolol versus timolol. A six-month double-blind comparsion. Arch Ophthal 104: 46
49. Thomas JV, Epstein DL (1981) Timolol and epinephrine in primary open angle glaucoma. Transient additive effects. Arch. Ophthal 99: 91–95
50. Topper JE, Brubaker RF (1985) Effects of timolol, epinephrine and acetazolamide on aqueos flow during sleep. Invest. Ophthal Vis Sci 26: 1315–1319
51. Tsoy EA, Meekins BB, Shields MB (1986) Comparison of two treatment schedules for combined timolol and Dipivefrin therapy. Am J Ophthal 102: 320–324
52. Urner-Bloch U, Aeschlimann JE, Gloor BP (1980) Treatment of chronic simple glaucoma with adrenaline/guanethidine combination at three different dosages (comparative double blind study). A. v. Graefe's Arch Klin Exp Ophthal 213: 175–185
53. Vogel R, et al (1989) Changing therapy from timolol to betaxolol. Arch Ophthal 107: 1303
54. Weinreb RN, Ritch R, Kushner FH (1986) Effect of adding betaxolol to dipivefrin therapy. Am J Ophthal 101: 196–198
55. Weinreb RN, Van Buskirk EM, Cherniack R, Drake MM (1988) Long-term betaxolol therapy in glaucoma patients with pulmonary disease. Am J Ophthal 106: 162–167
56. Weinreb RN et al (1990) A double-masked three-month comparison between 0,25 % betaxolol suspension and 0,5 % betaxolol ophthalmic solution. Am J Ophthal 110: 189–192

Korrespondenzadresse

Professor Dr. med. Dr. jur. Eugen Gramer
Universitätsaugenklinik Würzburg, Josef-Schneider-Straße 11, D-8700 Würzburg

Das nasale Gesichtsfeld bei Glaukom

Eine klinische Studie zur glaukomspezifischen Perimetrie

E. Gramer und M. Knaut-Spaeth

Zusammenfassung

Ob die Glaukomtherapie individuell ein ausreichendes therapeutisches Augeninnendruckniveau erreicht hat, kann nur retrospektiv geprüft werden, wenn eine Progredienz des Gesichtsfeldausfalls ausgeschlossen ist. Ein glaukomspezifisches computerperimetrisches Untersuchungsprogramm ist daher Voraussetzung für eine adäquate Therapiebeurteilung. In wie weit das nasale periphere Gesichtsfeld dazu computerperimetrisch geprüft werden sollte, wird untersucht.

70 Augen von 70 Patienten mit Glaukom ohne Hochdruck, Glaucoma chronicum simplex und Pigmentglaukom der Stadien I und II nach Aulhorn wurden mit dem Programm G1 des Octopus Perimeters 201 unter der Fragestellung untersucht, wie häufig nasale Gesichtsfeldausfälle im zentralen und peripheren Gesichtsfeld vorliegen:

1. 56 von 70 Augen (80 %) zeigten parazentrale Skotome und gleichzeitig Gesichtsfeldausfälle im Bereich des nasalen Sprungs zwischen 2° und 56° Exzentrizität.
2. 4 von 70 Augen (5,7 %) zeigten isolierte nasale Skotome außerhalb 26° Exzentrizität. Bei ausschließlicher Untersuchung des zentralen Gesichtsfeldes werden bei 5,7 % der Glaukompatienten (Glaukomstadium I und II) die Gesichtsfeldausfälle nicht aufgedeckt. Eine Perimetrie der peripheren nasalen Gesichtsfelder mit der schwellenbestimmenden Untersuchungsmethode (Normalversion) ist erforderlich.
3. Ein neues glaukomspezifisches Untersuchungsprogramm (GG-Programm) wird vorgestellt, welches das zentrale Gesichtsfeld mit 115 Prüfpunkten und auch das periphere nasale Gesichtsfeld mit 18 Prüfpunkten bei glaukomspezifischer Prüfpunktanordnung schwellenbestimmend untersucht.

Das Ziel der Glaukomtherapie liegt in der Senkung des Augeninnendrucks auf ein Druckniveau das einen Erhalt des Gesichtsfeldes sichert.

Ob die Glaukomtherapie individuell ein ausreichendes therapeutisches Augeninnendruckniveau erreicht hat, kann nur retrospektiv geprüft werden,

Gramer/Kampik (Hrsg.) Pharmakotherapie am Auge
© Springer-Verlag Berlin Heidelberg 1992

wenn eine Progredienz des Gesichtsfeldausfalls ausgeschlossen ist. Ein glaukomspezifisches computerperimetrisches Untersuchungsprogramm ist daher Voraussetzung für eine adäquate Therapiebeurteilung. In wie weit das nasale periphere Gesichtsfeld dazu computerperimetrisch geprüft werden sollte, wird derzeit noch unterschiedlich beurteilt.

Bereits im Jahr 1909 beschrieb Rönne [67] den sogenannten nasalen Sprung im Gesichtsfeld als einen glaukomspezifischen Gesichtsfeldausfall. Auch in den Anfangsstadien gehen die glaukomatösen parazentralen Gesichtsfeldausfälle [31, 50] oft mit nasalen Skotomen im Bereich des zentralen und nasalen peripheren Sprungs einher und sind mit automatisierter statischer Rasterperimetrie heute besser erfaßbar [1, 4–8, 11–17, 20, 21, 25, 30, 32–45, 48, 49, 52–55, 57–61, 63, 65, 67–69, 71–77].

Für die weitere Entwicklung geeigneter computerperimetrischer glaukomspezifischer Untersuchungsprogramme ist es wichtig zu wissen, wie häufig bei Glaukom im Stadium I und II isoliert ein zentraler und wie häufig isoliert ein peripherer nasaler Gesichtsfeldausfall auftritt, und wie häufig nasale zentrale und nasale periphere Gesichtsfeldausfälle gleichzeitig mit parazentralen Gesichtsfeldausfällen vorkommen.

Ziel der Studie ist es daher, die Häufigkeit nasaler glaukomatöser Gesichtsfeldausfälle im zentralen und peripheren Gesichtsfeld mittels automatisierter Rasterperimetrie erneut zu untersuchen. Drei Fragestellungen (I.–III.) wurden untersucht:

I. Häufigkeit der Lage parazentraler und peripherer Skotome bei Glaukom

1. Wie häufig liegen bei Glaukom isolierte nasale Gesichtsfeldausfälle im peripheren Gesichtsfeld ausschließlich außerhalb 26° Exzentrizität vor? Diese isolierten Skotome würden bei ausschließlicher Untersuchung des zentralen Gesichtsfeldes dann nicht aufgedeckt werden.
2. Wie häufig liegen isolierte parazentrale Skotome bei Glaukom vor?
3. Wie häufig liegen parazentrale Gesichtsfeldausfälle in Kombination mit nasalen zentralen und/oder nasalen peripheren Gesichtsfeldausfällen vor? Ein häufiges gleichzeitiges Vorliegen nasaler peripherer und parazentraler Skotome würde eine in Rasterdichte und Prüfmethode gleichwertige Untersuchung des zentralen und peripheren nasalen Gesichtsfeldes indizieren, da eine sensitive Skotomsuche an gleichzeitig beiden Prädilektionsorten in einem Untersuchungsprogramm dann die Sensitivität der perimetrischen Untersuchung erhöhen würde.

II. Häufigkeit der Lage parazentraler und peripherer Skotome bei Glaukom ohne Hochdruck, Glaucoma chronicum simplex und Pigmentglaukom

Wie häufig liegen, getrennt für die verschiedenen Glaukomformen:

1. isolierte nasale Gesichtsfeldausfälle,
2. isolierte parazentrale Skotome und
3. parazentrale Gesichtsfeldausfälle in Kombination mit nasalen zentralen und/oder nasalen peripheren Gesichtsfeldausfällen vor?

III. Welche Anforderungen an Rasterdichte und Prüfmethode sind an ein glaukomspezifisches Prüfpunktraster zu stellen?

Ein neues glaukomspezifisches Untersuchungsprogramm (GG-Programm) wird vorgestellt.

Methode. 70 Augen von 70 Patienten mit glaukomatösen Gesichtsfeldausfällen bis Stadium II, davon 46 Patienten mit Glaucoma chronicum simplex, 11 Patienten mit Glaukom ohne Hochdruck und 13 Patienten mit Pigmentglaukom, die in früheren Untersuchungen mit dem Programm 31 des Octopus Perimeters 201 reproduzierbar zentrale Gesichtsfeldausfälle (Stadium I und II nach Aulhorn) aufwiesen, wurden mit dem Programm G1 des Octopus Perimeters 201 erneut untersucht, da bei diesem Programm gleichzeitig auch das periphere Gesichtsfeld, allerdings mit dem 2-Niveau-Test, geprüft wird [30, 45].

Einschlußkriterien: Alle Augen wiesen einen Fernvisus von 0,8 und besser, keine ausgeprägte Trübung der brechenden Medien und keine andere Erkrankung als Glaukom auf. Alle Augen zeigten eine maximale Ametropie von +/− 3 Dioptrien zum weitgehenden Ausschluß refraktionsbedingter Befundabweichungen. Untersucht wurden Patienten aller Altersgruppen; das mittlere Alter lag bei 47+/−3 Jahren.

Programm G1: Abbildung 1 zeigt die Prüfpunktanordnung des Programms G1. 59 Prüfpunkte liegen innerhalb 26° Exzentrizität mit einem nach zentral hin verdichteten Prüfpunktraster. Diese Prüfpunkte werden zweimal eingabeInd schwellenbestimmend untersucht um unter anderem daraus den CLV-Wert [30, 35] zu berechnen. 14 periphere Prüfpunkte liegen zwischen 34° und 56° Exzentrizität und werden mit dem sogenannten Zwei-Niveau-Test [30] geprüft.

Definition des Skotoms: Ein Skotom wurde an Hand des Differenzwertausdruckes definiert (vergleiche Abb. 7). Für Prüfpunkte innerhalb 26° Exzentrizität wurde eine pathologische Befundabweichung entsprechend der Definition von Gloor et al. [33, 34] dann angenommen, wenn eine Abweichung von 5−9 dB in mindestens zwei benachbarten Prüfpunkten oder in drei und mehr nicht benachbarten Prüfpunkten vorlag oder wenn eine Abwei-

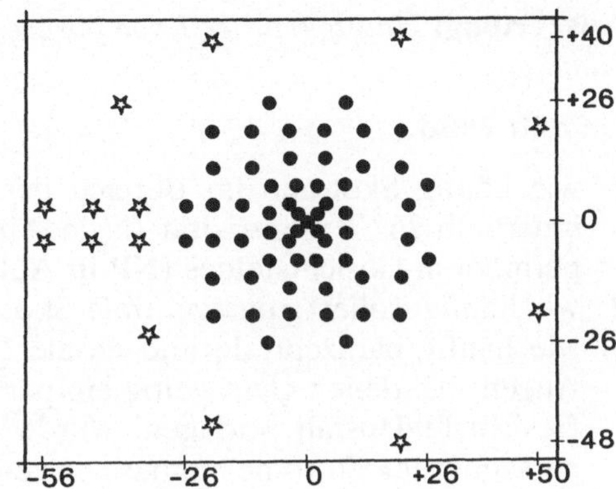

Abb. 1. Prüfpunktanordnung des Programms G1. * = Prüfpunkte, untersucht mit dem 2-Niveau-Test. ● = Prüfpunkte, untersucht durch Schwellenbestimmung

chung von 10 dB oder mehr in mindestens einem Prüfpunkt vorlag. Eine Abweichung in einem Prüfpunkt von 5–9 dB wurde nicht als pathologisch bewertet. In den Prüfpunkten des peripheren nasalen Gesichtsfeldes (vergleiche Bereich NP in Abb. 2) wurde ein relativer oder absoluter Ausfall in einem Prüfpunkt oder mehr als pathologisch eingestuft.

Definition des nasalen zentralen und nasalen peripheren Gesichtsfeldbereiches: Die Prüfpunkte in den nasalen zentralen Gesichtsfeldbereichen (N) und den nasalen peripheren Gesichtsfeldbereichen (NP) sind in Abb. 2 dargestellt. Beim Programm G1 liegen im Bereich des peripheren nasalen Gesichtsfeldes 8 Prüfpunkte (vergleiche Bereich NP in Abb. 2) und im Bereich des zentralen nasalen Gesichtsfeldes 20 Prüfpunkte (vergleiche Bereich N in Abb. 2). Die nasalen Prüfpunkte befinden sich in einem Bereich bis 45° oberhalb und unterhalb des 0°-Meridians.

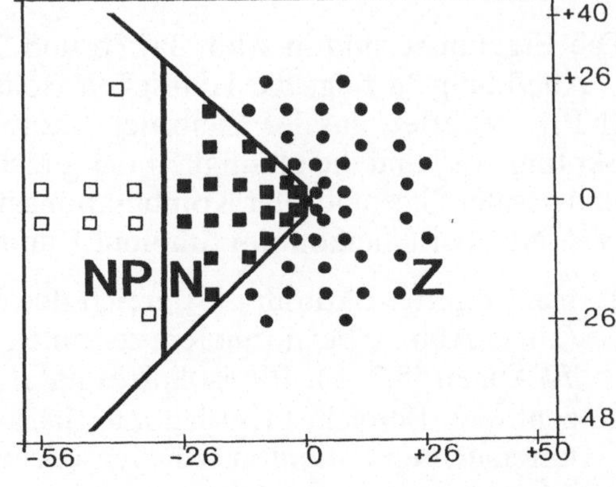

Abb. 2. Prüfpunkte des Programms G1 im nasalen peripheren Gesichtsfeldbereich (NP, offene Quadrate) und im nasalen zentralen Gesichtsfeld (N, geschlossene Quadrate). Die Häufung von isolierten Skotomen in diesen Bereichen und in Kombination mit Skotomen im parazentralen Gesichtsfeldbereich (Z, geschlossene Kreise) wird untersucht

Auswertung: *Häufigkeit der Lage parazentraler und peripherer Skotome bei Glaukom*

Geprüft wurde

1. wie häufig Skotome im Bereich des nasalen zentralen Gesichtsfeldes innerhalb 26° Exzentrizität (N in Abb. 2) und im Bereich des nasalen peripheren Gesichtsfeldes (NP in Abb. 2) vorlagen,
2. wie häufig isolierte parazentrale Skotome (Z in Abb. 2) vorlagen,
3. wie häufig parazentrale und nasale Skotome *gleichzeitig* vorlagen: für Augen, bei denen gleichzeitig ein parazentrales Skotom und ein nasaler Gesichtsfeldausfall vorlagen, wurde die Häufigkeit der Kombination parazentraler Skotome mit nasalen zentralen Ausfällen (vergleiche Z + N in Abb. 2, 3b) bzw. mit nasalen peripheren Ausfällen (vergleiche Z + NP in Abb. 2, 3b) und die Häufigkeit von parazentralen Gesichtsfeldausfällen mit nasalen zentralen sowie nasalen peripheren Ausfällen (vergleiche Z + N + NP in Abb. 2, 3b) untersucht. Diese drei Kombinationsmöglichkeiten zentraler Ausfälle mit peripherem Ausfall werden zusätzlich zusammengefaßt (vergleiche Z + N, Z + NP, Z + N + NP, in Abb. 2, 3a).
Damit soll die Gesamthäufigkeit nasaler Ausfälle bei gleichzeitigem Vorliegen parazentraler Skotome untersucht werden.

Häufigkeit der Lage parazentraler und peripherer Skotome bei Patienten mit Glaukom ohne Hochdruck, Glaucoma chronicum simplex und Pigmentglaukom

Die unter 1–3 genannten Fragestellungen wurden getrennt nach Glaukomformen untersucht. Damit soll geprüft werden, ob Unterschiede in der Lage der Skotome bestehen.

Ergebnis

I. Häufigkeit der Lage parazentraler und peripherer Skotome bei Glaukom

Die Ergebnisse sind in Abb. 3a, 3b und Tabelle 1 und 2 dargestellt.

Abbildung 3a zeigt die Häufigkeit isolierter nasaler peripherer Skotome (NP), isolierter nasaler zentraler Skotome (N), isolierter parazentraler Skotome (Z) und die Häufigkeit des gleichzeitigen Auftretens parazentraler und nasaler Skotome aller Kombinationsmöglichkeiten (Z + N, Z + NP, Z + N + NP) bei Glaukom im Stadium I und II.

1. Ein isoliertes Skotom im Bereich des nasalen peripheren Gesichtsfeldes (NP in Abb. 2) bei normalem zentralen Gesichtsfeld fand sich bei vier von 70 Augen (5,7 %). Ein isoliertes nasales Skotom im Bereich des nasalen zentralen Bereiches (N) lag innerhalb 26° Exzentrizität bei keinem der untersuchten Patienten vor (vergleiche Abb. 3a und Tabelle 1).

Tabelle 1. Häufigkeit der Lage der Skotome bei 70 Augen von 70 Patienten mit glaukomatösen Gesichtsfeldausfällen der Stadien I und II, untersucht mit dem Programm G1

Lokalisation (Exzentrizitätsbereich)	Isolierte nasale Skotome	Isolierte parazentrale Skotome	Parazentrale Skotome mit nasalen Skotomen
2°–26°	0	10 (= 14,3 %)	5 (= 7,1 %)
34°–56°	4 (= 5,7 %)		9 (= 12,9 %)
2°–56°			42 (= 60,0 %)
			56 (= 80,0 %)

2. Isolierte parazentrale Gesichtsfeldausfälle (Z) innerhalb 26° Exzentrizität ohne gleichzeitigem Vorliegen einer nasalen Gesichtsfeldveränderung (N oder NP) fanden sich bei 10 von 70 Augen (14,3 %). (Vergleiche Tabelle 1, Mitte)
3. 56 Augen (80 %) zeigten parazentrale Skotome (Z) und gleichzeitig Gesichtsfeldausfälle im Bereich des nasalen Sprungs im Exzentrizitätsbereich von 2°–56° (N + NP). (Vergleiche Tabelle 1, rechts) Das gleichzeitige Auftreten eines parazentralen Skotoms mit einem nasalen Gesichtsfeldausfall ist somit der häufigste Gesichtsfeldausfall. Abbildung 3b und Tabelle 1 (rechts) zeigen die Lage (Exzentrizität) der Skotome bei den 56 Augen mit parazentralem Skotom und gleichzeitigem nasalen Gesichtsfeldausfall: die nasalen Skotome lagen bei 5 Augen (7,1 %) nasal innerhalb 26° Exzentrizität, bei 9 Augen (12,9 %) nasal zwischen 34° und 56° Exzentrizität und bei 42 Augen (60 %) lagen die pathologischen Veränderungen nasal im Bereich von 2°–56° Exzentrizität. Bei Vorliegen parazentraler Skotome ist somit im Stadium I und II der gesamte nasale Bereich von 2°–56° Exzentrizitätsbereich bei 42 von 70 Augen (60 %) pathologisch verändert.

II. Häufigkeit der Lage parazentraler und peripherer Skotome bei Glaukom ohne Hochdruck, Glaucoma chronicum simplex und Pigmentglaukom

Tabelle 2 zeigt, getrennt für die verschiedenen Glaukomformen, bei vergleichbarem Erkrankungstadium (I und II), die absolute und relative Häufigkeit parazentraler Skotome kombiniert mit nasalen Ausfällen bei Glaukom ohne Hochdruck, Glaucoma chronicum simplex und Pigmentglaukom (Tabelle 2).

1. Isolierte periphere nasale Skotome (34°–56° Exzentrizität) fanden sich nicht bei Glaukom ohne Hochdruck, beim Glaucoma chronicum simplex

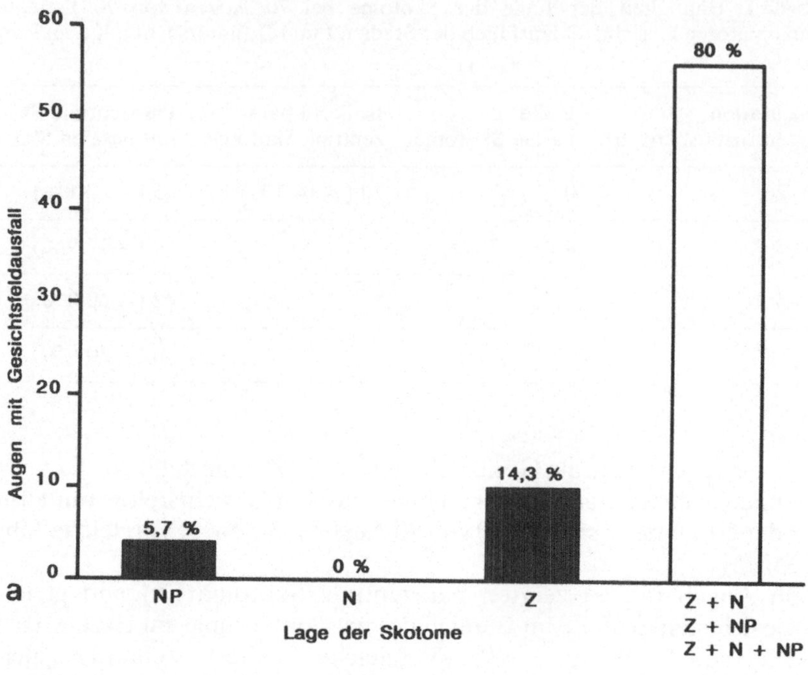
60
50
40
30
20
10
0
Augen mit Gesichtsfeldausfall
80 %
14,3 %
5,7 %
0 %
a
NP
N
Z
Z + N
Z + NP
Z + N + NP
Lage der Skotome

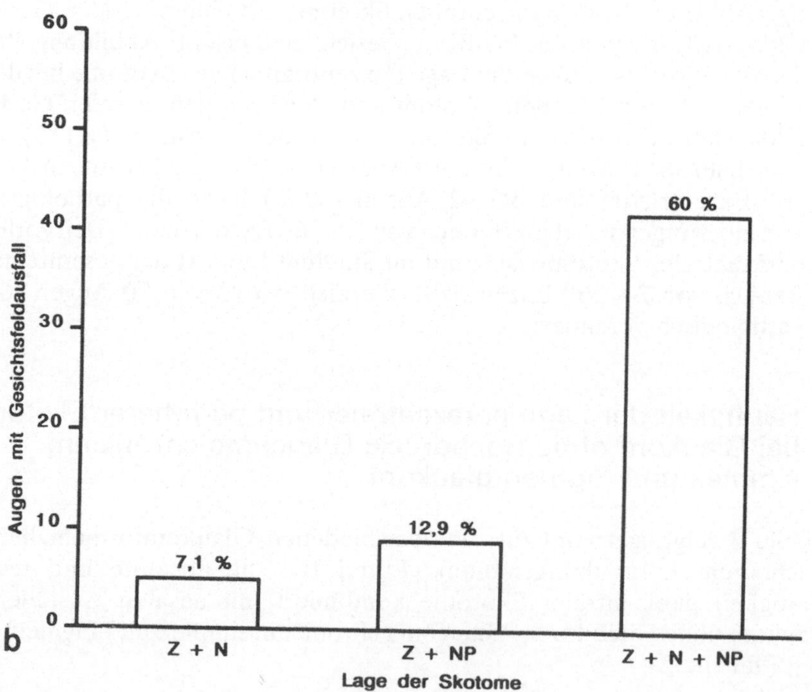
60
50
40
30
20
10
0
Augen mit Gesichtsfeldausfall
60 %
12,9 %
7,1 %
b
Z + N
Z + NP
Z + N + NP
Lage der Skotome

Tabelle 2. Absolute und relative Häufigkeit der Lage von isolierten nasalen Skotomen, von isolierten parazentralen Skotomen und von parazentralen Skotomen mit nasalem Ausfall bei Glaukom ohne Hochdruck, Glaucoma chronicum simplex und Pigmentglaukom mit Gesichtsfeldausfällen bis Stadium II

Lokalisation (Exzentrizitätsbereich)	Glaukom ohne Hochdruck $n=11$	Glaucoma chronicum simplex $n=46$	Pigmentglaukom $n=13$
Isolierte nasale Skotome			
2°–26°	0	0	0
34°–56°	0	2 (4,3 %)	2 (15,4 %)
Isolierte parazentrale Skotome	1 (9,1 %)	7 (15,2 %)	2 (15,4 %)
Parazentrales Skotom mit nasalem Ausfall in den Exzentrizitätsbereichen			
2°–26°	1 (9,1 %)	4 (8,7 %)	0
34°–56°	2 (18,2 %)	5 (10,9 %)	2 (15,4 %)
	7 (63,7 %)	28 (60,9 %)	7 (53,8 %)
2°–56°	10 (90,9 %)	37 (80,5 %)	9 (69,2 %)

bei 4,3 % und beim Pigmentglaukom bei 15,4 %. (Vergleiche Tabelle 2, oben)

2. Isolierte parazentrale Gesichtsfeldausfälle lagen bei Glaukom ohne Hochdruck bei 9,1 %, bei Glaucoma chronicum simplex bei 15,2 % und beim Pigmentglaukom bei 15,4 % vor. (Vergleiche Tabelle 2, Mitte)

3. Das gleichzeitige Vorliegen parazentraler Skotome und nasaler Ausfälle ist bei Glaukom ohne Hochdruck mit 90,9 % größer als bei Glaucoma chronicum simplex mit 80,5 % bzw. bei Pigmentglaukom mit 69,2 %.

Abb. 3a. Häufigkeit der Lage der Skotome bei 70 Augen von 70 Patienten mit glaukomatösen Gesichtsfeldausfällen bis Stadium II. NP = nasale periphere Skotome (isoliert) 34°–56° Exzentrizität), N = nasale zentrale Skotome (isoliert) (2°–26° Exzentrizität), Z = parazentrale Skotome (isoliert), Z + N, Z + NP, Z + N + NP = Summe aller parazentraler Skotome mit gleichzeitigem Vorliegen nasaler zentraler und nasaler peripherer Skotome.
80 % aller glaukomatösen Gesichtsfeldausfälle bis Stadium II zeigen gleichzeitig parazentrale und nasale Gesichtsfeldausfälle.
Abb. 3b. Häufigkeit der Lage der Skotome bei den 56 Augen von 56 Patienten mit glaukomatösen Gesichtsfeldausfällen bis Stadium II, die gleichzeitig parazentrale und nasale parazentrale und periphere Skotome aufweisen.
Z + N = Kombination von parazentralen Skotomen mit nasalen zentralen Skotomen (2°–26° Exzentrizität), Z + NP = Kombination von parazentralen Skotomen mit nasalen peripheren Skotomen (34°–56° Exzentrizität), Z + N + NP = Kombination von parazentralen Skotomen mit nasalen zentralen sowie nasalen peripheren Skotomen (2°–56° Exzentrizität)

Beim Glaukom ohne Hochdruck ist somit eine gleichzeitige Schädigung des zentralen Gesichtsfeldes und des nasalen peripheren Bereiches häufiger. (Vergleiche Tabelle 2, unten).

Diskussion

Häufigkeit der Lage parazentraler und peripherer Skotome bei Glaukom

1. In der Literatur wird über Häufigkeiten für isolierte nasale Skotome innerhalb 30° bis zu 22 % [17] berichtet. Das zentrale nasale Gesichtsfeld muß daher mit hoher Rasterdichte geprüft werden, da der nasale Bereich insgesamt am häufigsten geschädigt ist, wie auch unsere früheren Untersuchungen zur Topographie der Gesichtsfeldausfälle gezeigt haben [37, 38, 40, 41, 44] (Abb. 4).
Bei ausschließlicher Untersuchung des zentralen Gesichtsfeldes bis 30° Exzentrizität werden jedoch, wie die vorliegenden Untersuchungen zeigen, bei 5,7 % aller Patienten mit Glaukom bis Stadium II Gesichtsfeldausfälle in der Peripherie übersehen und somit ein falsch negativer Befund bei 5,7 % der Patienten erhoben. Über isolierte periphere Gesichtsfeldausfälle bei normalem zentralen Gesichtsfeld werden von LeBlanc bei 12,6 %, von Werner et al bei 9,1 %, von Dannheim bei 4 %, von Phelps et al. bei 3,6 % und 4,3 % und von Caprioli et al bei 11 % der untersuchten Augen berichtet, wobei überwiegend frühe glaukomatöse Gesichtsfeldschäden untersucht wurden. Werner et al. [75] fand bei Langzeitbeobachtung von 22 Augen, die in früheren Untersuchungen als gesund eingestuft worden waren, daß diese bei 45,5 % als erste Glaukomzeichen isolierte nasale Skotome bis 60° Exzentrizität aufwiesen. Eine glaukomspezifische Untersuchung muß daher auch den peripheren nasalen Bereich mit hoher Rasterdichte und schwellenbestimmender Untersuchungsmethode [13] prüfen.
2. Isolierte parazentrale Skotome im temporalen Bereich (Z) fanden wir bei 14,3 % der untersuchten Augen. Dieser Bereich ist somit relativ selten geschädigt. Dies stimmt auch mit unseren früheren Ergebnissen aus Untersuchungen zur Topographie glaukomatöser Gesichtsfeldschäden überein, untersucht in Häufigkeitsverteilungen absoluter und relativer Ausfälle [37, 38, 39, 44] und quantitativ untersucht mit Programm Delta bei 451 Augen [40, 41].
3. Wie die vorliegende Studie (vergleiche Tabelle 1, Abb. 3a, b) zeigt, ist das gleichzeitige Auftreten von parazentralen Skotomen und Ausfällen im nasalen Gesichtsfeldbereich (von 2°–56° Exzentrizität) mit insgesamt 80 % sehr häufig. Für die *Größenerfassung* des Skotoms (bis Stadium II) ist somit eine quantifizierende Untersuchung des nasalen peripheren Gesichtsfeldes erforderlich. Dies stimmt mit unseren früheren Untersuchungen zur Form der Skotome bis Stadium II überein: bei Auswertung

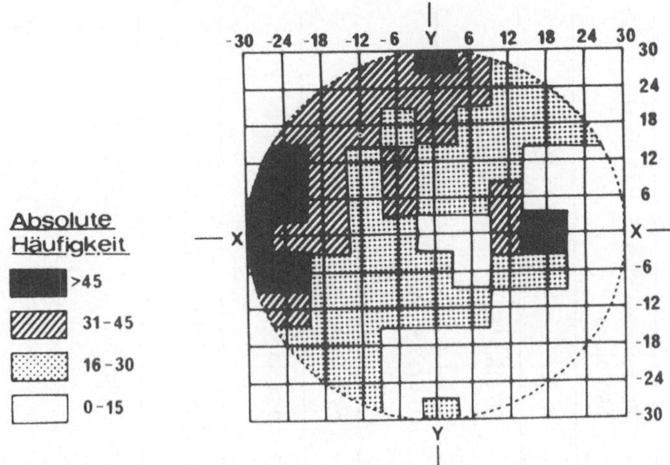

Abb. 4. Häufigkeitsverteilung absoluter glaukomatöser Gesichtsfeldausfälle bis Stadium II bei 301 Augen in den Prüfpunkten des Octopus-Programms 31 bei Glaucoma chronicum simplex aller Drucklagen, dargestellt für ein rechtes Auge. Die Meßpunkte mit einem Rasterabstand von 6° liegen jeweils in den Schnittpunkten der durch die Abbildung gezogenen Linien. Im Schnittpunkt der X- und Y-Achse liegt der Fixationspunkt. Meßpunkte in den schwarz gezeichneten Flächenarealen weisen am häufigsten, im schraffiert gezeichneten Bereich am zweithäufigsten absolute Ausfälle auf [44]. Die Ausfälle liegen häufiger in der oberen Gesichtsfeldhälfte

von 214 Gesichtsfeldbefunden (Programm 31, Prüffeldgröße 30°, Octopus-Perimeter 201) mit Gesichtsfeldausfällen ebenfalls des Stadium I und II zeigte sich bei 75,2 % eine Kombination zentraler Skotome mit peripheren Gesichtsfeldeinbrüchen (40–44). Armaly fand 18,9 %, LeBlanc 31,6 %, Werner et al. 4,5 %, Drance et al. 51,4 %, Werner et al. in einer späteren Untersuchung 69,0 %, Dannheim 37 %, Phelps et al. 4,9 % und 13,8 %, Caprioli et al. 34,8 % und LeBlanc et al. in einer späteren Studie 83 % parazentrale Skotome mit gleichzeitigem Vorliegen nasaler Skotome bis 60° Exzentrizität bei kinetischer und/oder statischer Untersuchung glaukomatös geschädigter Augen unterschiedlicher Stadien (vergleiche Tabelle 3). Eine Kombination parazentraler Skotome mit nasalen Skotomen innerhalb 30° Exzentrizität fanden wir in der vorliegenden Studie bei 7,1 % von 70 Augen (vergleiche Tabelle 1). Dieses Ergebnis stimmt mit dem von Phelps et al. überein, der bei 8,5 % von 94 Patienten mit Glaukom ohne Hochdruck parazentrale Skotome mit gleichzeitigem Vorliegen nasaler Skotome innerhalb 30° fand. Aulhorn et al. fand 17,5 %, Werner et al. 27,3 %, Zingirian et al. 32 %, Hart et al. 54 % und Phelps et al. bei Patienten mit Glaucoma chronicum simplex 21,9 % parazentrale Skotome und gleichzeitig nasale Skotome bis 30° Exzentrizität. Dies macht die Notwendigkeit einer glaukomspezifischen Untersuchung mit hoher Rasterdichte im zentralen Gesichtsfeldbereich

Tabelle 3. Häufigkeit von nasalen Skotomen mit verschiedenen Geräten unterschiedlicher Glaukomstadien

Autor	Perimeter	Stadium	Isolierte nasale Skotome		Parazentrale Skotome mit nasalen Skotomen	
Exzentrizitätsbereich			< 30°	30°–60°	< 30°	30°–60°
Armaly [6] n = 196	Goldmann	I–III nach Aulhorn	5 (4,7 %)	(bis 50°)	20 (18,9 %)	(bis 50°)
Aulhorn et al. [7] n = 1561	Goldmann Tübinger	Beginnend bis fortgeschritten	7 (0,45 %)		273 (17,5 %)	
LeBlanc [59] n = 79	Goldmann	Frühe Stadien		10(12,6 %)	25 (31,6 %)	(bis 60°)
Werner et al. [74] n = 22	Goldmann Tübinger	Frühe Stadien	10 (45,5 %)	2 (9,1 %) (bis 60°)	6 (27,3 %)	1 (4,5 %)
Drance et al. [21] n = 35	Goldmann	Frühe Stadien	7 (20 %)	(bis 60°)	18 (51,4 %)	(bis 60°)
Werner et al. [74] n = 87	Goldmann	Frühe Stadien	17 (19,5 %)	(25°–50°)	60 (69 %)	(25°–50°)
Zingirian et al. [77] n = 25	Goldmann	Frühe Stadien	5 (20 %)		8 (32 %)	
Dannheim [17] n = 100	Tübinger, Roden-stock-Peristat und Octopus 201	I–III nach Aulhorn	22 (22 %)	4 (4,0 %)		37 (37 %)
Gramer et al. [38] n = 214	Octopus 201	I–II nach Aulhorn	8 (3, 7 %)		161 (75,2 %)	(mit peripherhen Einbrüchen)

Tabelle 3 (Fortsetzung)

Autor	Perimeter	Stadium	Isolierte nasale Skotome		Parazentrale Skotome mit nasalen Skotomen	
Hart et al. [47] n = 98	Goldmann	Frühe Stadien			53 (54 %)	
Phelps et al. [64] n = 224 POAG n = 94 LTG	Goldmann	Beginnende und frühe Stadien („mild", „modera-te")	12 (5,4 %) 7 (7,4 %)	8 (3,6 %) 4 (4,3 %)	49 (21,9 %) 8 (8,5 %)	11 (4,9 %) 13 (13,8 %)
Caprioli et al. [13] n = 178	Octopus	Glaukomverdacht, beginnende u. fort-geschrittene Stadien	19 (11 %)		62 (34,8 %)	
LeBlanc et al. [61] n = 96	Goldmann	Frühe Stadien			80 (83 %)	

und der quantitativen Untersuchung auch des nasal-peripheren Gesichtsfeldes, wie im folgenden vorgeschlagen, deutlich.

II. Häufigkeit der Lage parazentraler und peripherer Skotome bei Glaukom ohne Hochdruck, Glaucoma chronicum simplex und Pigmentglaukom

1. In der vorliegenden Studie waren beim Pigmentglaukom isolierte periphere nasale Skotome auffallend häufig. Bei augendruckabhängigem Glaukomschaden scheinen somit isolierte periphere Ausfälle, soweit bei der relativ kleinen Fallzahl beurteilbar, häufiger vorzukommen. Unsere früheren Untersuchungen zur Topographie glaukomatöser Gesichtsfeldausfälle innerhalb 30° Exzentrizität zeigten bei Glaukom ohne Hochdruck bereits im Anfangsstadium sehr tiefe Skotome [40, 41], die im Stadium II häufiger in der unteren Gesichtsfeldhälfte lagen verglichen zum Glaucoma chronicum simplex und häufiger in der nasalen Gesichtsfeldhälfte lagen [40, 41, 44]. Sowohl beim Glaukom ohne Hochdruck, Glaucoma chronicum simplex als auch beim Pigmentglaukom war die nasale Gesichtsfeldhälfte häufiger betroffen als die temporale. Augen mit Pigmentglaukom und Glaucoma chronicum simplex mit hohen Augeninnendruckwerten zeigten jedoch häufiger eine Tendenz zu einem diffusen Gesichtsfeldausfall, also zu einer frühzeitigen Schädigung auch peripherer Gesichtsfeldbereiche. Auch in der vorliegenden Studie wurden mehr nasale Gesichtsfeldausfälle bei Glaukom ohne Hochdruck gefunden als bei Glaucoma chronicum simplex und Pigmentglaukom innerhalb 30° Exzentrizität, was die früheren, mit Programm 31/Delta erhobenen Ergebnisse [40] bestätigt.
2. Isolierte parazentrale Skotome entsprechend der in Abb. 2 gezeigten Definition wurden in der vorliegenden Studie etwa gleich häufig bei Glaucoma chronicum simplex und Pigmentglaukom gefunden, seltener dagegen bei Glaukom ohne Hochdruck. Diese Unterschiede sind unter anderem, wie an anderer Stelle ausführlich besprochen [40], mit einem unterschiedlichen Anteil vaskulärer Risikofaktoren zu erklären.
3. Das gleichzeitige Vorliegen parazentraler und nasaler peripherer Skotome ist bei Glaukom ohne Hochdruck mit 90,9 % größer als bei Glaucoma chronicum simplex mit 80,5 % bzw. Pigmentglaukom mit 69,2 %. Bei Glaukom ohne Hochdruck ist somit das zentrale Gesichtsfeld und gleichzeitig der nasale periphere Bereich häufiger geschädigt, was wiederum unsere früheren Ergebnisse [40] mit dem jetzt verwendeten G 1-Prüfpunktraster bestätigt. Diese Ergebnisse machen zusammen mit den Untersuchungsergebnissen zur stadienabhängigen Topographie aller Skotome bei unterschiedlichen Glaukomformen deutlich, daß auch das unten beschriebene glaukomspezifische Prüfpunktraster (GG-Programm) auf alle Glaukomformen anwendbar ist.

III. Welche Anforderungen an Rasterdichte und Prüfmethode sind an ein glaukomspezifisches Prüfpunktraster zu stellen?

Die obigen Ausführungen sowie auch frühere Untersuchungen zur Bedeutung der Rasterdichte bei der Computerperimetrie des Glaukoms [42, 43] zeigen, daß für die Glaukomperimetrie ein spezifisches Prüfpunktraster erforderlich ist, das im Bereich bis ca. 20° Exzentrizität mit einem Raster von 4,2° untersuchen sollte [21, 37, 42, 77]. Durch die Verdichtung des Rasters im Zentrum, insbesonders in der Makularegion, gibt das Programm G1 [30] zusätzliche Informationen zu diesem Bereich.

Es stellt sich die Frage, inwieweit die Berechnung der Indices [27, 28, 33, 69] im Programm G1 den zusätzlichen Zeitaufwand einer Doppelbestimmung in den 59 Prüfpunkten in einem entsprechend erhöhten diagnostischen Aussagewert bei der Routineperimetrie rechtfertigt. Ist es für die Routineperimetrie sinnvoll, die Zeit in eine zweimalige stellenbestimmende Untersuchung aller zentralen Prüfpunkte zur Berechnung der Indices zu investieren oder sollte die Untersuchungszeit, die letztlich durch die Belastbarkeit des Patienten begrenzt wird, nicht besser in eine Erhöhung der Prüfpunktzahl und damit Erhöhung der räumlichen Auflösung investiert werden? Auf eine Doppelbestimmung der Lichtunterschiedsempfindlichkeit in allen Prüfpunkten kann verzichtet werden, nicht jedoch auf die zeitlich aufwendige eingabelnde schwellenbestimmende Untersuchungsmethode in jedem Prüfpunkt, die für die Skotomtiefendarstellung in der Glaukomperimetrie unerläßlich ist. Die quantitative Tiefenauslotung ist erforderlich, da trotz Druckregulierung sich verschlechternde Gesichtsfelder vorwiegend eine Tiefenzunahme der Skotome zeigen [41]. Nur mit einer schwellenbestimmenden Untersuchungsmethode kann diese Tiefenzunahme in der erforderlichen Sensitivität langzeitkontrolliert werden. Wird auf eine Doppelbestimmung in den einzelnen Prüfpunkten verzichtet, so kann bei gleichem Zeitaufwand etwa die doppelte Anzahl an Prüfpunkten schwellenbestimmend untersucht werden. Wir schlagen daher ein neues Prüfpunktraster vor mit erhöhter Prüfpunktzahl und glaukomspezifischer Prüfpunktanordnung unter Beibehaltung der schwellenbestimmenden Untersuchungsmethode nach der Normalversion (Abb. 5).

Für die Erstuntersuchung des Patienten mit Glaukomverdacht, die im allgemeinen in der Praxis des niedergelassenen Augenarztes erfolgt, bietet dieses neue dichtere Prüfpunktraster in einer mit dem Programm G1 vergleichbaren Untersuchungszeit eine höhere räumliche Auflösung als das Programm 31 oder 32 oder G1, wie Abb. 6 zeigt.

Sogenannte Schnelltests des Gesichtsfeldes bei Glaukomverdacht mit überschwelligen Prüfmethoden sind als Ausgangswert für eine Langzeitbeobachtung nicht ausreichend. Bei Glaukomverdacht sollte von Anfang an mit hoher Sensitivität, also mit einer hohen Rasterdichte, eingabelnder Prüfmethode und glaukomspezifisch ausreichender Prüffeldgröße [36, 40] unter-

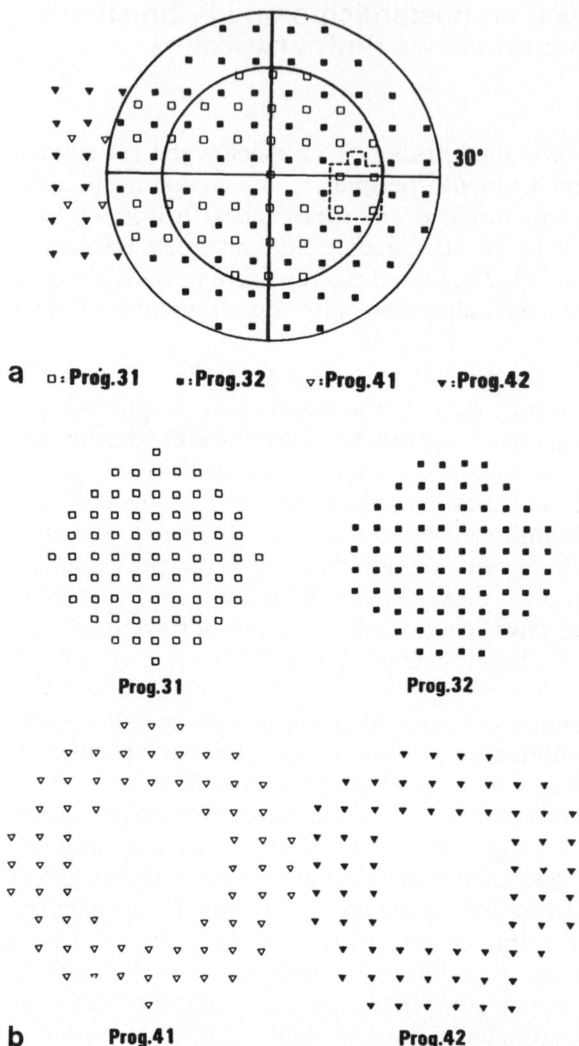

Abb. 5a. Glaukomspezifisches Prüfpunktraster (GG-Programm). Das zentrale Gesichtsfeld wird im Bjerrumbereich einschließlich des Bereichs des blinden Flecks mit einem Prüfpunktraster von 4,2° bei paraxialer Prüfpunktanordnung nasal bis 30° und nach oben und unten bis 24° untersucht. Weiter peripher wird das zentrale Gesichtsfeld mit einem 6°-Raster schwellenbestimmend untersucht. Außerhalb 30° erfolgt im Bereich des nasalen Sprungs ebenfalls eine schwellenbestimmende Untersuchung mit einem 8,4° beziehungsweise 12°-Raster.

b Prüfpunktraster der Programme 31, 32, 41, 42. Mit dem GG-Prüfpunktraster werden in einem Untersuchungsgang die glaukomrelevanten Netzhautorte untersucht, zu deren Erfassung sonst vier getrennte Untersuchungen mit den Programmen 31, 32, 41 und 42 mit insgesamt 279 Prüfpunkten nötig wären. Bei schwellenbestimmender Untersuchung nach der Normalversion lassen sich so durch Verzicht auf Doppeluntersuchungen diese 133 Testpunkte in einer mit dem Programm G1 vergleichbaren Untersuchungszeit mit höherem Auflösungsvermögen prüfen

sucht werden. Eine Befunddarstellung, die das Ergebnis in einem einzelnen, übersichtlichen Befundausdruck darstellt [42], wäre sinnvoll.

Wie die Ergebnisse dieser Studie zeigen, lagen die meisten Skotome gleichzeitig parazentral und nasal vor wobei sie nasal häufiger nasal peripher (12,9 %) als nasal zentral (7,1 %) auftraten (vergleiche Tabelle 1). Die isoliert vorkommenden nasalen Skotome lagen nur peripher. Wir haben daher ein neues Prüfpunktraster entwickelt, bei dem die Anordnung der Prüfpunkte sich an unseren Untersuchungen zur Topographie der Gesichtsfeldausfälle aller Stadien und Glaukomformen [38, 39, 40, 44], der Häufigkeitsverteilung der Skotome durch Einzelprüfpunktauswertung [38, 44] sowie früheren Untersuchungen zur Rasterdichte [37, 42] und Untersuchungen zum Informationsgehalt der Prüfpunktraster der Programme G1 und 31 des Octopusperimeters 201 [43] orientiert.

Anordnung und Zahl der Prüfpunkte im neuen Raster. Abbildung 5a zeigt das neue Prüfpunktraster (GG-Programm). Im Bereich von 0–24° nach oben und unten sowie bis 30° nach nasal wird das zentrale Gesichtsfeld mit einem homogenen 4,2°-Raster untersucht. Frühere Untersuchungen mit dem dichten Raster des Competer [39], das eine hohe Prüfpunktdichte, jedoch mit kreisförmiger Anordnung der Prüfpunkte aufweist, haben die Sensitivität des homogenen Rasters im zentralen Bereich bis 25° gezeigt [39]. Zingirian et al, [77] sowie Drance et al, [21] fanden bei Augen gesunder Probanden einen nasalen Sprung mit einem Abstand kleiner 4° bzw. kleiner 5°. Bei Untersuchung des Gesichtsfeldes mit einem engeren Raster als 4,2° könnte sich möglicherweise ein falsch positiver Befund ergeben. Das hier

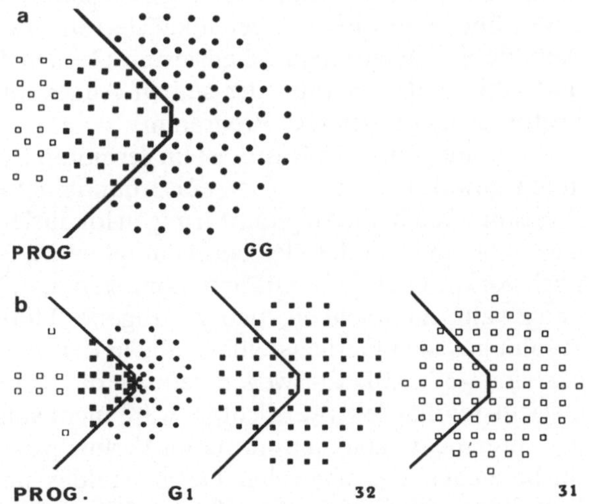

Abb. 6a. Darstellung des *nasalen* Prüffeldes bei verschiedenen Programmen. Im GG-Programm (Abb. 6a) werden insgesamt 54 Prüfpunkte im nasalen Gesichtsfeldbereich bis 45° Exzentrizität getestet (unten). Im Programm G1 (unten links) werden nasal insgesamt 28 Prüfpunkte bis 56° Exzentrizität, im Programm 32 (unten Mitte) werden 22 und im Programm 31 (unten rechts) werden 21 Prüfpunkte bis 30° Exzentrizität untersucht (Abb. 6b)

gewählte kartesische 4,2 % -Raster bietet eine hohe Wahrscheinlichkeit zur Erfassung von Form und Größe des Skotoms, wie unsere Untersuchungen mit dem Testskotom „blinder Fleck" belegen [41]. Prüfpunktraster mit kreisförmiger Anordnung oder mit linearer „sternförmiger" Anordnung führen zu einer erheblichen Gestaltungstransformation, da das ausgedruckte Skotombild durch die vorgegebene Lage der Prüfpunkte stärker beeinflußt wird als durch das neutrale 4,2° -Raster. Wegen der in der nasalen Gesichtsfeldhälfte bei allen Glaukomformen häufiger vorliegenden Ausfälle wurde nach nasal bis 30° Exzentrizität ein 4,2°-Raster gewählt, während wir nach unten, oben und temporal von 24° bis 30° ein 6°-Raster für ausreichend erachten. Untersuchungen zur Topographie frühglaukomatöser Gesichts-feldausfälle bis Stadium II [37, 38, 44, 63] zeigen, daß der temporal untere Quadrant am seltensten glaukomatöse Ausfälle ausweist. Im nasalen Bereich ober- und unterhalb des 0°-Meridans liegen jedoch am häufigsten Ausfälle vor und entsprechend liegen in diesem Bereich die meisten Prüfpunkte. Abbildung 6 zeigt die Zahl und Anordnung der Prüfpunkte verschiedener Programme. Der nasale Bereich wurde zum besseren Vergleich der hier liegenden Prüfpunktzahl abgegrenzt. Mit dem GG-Programm (vergleiche Abb. 5a, Abb. 6a, Abb. 8) wird der nasale Bereich innerhalb 30° mit 36 und weiter peripher zusätzlich mit 17 Prüfpunkten schwellenbestimmend geprüft. Mit Programm G1 werden bis 30° nasal in 20 Prüfpunkten Schwellenbestimmungen ausgeführt und weiter peripher in 8 Prüfpunkten mit dem Zwei-Niveau-Test untersucht. Mit Programm 32 wird in 22 und mit Programm 31 in 21 Prüfpunkten schwellenbestimmend der nasale Bereich bis 30° geprüft (vergleiche Abb. 6b). Die nasal somit weitaus höhere Raster-dichte des GG-Programms im Vergleich zum Beispiel zum Programm G1 läßt eine höhere Sensitivität bei lokalisierten Gesichtsfeldausfällen erwarten. Abbildung 7 zeigt einen lokalisierten Gesichtsfeldausfall im Programm G1 und Abb. 8 den Befund des selben Auges im Differenzwertausdruck der Prototypversion des GG-Programms.

Das homogene 4,2°-Raster ist im gesamten Bjerrumbereich nach oben und unten gewahrt, so daß Nervenfaserbündeldefekte im oberen und unteren Bjerrumbereich, die zu punktförmigen lokalisierten Ausfällen führen und die lagemäßig in etwa der gleichen Häufigkeit im gesamten oberen Bjerrumbe-reich vorkommen [37], mit dem homogenen 4,2°-Raster eine hohe Aufdek-kungswahrscheinlichkeit haben. Eigene Untersuchungen belegten, daß absolut gesehen Gesichtsfeldausfälle in der oberen Gesichtsfeldhälfte häufi-ger sind [37, 40]. Deswegen jedoch die Prüfpunkte nur in der oberen Gesichtsfeldhälfte zu verdichten, wäre nicht sinnvoll. Eigene quantifizieren-de Untersuchungen zum mittleren Verlust pro Testpunkt in den Exzentrizi-tätsbereichen des zentralen Gesichtsfeldes unter Wahl der willkürlichen Einteilung von 0° bis 10°, 10° bis 20° und 20° bis 30° ergaben, daß im Glaukomstadium II bis IV, definiert nach dem Gesamtverlust im Gesichts-feld, der Exzentrizitätsbereich von 10° bis 20° besonders häufig Ausfälle aufweist [40]. Zur Erfassung der Skotomtiefe muß daher der gesamte Bereich bis 25°, wie im vorliegenden Prüfpunktraster realisiert, nasal des blinden

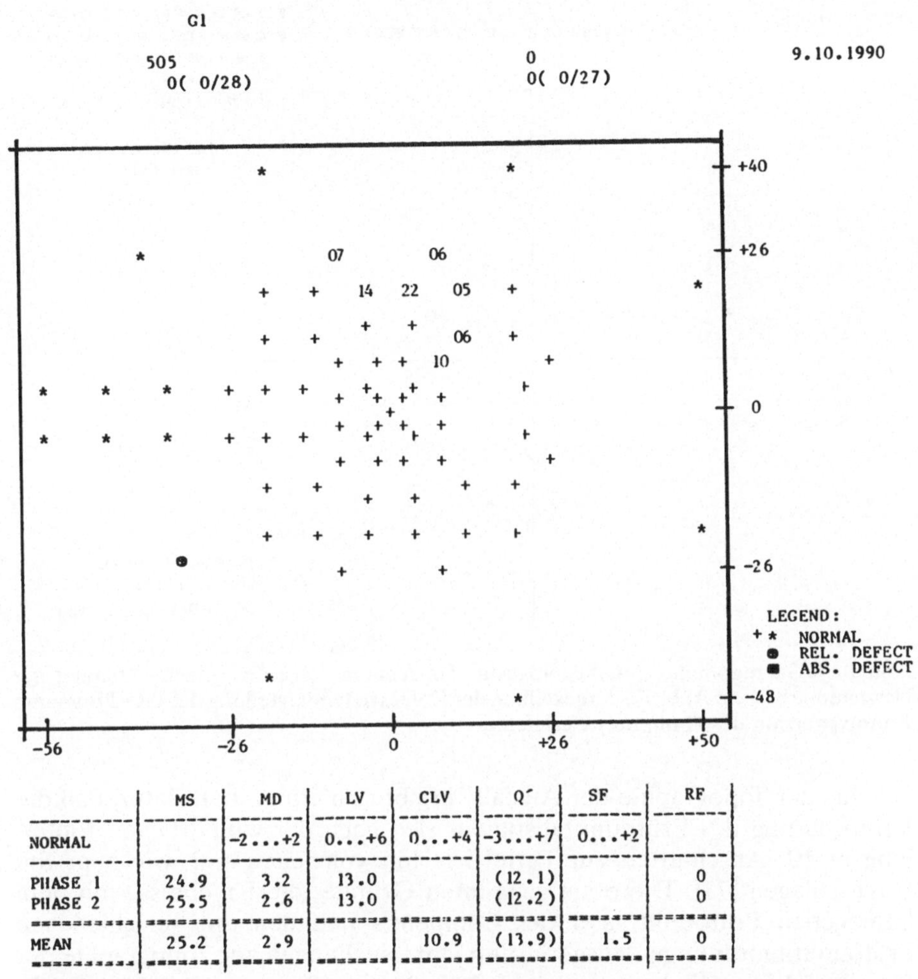

	MS	MD	LV	CLV	Q´	SF	RF
NORMAL		-2...+2	0...+6	0...+4	-3...+7	0...+2	
PHASE 1	24.9	3.2	13.0		(12.1)		0
PHASE 2	25.5	2.6	13.0		(12.2)		0
MEAN	25.2	2.9		10.9	(13.9)	1.5	0

Abb. 7. G1-Programm: Gesichtsfeldausfall am rechten Auge bei einem Patienten mit Netzhautnarbe, ausgedruckt in der Defekttiefendarstellung des G1-Programms

Flecks und nach nasal im Verlauf des 0°-Meridians bis 30° mit hoher Rasterdichte untersucht werden. Die dem Prüfpunktraster zugrundeliegenden Untersuchungen zur Topographie der Gesichtsfeldausfälle wurden auch mit anderen Prüfpunktrastern am Competer bestätigt [39] und korrelieren auch mit den glaukomatösen Papillenveränderungen [37 mit weiteren Literaturhinweisen). Unbestritten ist ein zur Peripherie hin größer werdender Prüfpunktabstand sinnvoll entsprechend der peripher größeren rezeptiven Felder, da die Untersuchung der Peripherie mit engem Prüfpunktraster einen nur noch verhältnismäßig geringen zusätzlichen Informationsgewinn erbringt. Offen ist, ab welchem Exzentrizitätsbereich eine Vergrößerung des Prüfpunktabstandes zu empfehlen ist. Weder morphologisch noch funktio-

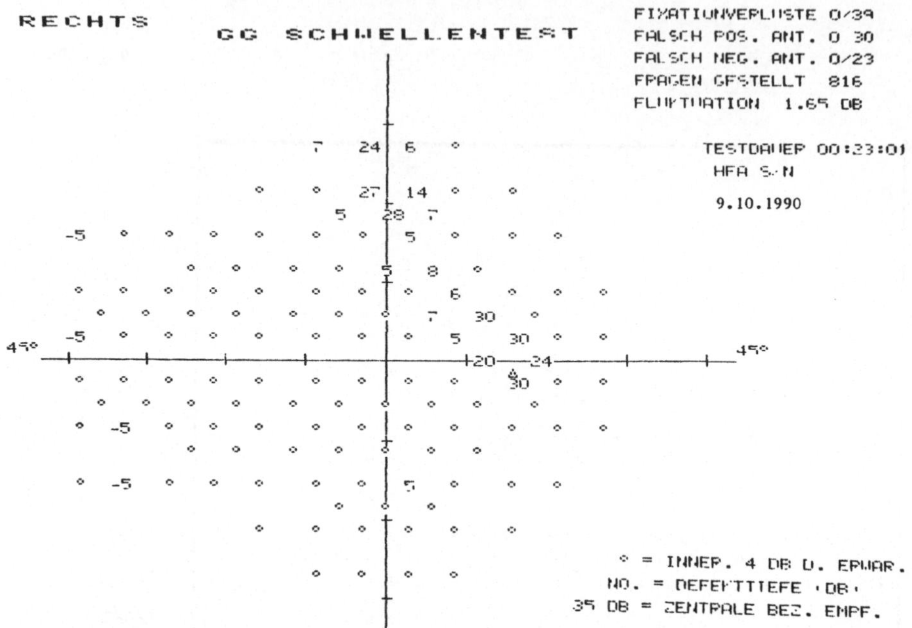

Abb. 8. GG-Programm: Gesichtsfeldausfall am rechten Auge des selben Patienten mit Netzhautnarbe (wie Abb. 7), dargestellt in der Defekttiefendarstellung der GG-Programm Prototypversion des Humphrey-Perimeters

nell aus der Topographie der Ausfälle ergibt sich ein Anhalt dafür, daß die Vergrößerung des Prüfpunktabstandes sich nach der willkürlichen Einteilung in 10°-Abschnitten zur Peripherie hin vollziehen soll, wie zum Teil vorgeschlagen [73]. Die oben genannten Gründe, die Ergebnisse mit dem homogenen Prüfpunktraster des Competers und den mit verschiedenen Prüfpunktanordnungen ausgeführten Untersuchungen zur Topographie der Gesichtsfeldausfälle legen nahe, daß eine Vergrößerung des Prüfpunktabstandes erst ab 20° bis 25° Exzentrizität beginnen sollte. Die Untersuchungen zur Topographie der Ausfälle bei verschiedenen Glaukomarten und verschiedenen Glaukomstadien zeigen ferner, daß die punktförmigen Ausfälle prinzipiell im gesamten zentralen Gesichtsfeld auftreten können, wobei abhängig davon, ob es sich um einen vorwiegend augeninnendruckabhängigen oder vorwiegend augeninnendruckunabhängigen, also vaskulären Glaukomschaden handelt, die Lage und Tiefe der Skotome quantitative Unterschiede aufweisen [40]. So zeigen Augen mit Glaucoma chronicum simplex und hohen Augeninnendruckwerten sowie Augen mit Pigmentglaukom eine mehr gleichmäßige Verteilung der Ausfälle in oberer und unterer Gesichtsfeldhälfte, also einen mehr diffusen Gesichtsfeldschaden [40, 64]. Dieser ist wiederum mit einem im zentralen Gesichtsfeld einheitlich dichten Raster besser erfaßbar. Das vorgeschlagene Raster (vergleiche Abbildung 5a, 8) läßt daher erwarten, daß die glaukomatösen Gesichtsfeldausfälle aller Glaukomformen gleichermaßen erfaßt werden und es somit ein für alle Glaukomformen anwendbares, glaukomspezifisches Raster darstellt. Bei der Anordnung der Prüfpunkte wurde eine, bezogen auf die X-Achse, paraxiale Prüfpunktanordnung gewählt. Eine Ausnahme bilden die Prüfpunkte im Bereich des blinden Flecks und des zentralen Prüfpunktes zur Ermittlung der Makulafunktion. Prüfpunkte unmittelbar auf der X-Achse, die der Raphe des Nervenfaserverlaufs [9, 50, 54] entspricht, sind für die Aufdeckung von Nervenfaserbündeldefekten nicht sinnvoll. Die Prüfpunktanordnung des neuen Rasters (vergleiche Abbildung 5a) wurde hinsichtlich der Koordinatenlage der Einzelprüfpunkte so gewählt, daß es sich aus Prüfpunkten der bisherigen Standardprogramme der Octopus-Perimeter (Programm 31, 32, 41, 42) bzw. der Humphrey-Perimeter (Programm THR 30-1, 30-2, 60-1, 60-2) zusammensetzt (vergleiche Abbildung 5b). Das bisher bewährte und für die Glaukomperimetrie wegen seiner paraxialen Lage der Prüfpunkte am meisten verwendete Untersuchungsprogramm 32 bzw. 30-2 ist im GG-Prüfpunktraster mit allen Prüfpunkten enthalten. Die Programmierung des Untersuchungsablaufs des GG-Programms sollte so erfolgen, daß die zum 6°-Raster des Programms 32 bzw. 30-2 gehörenden 72 Prüfpunkte zuerst untersucht werden. Für den Fall einer Unterbrechung des Untersuchungsprogramms ist dann zumindest eine Verwertbarkeit dieser Befunde und auch ein Ausdruck der Ergebnisse entsprechend dem Programm 32 möglich. Ferner hat dies den Vorteil, daß vom Programm 32 bzw. 30-2 ein problemloser Übergang zum GG-Programm im Rahmen von Verlaufsbeobachtungen möglich ist und somit trotz Anwendung dieses glaukomspezifischen Rasters eine Kontinuität der Verlaufskontrolle innerhalb dieser identischen Testorte gegeben ist. Die Prüfpunkte des GG-Programms könnten so auch in zeitlich getrennten Schritten geprüft werden: An einem Tag die Prüfpunkte des Programms 32 und in einem weiteren Schritt die Ergänzung zum GG-Programm durch Untersuchung der restlichen Prüfpunkte. Bei dem vorgeschlagenen GG-Prüfpunktraster werden insgesamt 133 Prüfpunkte untersucht, wobei 115 Prüfpunkte innerhalb 30° Exzentrizität liegen und mit zusätzlich insgesamt 18 Prüfpunkten das periphere Gesichtsfeld im nasalen Bereich mit ebenfalls schwellenbestimmender Untersuchungsmethode geprüft wird. Beim Programm G1 werden in Anbetracht der dort ausgeführten Doppelbestimmung 59 Prüfpunkte zweimal untersucht, also 118 Schwellenbestimmungen im zentralen Gesichtsfeld ausgeführt. Zusätzlich werden 14 Prüfpunkte im 2-Niveau-Test peripher untersucht (vergleiche Abb. 1). Die Gesamtzahl der Schwellenbestimmungen unterscheidet sich somit zwischen dem Programm G1 und dem neuen GG-Programm-Raster nur unwesentlich. Da beim Programm G1 über besondere Probleme der Patientenmitarbeit nicht berichtet wird, erscheint die für das glaukomspezifische Gesichtsfeldprogramm (GG-Programm) gewählte Prüfpunktzahl hinsichtlich der Untersuchungszeit durchaus praktikabel. In diesem Zusammenhang ist interessant, daß der in unserer früheren Studie [43] ausgeführte Phasenvergleich im Programm G1 keinen Hinweis auf einen Ermüdungseffekt ergab, was wiederum für die Anwendbarkeit der Zahl der vorgeschlagenen Schwellenbestimmungen spricht. Hinzu kommt, daß nach Prüfung der 115 Prüfpunkte im Zentrum bis 30° durch die dann notwendige Abnahme des Korrekturglases eine Ruhepause für den Patienten entsteht und erst anschließend die 18 peripheren Prüfpunkte schwellenbestimmend untersucht werden.

Prüffeldgröße. Die Prüffeldgröße unseres glaukomspezifischen Rasters beträgt nach oben, unten und temporal 30° Exzentrizität und nach nasal 45°. Wegen der altersabhängigen Verkleinerung des nasalen Gesichtsfeldes [19, 22, 23], und der senilen Ptosis, welche besonders das obere periphere Gesichtsfeld einengt, scheint der Bereich bis 45° Exzentrizität weniger artefaktgefährdet zu sein [43] als bis 56°, wie er im Programm G1 [30] geprüft wird. Bis 45° Exzentrizität sind weniger falsch negative oder falsch positive Antworten zu erwarten.

Nasale Peripherie außerhalb des 30°-Gesichtsfeldes. Der nasale Bereich wird in Anbetracht der in dieser Studie übereinstimmend mit anderen (Tabelle 3) [18, 24, 25, 62, 70] Arbeiten festgestellten häufigen Schädigung des nasalen Bereichs auch außerhalb 30° schwellenbestimmend untersucht. Für die Untersuchung der nasalen Peripherie verwenden wir Prüfpunkte aus den Programmen 41 und 42 (entsprechend den Programmen P 30/60-1-THR und P 30/60-2-THR des Humphrey Perimeters FA-610). Eine Kombination dieser Programme ergibt eine Auflösung von 8,4°, so daß wir durch Kombination dieser Prüfpunkte in der Nähe des 0°-Meridians im Bereich des nasalen Sprungs ein 8,4°-Raster erhalten und etwas weiter ober- und unterhalb der Horizontalen unter Verwendung einzelner Punkte des Programms 42 ein 12°-Raster anwenden. Von 30–45° erfolgt also im Bereich des peripheren nasalen Sprungs ebenfalls eine schwellenbestimmende Untersuchung mit einem 8,4° bzw. 12°-Raster. Viele Autoren schlagen für die Untersuchung des zentralen Gesichtsfeldes statische Methoden vor und für das nasale periphere Feld zunächst kinetische [60, 62, 70], um bei Entdeckung einer Veränderung nasal peripher anschließend ebenfalls statisch und damit genauer zu untersuchen. Daß eine qualitative Untersuchung der nasalen Peripherie nicht ausreichend sensitiv genug ist, zeigen die Untersuchungen von Caprioli et al. [13]. Er fand bei quantitativer schwellenbestimmender Untersuchung in 40 Testpunkten innerhalb 32°–54° Exzentrizität Skotome, die bei qualitativer Untersuchung im nasalen Bereich übersehen wurden. Unsere Untersuchungen zur Topographie zeigen im nasalen Gesichtsfeldbereich bei Glaukom ohne Hochdruck und Glaucoma chronicum simplex [37] häufig Ausfälle im nasalen Bereich, so daß gerade hier eine Erweiterung des Prüffeldes nach peripher bei schwellenbestimmender Untersuchung notwendig ist. In der Literatur werden über Häufigkeiten isolierter nasaler Skotome außerhalb 30° Exzentrizität bis 12,6% bei Untersuchung frühglaukomatöser Augen berichtet (vergleiche Tabelle 3). Der nasale Sprung ist somit ein wichtiger Indikator zum einen für frühe glaukomatöse Gesichtsfeldveränderungen, zum anderen zum zusätzlichen Ausschluß eines zentralen Gesichtsfeldausfalles [3, 10], da bei Untersuchung des Zentrums wie der nasalen Peripherie wegen der bei 80 Prozent kombinierten Skotome mit hoher Rasterdichte und schwellenbestimmender statischer Untersuchungsmethode sich die Wahrscheinlichkeit der Aufdeckung einer glaukomatösen Veränderung erhöht. Die Aufnahme weiterer Prüfpunkte in der Peripherie oder auch im Zentrum, die in einem Untersuchungsgang geprüft werden, erscheint nicht empfehlenswert, da das Konzentrationsvermögen der meist älteren Glaukompatienten möglicherweise überfordert wird und der Vorteil eines noch größeren Auflösungsvermögens durch den Nachteil einer höheren Zahl mitarbeitsbedingter falsch positiver und falsch negativer Antworten wieder eingeschränkt würde. Die mit zunehmender zeitlichen Belastung des Patienten möglicherweise auftretende Häufung von Fixationsabweichungen wird bei Geräten mit automatischer Fixationskontrolle (Octopus-Perimeter) dadurch korrigiert, daß die während einer Fixationsabweichung dargebotenen Stimuli annuliert und erneut dargeboten werden. Dadurch wird auch bei hoher Prüfpunktzahl der Anteil mitarbeitsbedingter Fehler korrigiert.

Untersuchung des blinden Flecks. Der Bereich des blinden Flecks wird mit insgesamt 6 Prüfpunkten (in Abb. 5a umrandet dargestellt) untersucht. Die Untersuchungen zur Aufdeckung des „Testskotoms" blinder Fleck durch Kombination der Programme 31 und 32 zeigten, daß diese Prüfpunktdichte für die Aufdeckung des blinden Flecks geeignet ist [42] und belegt gleichzeitig, daß die gewählte Rasterdichte von 4,2° im zentralen Gesichtsfeld eine Aufdeckung absoluter Skotome von der Größe des blinden Flecks als absolutes Skotom weitgehend sicherstellt. Bei alleiniger Untersuchung mit einem 6°-Raster werden Skotome von der Größe des blinden Flecks in etwa der Hälfte aller Untersuchungen nur am Rande angeschnitten und somit fälschlicherweise als relative Skotome dargestellt [37, 42]. Die Perimetrie des blinden Flecks hat glaukomspezifisch keine gesicherte Bedeutung [39], doch dient sie als Qualitätssicherung für den Gesamtbefund. Die Aussagen von Gesichtsfeldbefunden, die das physiologische absolute Skotom nicht aufdecken, müssen fraglich erscheinen. Auch Lageveränderungen des blinden Flecks durch hohe Brillenkorrekturwerte oder durch ein absolutes Zentralskotom sollten beachtet werden. Die Verlagerung des blinden Flecks kann somit eine exzentrische Fixation bei Zentralskotom anzeigen, wobei differentialdiagnostisch die refraktionsbedingten Größe- und Lageveränderungen berücksichtigt werden müssen [38].

Befundausdruck. Die klinisch bewährte Differenzwertdarstellung kann mit dem neuen Prüfpunktraster problemlos beibehalten werden. Dadurch ergeben sich keine Interpretationsschwierigkeiten im neuen Befundausdruck. Abbildung 8 zeigt einen Befundausdruck der GG-Programm-Prototypversion.

Standardisierung. Die Benutzung eines einheitlichen Prüfpunktrasters in verschiedenen automatischen Perimetern könnte der notwendigen Standardisierung der Prüfpunktanordnung bei der Glaukomperimetrie gerecht werden und so zu einer besseren Vergleichbarkeit der mit unterschiedlichen Geräten erhobenen Befunde beitragen. Aufgrund der unterschiedlichen Umfeldleuchtdichten sind die Defekttiefen in den Einzelprüfpunkten quantitativ auch zwischen Octopus Perimeter und Humphrey-Perimeter nicht vergleichbar, doch erleichtert die einheitliche Befunddarstellung im Differenzwertausdruck den Vergleich verschiedener Gesichtsfeldbefunde. Eine einheitliche Größe des Ausdrucks bei verschiedenen Geräten wäre sinnvoll, da dann die Befundausdrucke zur Verlaufskontrolle übereinandergelegt werden können. Dies ermöglicht eine bessere Beurteilung der Befundänderung. Eine zusätzliche Untersuchung bei z.B. Einweisung des Patienten in die Klinik oder bei Arztwechsel könnte wegen der besseren Vergleichbarkeit der Vorbefunde entfallen. Dies erspart Zeit und Kosten. Das hier vorgeschlagene neue Prüfpunktraster wird den von der Standardisierungskommission der International Perimetric Society (Aulhorn, Campos, Dannheim, Durst, Fankhauser, Flammer, Gramer, Zingirian) am 24.10.1987 in Bern erarbeiteten Empfehlungen gerecht. Die dabei empfohlene Untersuchung des zentralen Gesichtsfeldes mit mindestens 100 Prüfpunkten wird ebenfalls von dem neuen glaukomspezifischen Raster erfüllt.

Um den diagnostischen Wert dieses neuen GG-Programms im Vergleich zu bisher verwendeten Prüfpunktrastern zu belegen, sind weitere kontrollierte Studien erforderlich. Es wird sich dann zeigen, ob das 8,4° bzw. 12°-Raster zur weiteren Aufdeckung glaukomatöser Defekte in der nasalen Peripherie bis 45° ausreicht oder ob, wie Caprioli et al. beschrieb [13] ein noch engeres Raster, welches nasal noch weiter peripher reicht, notwendig ist.

Literatur

1. Anderson DR (1982) Testing the field of vision. Visual field loss in glaucoma, Mosby, St. Louis, pp 108–115
2. Airaksinen PJ, Drance SM, Douglas GR, Mawson DK, Nimienen H (1984) Diffuse and localized nerve fiber loss in glaucoma. Am J Ophthalmol 98: 566–571
3. Armaly MF (1969) Cup/disc ratio in early open-angle glaucoma. Doc Ophthalmol DR. Junk, The Hague, pp 526–533
4. Armaly MF (1969) The visual field defect and ocular pressure level in open angle glaucoma. Invest Ophthalmol 8: 105
5. Armaly MF (1969) Ocular pressure and visual fields, a ten-year follow-up study. Arch Ophthalmol 81: 25–40
6. Armaly MF (1972) Selective perimetry for glaucomatous defects in ocular hypertension. Arch Ophthalmol 87: 518–524
7. Aulhorn E, Harms H (1967) Early visual field defects in glaucoma. Glaucoma Symposium, Karger, New York, pp 151–186
8. Aulhorn E, Karmeyer H (1977) Frequency distribution in early glaucomatous visual field defects. Docum Ophthalmol Proc Series 14: 75–83
9. Bair HL (1940) Some fundamental physiological principles in the study of the visual field. Arch Ophthalmol 24: 10

10. Bigger JF, Becker B (1971) Cataracts and open angle glaucoma: The effect of cataract extraction on visual fields. Am J Ophthalmol 71: 335–340
11. Blum G, Gates LK, James BR (1959) How important are the peripheral fields? Arch Ophthalmol 61: 1, 8
12. Caprioli J, Sears M (1986) Patterns of early visual field loss in open angle glaucoma. Docum Ophthalmol Proc Series 49: 307–315
13. Caprioli J, Spaeth GL (1985) Static threshold examination of the peripheral nasal visual field in glaucoma. Arch Ophthalmol 103: 1150–1154
14. Coughlan M, Friedmann AL (1981) The frequency distribution of early visual field defects in glaucoma. Doc Ophthalmol The Hague Proc Series 26: 345–349
15. Damgaard-Jensen L (1977) Vertical steps in isopters at the hemiopic border – in normal and glaucomatous eyes. Acta Ophthalmol 55: 11–122
16. Damgaard-Jensen L (1977) Demonstration of peripheral hemianopic border steps by static perimetry. Acta Ophthalmol 55: 815–818
17. Dannheim F (1981) Patterns of visual field alterations for luminal and supraluminal stimuli in chronic simple glaucoma. Doc Ophthalmol 26: 97–102
18. De Oliveira-Rassi M, Shields MB (1982) Crowding of the peripheral nasal isopters in glaucoma, Am J Ophthalmol 94: 4–10
19. Drance SM (1967) Studies on the effects of age on the central and peripheral isopters of the visual field in normal subjects. Am J Ophthalmol 63: 1667
20. Drance SM (1969) The early field defects in glaucoma. Invest Ophthalmol 8: 84–91
21. Drance SM, Fairclough M, Thomas B, Douglas GR, Susanna R (1979) The early visual field defect in glaucoma and the significance of nasal steps. Docum Ophthalmol Proc Series 19: 119
22. Fisher RF (1967) The influences of orbital contours and lid ptosis on the size of the peripheral visual field. Vision Res 7: 671
23. Fisher RF (1986) The variations of the peripheral visual fields with age. Docum Ophthalmol 14: 41–67
24. Flammer J (1985) Psychophysics in glaucoma. A modified concept of the disease. Proc of the European Glaucoma Society, Helsinki 1984, 11–17
25. Flammer J (1987) Das Glaukomgesichtsfeld. Augenärztliche Fortbildung 10 (Nrs. 3): 103–108
26. Flammer J, Drance SM, Augustiny L, Funkhouser A (1985) Quantification of glaucomatous visual field defects with automated perimetry. Ophthalmol Vis Sci 16: 176–181
27. Flammer J, Drance SM, Funkhouser A, Augustiny L (1984) Differential light threshold in automated static perimetry. Arch Ophthalmol 102: 876
28. Flammer J, Drance SM, Zulauf M (1984) Differential light threshold. Short- and long-term fluctuation in patients with glaucoma, normal controls, and patients with suspected glaucoma. Arch Ophthalmol 102: 704
29. Flammer J, Eppler E, Niesel P (1982) Die quantitative Perimetrie beim Glaukompatienten ohne lokale Gesichtsfelddefekte. Graefes Arch Clin Exp Ophthalmol 219: 92
30. Flammer J, Jenni F, Bebie H (1987) The Octopus glaucoma program G1. Glaucoma 9/2: 67–72
31. Forbes M (1966) Influence of miotics on visual fields in glaucoma. Invest Ophthalmol 5: 139–145
32. Furuno F, Matsuo H (1979) Early stage progression in glaucomatous visual field changes. Doc Ophthalmol Proc Series 19: 247–253
33. Gloor B, Stürmer I, Vockt B (1984) Recent advances in the study of glaucomatous field defects using the Octopus automated perimeter. Klin Monatsbl Augenheilkd 184: 249–253
34. Gloor B, Gloor, E (1986) Die Erfaßbarkeit glaukomatöser Gesichtsfeldausfälle mit dem automatischen Perimeter Octopus. Kin Mbl Augenheilkd 188: 33–38
35. Glowazki A, Flammer J (1986) Is there a difference between glaucoma patients with rather localized visual field damage and patients with more diffuse visual field damage? Docum Ophthalmol Proc Series 49: 317–320

36. Gramer E (1985) Lesen von Gesichtsfeldbefunden bei der automatischen Perimetrie. Z prakt Augenheilkd 6: 353–364
37. Gramer E (1987) Gesichtsfeldveränderungen bei Glaukom. In: G.K. Krieglstein (ed.), Das chronische Glaukom – Zeitgemäße Diagnostik und Therapie, S. 19–60, Augenspiegel-Verlag Ratingen
38. Gramer E, Gerlach R, Krieglstein GK, Leydhecker W (1982) Zur Topographie früher glaukomatöser Gesichtsfeldausfälle bei der Computerperimetrie. Klin Monatsbl Augenheilkd 180: 515–523
39. Gramer E, Gerlach R, Krieglstein GK (1982) Zur Sensititivität des Computerperimeters Competer bei frühen glaukomatösen Gesichtsfeldausfällen. Eine kontrollierte Studie. Klin Mbl Augenheilkd 180: 203–209
40. Gramer E, Althaus G (1987) Quantifizierung und Progredienz des Gesichtsfeldschadens bei Glaukom ohne Hochdruck Glaucoma chronicum simplex und Pigmentglaukom. Eine klinische Studie mit dem Programm Delta des Octopus-Perimeters 201. Klin Mbl Augenheilkd 191: 184–198
41. Gramer E, Althaus G, Leydhecker W (1986) Topography and progression of visual field damage in low tension glaucoma, open angle glaucoma and pigmentary glaucoma with the program Delta of the Octopus Perimeter 201. Doc Ophthalmol Proc Series 49: 349–363
42. Gramer E, Althaus G, Leydhecker W (1986) Die Bedeutung der Rasterdichte bei der computergesteuerten Perimetrie. Eine klinische Studie. Z prakt Augenheilkd 7: 197–202
43. Gramer E, Knaut-Spaeth M (1990) Glaukomspezifische Untersuchung des Gesichtsfeldes. Eine klinische Studie zum Informationsgehalt der Programme G1 und 31 des Octopus-Perimeters 201. In: E. Gramer (Hrsg) Glaukom – Diagnostik und Therapie. Seite 38–59. Enke Verlag Stuttgart
44. Gramer E, Mohamed J, Krieglstein GK (1982) Der Ort von Gesichtsfeldausfällen bei Glaucoma simplex, Glaukom ohne Hochdruck und ischämischer Neuropathie. Indikation zur vasoaktiven Therapie. In: Krieglstein GK, Leydhecker W (Hrsg): Medikamentöse Glaukomtherapie: 59–72
45. Haas AL, LeBlanc RP, Schneider UC (1989) The significance of peripheral suprathreshold measurements in the Octopus program G1. Perimetry Update, Proc of the VIIIth international perimetric society meeting (ed by Heijl A:) 425–430, Kugler & ghedini, Amsterdam, Milano
46. Harrington DO (1981) The visual fields. Mosby, St. Louis
47. Hart WM, Becker B (1982) The onset and evolution of glaucomatous visual field defects. Am Acad Ophthalmol 89: 268–279
48. Heijl A, Drance SM (1981) A clinical comparison of three computerized automated perimeters in the detection of glaucoma defects. Doc Ophthalmol Proc Series 26: 43–48
49. Heijl A, Lundquist L (1984) The location of the earliest glaucomatous visual field defects documented by automatic perimetry. Doc Ophthalmol Proc Series 35: 135–138
50. Heilmann K (1972) Augendruck, Blutdruck und Glaukomschaden. In: Bücherei des Augenarztes, Nr. 61, ed by Hollwich F. Enke Verlag Stuttgart
51. Hollows FC, Graham PA (1966) Intra-ocular pressure, glaucoma, and glaucoma suspects in a defined population. Brit J Ophthal 50: 570–586
52. Jenni F, Flammer J (1986) Experience with the reability parameters of the Octopus automated perimeter. Doc Ophthalmol Proc Series 49: 601–603
53. Jenni F, Hirsbrunner HP, Fankhauser F (1989) The nasal step in the normal and glaucomatous visual field. Perimetry Update. Proc of the VIIIth perimetric society meeting (ed by Heijl): 305–311, Kugler & ghedini, Amsterdam, Milano
54. Katsumori N, Mizokami A (1989) Clinicopathological studies of the retinal nerve fiber layer in early glaucomatous visual field damage. Perimetry Update. Proc of the VIIIth perimetric society meeting (ed by Heijl): 289–295, Kugler & ghedini, Amsterdam, Milano

55. Kitazawa Y, Tarahashi O, Ohiwa J (1979) The mode of development and progression of field defects in very early glaucoma. A follow- up study. In: 3rd international visual field symposium ed by Greve, Heijl: 211–221, Junk Publishers, Dordrecht
56. Kommerell G (1969) Binasale Refraktionsskotome. Klin Monatsbl Augenheilkd 154: 85–88
57. Lachenmayer B (1987) Glaukomüberwachung in der Praxis mittels automatisierter Perimetrie. Augenärztliche Fortbildung 10 (Nr. 3): 88–96
58. Langerhorst CT, Van den Berg TJTP, Greve EL (1989) Fluctuation and general health in automated perimetry in glaucoma. Perimetry Update. Proc of the VIIIth perimetric society meeting, ed by Heijl: 159–164, Kugler & ghedini, Amsterdam, Milano
59. LeBlanc RP (1976) Peripheral nasal field defects. Doc Ophthalmol 14: 131
60. LeBlance RP, Becker B (1971) Peripheral nasal field defects. Am J Ophthalmol 72: 415–419
61. LeBlanc RP, Lee A, Baxter M (1985) Peripheral nasal field defects. Doc Ophthalmol Proc Series 42: 377–381
62. MillerKN, Shields MB, Ollie AR (1989) Automated kinetic perimetry with two peripheral isopters in glaucoma. Arch Ophthalmol 107: 1316–1320
63. Nicholas SP, Werner EB (1980) Location of early glaucomatous visual field defects. Can J Ophthalmol 15: 131–133
64. Phelps CD, Hayreh SS, Montague PR (1982) Visual fields in low-tension glaucoma, primary open angle glaucoma, and anterior ischemic optic neuropathy. Fifth International Visual Field Symp ed by Greve and Heijl: 113–124, Junk Publishers, Dordrecht
65. Portney GL, Krohn MA (1978) The limitations of kinetic perimetry in early scotoma detection. Am Acad Ophthalmol Otolaryngol 85: 287–293
66. Rock WJ, Drance SM, Morgan RW (1971) A modification of the Armaly visual field screening technique for glaucoma. Can J Ophthalmol 6: 283–292
67. Rönne H (1909) über das Gesichtsfeld beim Glaukom. Klin Monatsbl Augenheilkd 47: 12–33
68. Schulzer M, Mikelberg FS, Drance SM (1987) A study of the value of the central and peripheral isopters in assessing visual field progression in the presence of paracentral scotoma measurements. Brit J Ophthalmol 71: 422–427
69. Seamore C, LeBlanc R, Rubillowicz M, Mann C, Orr A (1988) The valua of indices in the central and peripheral visual fields for the detection of glaucoma. Am J Ophthalmol 106: 180–185
70. Stewart WC, Shields BM, Ollie AR (1988) Peripheral visual field testing by automated kinetic perimetry in glaucoma. Arch Ophthalmol 106: 202–206
71. Stürmer J, Gloor B, Tobler H (1984) Wie sehen Glaukomgesichtsfelder wirklich aus? Klin Monatsbl Augenheilkd 184: 390–393
72. Tate GW, Lynn JR Principles of quantitative perimetry in testing and interpreting the visual field
73. Weber J, Dobek K (1986) What is the most suitable grid for computer perimetry in glaucoma patients? Ophthalmologica Basel 192: 88–96
74. Werner EB, Beraskow J (1979) Peripheral nasal field defects in glaucoma. Trans Am Acad of Ophthalmol 86: 1875–1878
75. Werner EB, Drance SM (1977) Early visual field disturbances in glaucoma. Arch Ophthalmol 95: 1173–1175
76. Wirtschafter JD, Hard-Boberg AL, Coffmann SM (1984) Evaluation the usefulness in neuro- ophthalmology of visual field examinations peripheral to 30 degrees. Trans Am Ophthalmol Society 82: 329–357
77. Zingirian W et al. (1979) The nasal step in normal and glaucomatous visual fields. Can J Ophthalmol 14: 88–94

Korrespondenzadresse

Professor Dr. med. Dr. jur. Eugen Gramer
Universitätsaugenklinik Würzburg, Josef-Schneider-Straße 11,
D-8700 Würzburg

Cornea

Diagnosis of the Dry Eye

O. P. van Bijsterveld

Introduction

The causes of keratoconjunctivitis sicca (KCS) are manifold. Cicatricial, nutritional, neurogenic – both acquired and congenital – and exposure factors can be present alone or in any given combination. In this study, the evaluation of the clinical tests in keratoconjunctivitis sicca is limited to those forms of KCS that are caused by a decrease in the tear gland function, be it as a result of autoimmune inflammatory reactions or as a result of involution.

As in every day clinical practice the Schirmer I, the Rose bengal and the break-up time tests are by far the most commonly used, these tests will be reviewed in more detail. The lysozyme and the lactoferrin tests will be only very briefly assessed as they are actually laboratory tests, although in those clinics interested in dry eye problems, these tests are used as routine clinical procedures.

The Schirmer Test

In 1903 Schirmer [1] developed a clinical test to measure the amount of tear fluid produced in a certain time period. The interpretation of the test has been controversial. Schirmer believed that if wetting of the filter-paper strip was below 15 mm, keratoconjunctivitis sicca should be suspected. It is true that in early KCS – as judged by the concentration of tear proteins such as lysozyme and lactoferrin – values of 15 mm or more in wetting of the filter-paper strip can be observed, but taking this limit for the diagnosis of KCS would imply that 51 % of the normal population – judged by the concentration of tear proteins in the tear fluid – suffer from KCS.

Beetham [2], on the basis of his clinical experience, felt that wetting of less then 10 mm of the filter-paper strip was indicative for KCS. Again, in early KCS, as judged by the concentration of tear proteins in the tear fluid, values of 10 mm or more in wetting of the filter-paper strip can be observed, but taking this limit for the diagnosis of KCS implies that 35 % of the normal population – judged by the concentration of the tear proteins in the tear fluid – have dry eyes.

These limits between normality and disease were based on taking the

Gramer/Kampik (Hrsg.) Pharmakotherapie am Auge
© Springer-Verlag Berlin Heidelberg 1992

average minimal values of wetting of the filter-paper strip that were observed in persons without any functional symptoms. These are not meaningful limits and consequently divers and radical opinions on the merits of the Schirmer test were common. This neglect to set useful limits between normality and disease resulted also in a tendency to devise new tests based on the same principle that were supposed to be more accurate.

The correct way to set limits between normality and disease is to study the frequency distribution of Schirmer values in patients in whom there is no doubt that they are suffering from KCS on one hand, and those of a control population on the other hand [3]. By doing so, a considerable overlap of these distributions is apparent, indicating the weakness of the Schirmer test as a diagnostic test. In a test with high discriminatory power, the distribution of the studied parameter of the population with KCS and that of a control group have little overlap.

If the probability of misclassification for the Schirmer I test is balanced, that is to say choosing that limit of the Schirmer value in patients with KCS and control persons, at which an equal number of patients are wrongly diagnosed as being normal and vice-versa, then the optimal limit is 5.5 mm wetting of the filter-paper strip in 5 minutes. With this limit the probability of misclassification is 16 %; this means that 1 in every 6 patients is misclassified as normal and 1 in every 6 normal persons is considered to have KCS. This shows the Schirmer test to be not particularly good for the diagnosis of KCS. It is important to realise that this value of the Schirmer test, i.e. 5.5 mm wetting of the filter-paper strip to diagnose keratoconjunctivitis sicca does not represent a limit that patients with the dry eye state cannot exceed. The average of the Schirmer values in early cases of keratoconjunctivitis sicca will most certainly exceed the diagnostic limit of 5.5 mm wetting of the filter-paper strip, but these values cannot be used to diagnose the dry eye state with any certainty.

The Jones Test

Jones [4] separated tear secretion in reflex and basic secretion. Reflex secretion in his theory would be a function of the main lacrimal gland, while basic secretion would be a function of the accessory lacrimal glands of Wolfring and Krause. According to Jones, the Schirmer I test measures the reflex secretion as the filter-paper strip stimulates the trigeminal nerve. However, if the same test is performed after local anaesthesia the afferent stimulus originating from the conjunctiva is suppressed and the resultant wetting of the filter-paper strip would represent the "basic" secretion and would reflect the physiologic tear flow.

This concept of Jones has created considerable interest, especially because the idea emerged that studying the physiologic tear flow would most likely yield a new, relatively simple test to perform, or so it was hoped at least. Norn [5], however, pointed out that the lid margin with its cilia is more sensitive then the conjunctiva and this was also the view of Jordan and Baum [6]. Their study indicates that all tear production can be accounted for by reflex secretion in response to different magnitudes of stimulation.

Then the question should be raised whether the Schirmer test with anaesthesia really is better then the same test without anaesthesia. Based upon the study of the magnitudes of overlap of the frequency distributions of Schirmer values in patients with KCS and control persons with and without topical anaesthesia, it is apparent that the Schirmer test without anaesthesia has in fact a better discriminatory ability then the Schirmer test with anaesthesia, but clinically this difference is not significant.

The Rose Bengal Test

Rose bengal is a vital stain. It stains those cells that have a tendency to keratinisation such as one can expect to find in keratoconjunctivitis sicca, as well as in epithelial erosions. If the intensity of staining of both medial and lateral bulbar conjunctiva and of the cornea is scored, with each section scoring up to a maximum of three points, a total score of nine could be obtained [3]. In this way the frequency distribution of this parameter in persons with KCS and control persons can be established.

If one compares the frequency distributions of this parameter, it is at once apparent that the overlap is much smaller then with the Schirmer test. Under ideal circumstances the probability of misclassification is around 5 % at the score limit of 3.5 points. This means that one in every 20 patients is misclassified as normal and one in every twenty control persons is considered to have keratoconjunctivitis sicca.

The Rose bengal score is not very specific: patients with infectious conjunctivitis, allergic conjunctivitis, and other forms of chronic irritative conjunctivitis, will show an increased score. On the other hand, patients with early keratoconjunctivitis sicca who live and work in an air- and moisture conditioned environment will show a relatively low score. In all, a probability of misclassification of about 10 % can be expected.

Tearfilm Break-up Time

Another clinical test is the tear film break-up time [7]. This is defined as the time in seconds for the appearance of the first randomly distributed dry spot after a complete blink. If the break-up time is less then 10 seconds, it is considered pathologic. The break-up time is dependant upon a number of variables such as the concentration of fluorescein, age and the number of blinks.

The break-up time decreases with advancing age. This relationship is linear. With blinking, the break-up time initially increases and then decreases rather rapidly. The relation between the break-up time and the number of blinks in normal persons corresponds to a second degree curve. Because of all these variables the break-up time is not a good test to use for the diagnosis of keratoconjunctivitis sicca. For the diagnosis of tear film instability, however, it is the only test we have.

Tear Proteins

As early as 1922 Fleming reported the presence of lysozyme in the tear fluid [8]. Other proteins have also been reported, notably lactoferrin [9] and tear specific prealbumin [10, 11]. All these proteins are major components of the lacrimal fluid. Their presence under both normal and pathological conditions has been well documented [3, 8, 12–15]. The tear proteins are synthesized by the lacrimal gland [16]. In degenerations of the tear gland the concentration of the tear proteins in the lacrimal fluid decreases.

The most frequent cause of diminished tear gland function is age related involution, an uncertain diagnosis without biopsy of the tear gland. Less frequently degeneration of the tear gland is the result of auto-immune inflammatory reactions such as can be observed in Sjoegren's syndrome, characterized among other things by a lymphocytic cell infiltration in the lacrimal gland, that ultimately destroys the epithelial cells of that gland.

The diagnosis of Sjoegren's syndrome as an underlying disease of KCS is important as this syndrome can lead to many other ocular and also medical complications. As the routine ophthalmological investigation of the tear gland function is not particularly elaborate, it would be of considerable interest if differences could be demonstrated in the profile of the common parameters of tear function in patients with keratoconjunctivitis sicca associated with Sjoegren's Syndrome and in those in which there is no such association. Usually, the diagnosis of collagen disease is initially made by the medical department. Sometimes the dry eye state, however, precedes the symptoms of general involvement.

The various tear function parameters reflect different functions of the tear gland. In 1980 Gillette and associates [17] demonstrated that lysozyme was secreted both by the tubular and acinar structures of the lacrimal gland, in approximately equal amounts. The lysozyme tear fluid concentration, which we assayed by means of the agar diffusion technique using *Micrococcus lysodeikticus* as substrate [3], then looks like a good starting point to study the pattern of the other tear function parameters, which we did by selecting patients from both groups with comparable lysozyme tear fluid distributions.

The lactoferrin tear fluid concentration was assayed by means of the immunoprecipitation technique [14]. In Table 1 the lactoferrin tear fluid concentration is listed, together with the Schirmer values and the break-up-time between the groups.

The lactoferrin tear fluid concentration and the break-up time values were significantly lower in the Sjoegren group and the Schirmer values nearly so.

Table 1. Lactoferrin tear fluid concentration in mcg per ml, Schirmer values in mm wetting of the filter paper strip and tear film break-up time in seconds in patients with KCS, with (KCS-SJ) and without association of Sjoegren's syndrome (KCS-NSJ)

	Patients		
	KCS-SJ	KCS-NSJ	Significance
Lactoferrin concentration	478	799	P < 0.05
Schirmer values*	4	7	P < 0.10
Tear film break-up time	3	5	P < 0.025

* Shown here as median values.

However, none of these tests alone were able to differentiate between the two groups as the probability of misclassification for these single parameters was between 42 % and 50 %.

By combining the values of these parameters, as in a multivariate analysis, the probability of misclassification decreased markedly. For any individual patient the discriminant function value (DFV) can be arrived at by using the formula: DFV=(−0.083 * the millimeter diameter of lactoferrin precipitation) + (−0.0219 * the mm wetting of the filter paper strip in 5 minutes) + (−0.1414 * the break-up time in seconds). The higher the value, the more likely the KCS is to be associated with Sjoegren's disease and vice versa.

The various probabilities of misclassification at any given value are shown in Table 2. If for example one finds a discriminant function value of say −0.40 for a certain patient, then you can see that the probability of misclassification is 0 % for KCS Sjoegren, and for KCS-non Sjoegren 100 %, which strongly suggests that the dry eye state is associated with systemic involvement. For low values the reverse is true. You can also see that for intermediate values the association is not very close.

There is an immunohistological basis for our findings. Gillette et al. [17] demonstrated that lactoferrin was secreted in the acini but not in the tubuli. Tear fluid is also secreted for the most part in the acini, and it stands to reason that the break-up time has a relation to the tear protein concentration, secreted for about 70 % in the acini. There is also some histopathological basis for our findings. Chomette et al. [18] demonstrated that in Sjoegren's disease the lacrimal acini were destroyed early. Therefore, the lactoferrin tear fluid concentration, the Schirmer values and the break-up time analysed together can be of some help to differentiate between the Sjoegren and the non-Sjoegren patients in the dry eye state.

Table 2. The probabilities of misclassifying a patient with KCS with (*KCS-SJ*) and without (*KCS-NSJ*) associated Sjoegren's syndrome at various discriminant function values

KCS-SJ	Patients	KCS-NSJ
	Discriminant function value	
Probability of misclassification %	Equal or higher/ lower than	Probability of misclassification %
0	−0.40	100
20	−0.79	73
37	−1.19	33
53	−1.59	20
67	−1.99	3
73	−2.39	3
90	−2.79	0
100	−3.19	0

Summary

The clinical tests to diagnose keratoconjunctivitis sicca are weak, whereas the laboratory tests are very powerful, but there is no reason whatsoever to discard the present clinical tests. For example, finding a Schirmer test consistently lower than 5 mm is an easy way to strongly suspect a dry eye state. The level of tear fluid production can help one to determine the preferred viscosity of the tear substitute. Then: what test should be used other than the Rose bengal test to evaluate the over-all effect of the dry eye state on the external eye? What other test than the break-up time is there to evaluate tear film stability? There is no doubt that the laboratory tests will be used in the future as routine clinical procedures in addition to but not replacing the clinical tests, as the tear protein concentration, the Schirmer test values and the break-up time are important for the diagnosis of the dry eye state and, analysed together, they may be of value to differentiate between Sjoegren's and non-Sjoegren's keratoconjunctivitis sicca.

References

1. Schirmer O (1903) Studien zur Physiologie der Tränenabsonderung und Tränenabfuhr. Arch Ophthalmol 56: 197–291
2. Beetham WP (1935) Filamentary keratitis. Trans Am Acad Ophthalmol Soc 33: 413–417
3. van Bijsterveld OP (1969) Diagnostic tests in the sicca syndrome. Arch Ophthalmol 82: 10–14
4. Jones LT (1966) The lacrimal secretory system and its treatment. Am J Ophthalmol 62: 47–60

5. Norn MS (1973) Conjunctival sensitivity in normal eyes. Acta Ophthalmol 51: 58–66
6. Jordan A, Baum J (1980) Basic tearflow, does it exist? Ophthalmol 87: 920–930
7. Norn MS (1969) Dessication of the precorneal tear film. I Corneal wetting time. Acta Ophthalmol 47: 865–880
8. Fleming A (1922) On a remarkable bacteriolytic element found in tissues and secretions. Proc Soc Lond (B) 93: 306–317
9. Broekhuyse RM (1974) Tear lactoferrin: a bacteriostatic and complexing protein. Invest Ophthalmol 13: 550–554
10. Josephson AS, Wald A (1969) Enhancement of lysozyme activity by anodal tear protein. Proc Soc Exp Biol Med 131: 677–679
11. Janssen PT, van Bijsterveld OP (1983) The relations between tear fluid concentrations of lysozyme, tear-specific prealbumin and lactoferrin, Exp Eye Res 36: 773–779
12. Regan EF (1950) The lysozyme content of tears. Am J Ophthalmol 33: 600–605
13. Bonavida B, Sapse AT (1968) Human tear lysozyme: II Quantitative determination with standard Schirmer strips. Am J Ophthalmol 66: 70–76
14. Janssen PT, van Bijsterveld OP (1983) A simple test for lacrimal gland function: a tear lactoferrin assay by radial immunodiffusion. Graefe's Arch Clin Exp Ophthalmol 220: 171–174
15. Boersma MHG, van Bijsterveld OP (1987) The lactoferrin test for the diagnosis of keratoconjunctivitis sicca in clinical practice. Ann Ophthalmol 19: 152–154
16. Janssen PT, van Bijsterveld OP (1983) Origin and biosynthesis of human tear fluid proteins. Invest Ophthalmol 24: 623–630
17. Gillette TE, Allensmith MR, Greiner JV, Janusz M (1980) Histologic and immunohistologic comparison of main and accessory lacrimal tissue. Am J Ophthalmol 89: 724–730
18. Chomette G, Auriol M, Liotet S (1986) Ultrastructural study of the lacrimal gland in a case of Sjoegren's syndrome. Scand J Rheumatol (Suppl) 61: 71–75

Corresponding Address

O. P. van Bijsterveld, M.D., Ph.D.
Department of Ophthalmology, University Eye Hospital Utrecht.
P.O. Box 85500, NL-3508 G.A.-Utrecht, Niederlande

Changes in the Diagnostic Parameters During Keratoconjunctivitis Sicca (KCS) Therapy

N. Klaassen-Broekema and O. P. van Bijsterveld

Summary

In 35 patients with mild, moderate and severe Keratoconjunctivitis sicca (KCS) an association was found between treatment effect, break-up time value and Rose bengal score. Neither of these tests, used separately, was succesful as a clinically valuable predictor of treatment effect as the scatter, in score points, was too large. Analyzed together, however, as in a partial regression analysis, an adequate prediction is possible, which is clinically of some value.

Introduction

Selecting an optimal local treatment for any patient suffering from kerato-conjunctivitis sicca (KCS) is usually a matter of trial and error. This can be very frustrating for both, patient and doctor. We therefore, analyzed the changes in the diagnostic tests, such as the Schirmer test, the tearfluid lysozymeconcentration, the tearfilm break up time (BUT) and the Rose bengal (Rb) staining score during therapy with a non-fatty elastic carbopolymere tear substitute in 35 patients. The aim of this study was to develop a model to predict the subjective treatment effect of one particular therapy in any given patient with KCS.

Materials and Methods

35 patients, 29 males and 6 females suffering from KCS with an average age of 56.8 years, ranging from 30 to 78 years, were studied. After a complete routine ophthalmological examination, tear function tests were performed in all patients in the unanaesthetized eye before treatment and after 12 weeks of treatment. The treatment consisted of a non-fatty elastic carbopolymere with a dosage regimen of 1 drop in each eye 4 times a day or less if so desired. At the end of the treatment period the patient was asked to report the effect of the teargel: treatment gain was scored from + 1 to +5, treatment loss from −1 to −5.

Gramer/Kampik (Hrsg.) Pharmakotherapie am Auge
© Springer-Verlag Berlin Heidelberg 1992

The Schirmer test [1, 2] was carried out, using filter-paper strips of 5 × 35 mm (Whatman no. 41). The wetting of the strip was recorded after 5 minutes. Tear samples to estimate the tearfluid lysozyme concentration by the agar diffusion method [3, 4] were obtained by inserting a sterile Whatman no. 3 filter paper disc of 6 mm diameter in the cul-de-sac of the eye.

The break-up time of the tearfilm was determined according to the method of Norn [5]. Rose bengal in a 1 % solution was used to study the degree of corneal and conjunctival staining of the epithelium [3]. The intensity of staining of both medial and lateral conjunctiva and the cornea was scored, each section up to three points, so that a maximum score of nine could be obtained.

As we found no significant differences in tear function parameters between the right and the left eye, the values of the results of all tests of both eyes were averaged for a better estimate.

Results

In Fig. 1 the treatment effect expressed in patient scores is shown. It appeared that 25 patients (71 %) showed a subjective improvement, 6 patients (17 %) mentioned an increase in ocular discomfort after therapy, while 4 patients (11 %) didn't report any change at all.

In Table 1 the tear function parameters of the patient group before and after treatment are summarized. There was statistically no significant difference between pretreatment and posttreatment values of both the values

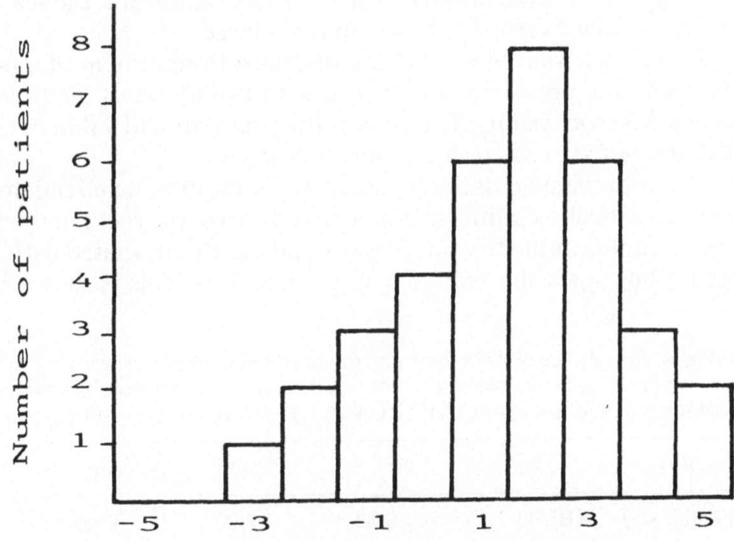

Fig. 1. The number of patients with the specified treatment gain or loss after twelve weeks of treatment

Table 1. Average values of tests with standard deviations at the beginning and after 12 weeks of treatment. OD and OS are averaged

Parameter	Treatment	Beginning (0)	End (12)	Sig.
Lysozyme[a]	Average	19.2	19.9	NS
	SD(n-1)	5.0	5.0	
Schirmer[b]	Average	6.4	4.8	NS
	SD(n-1)	9.3	7.5	
Break-up time[c]	Average	3.3	5.4	P<0.01
	SD (n-1)	2.9	3.1	
Rose bengal score[d]	Average	4.3	3.1	P<0.01
	SD(n-1)	2.3	1,7	

[a] Tearfluid concentration mm diameter lysis.
[b] mm wetting of the filterpaper strip in 5 minutes.
[c] In seconds.
[d] Score.

of the Schirmer test and the tearfluid lysozyme concentration, inspite of the fact that on the average there was statistically a significant amelioration of the eye condition.

Statistically a significant improvement of both the BUT and the Rb staining score after twelve weeks of therapy was found. The improvement in the BUT during treatment was significantly correlated with the treatment effect. Also, the time of the tearfilm break-up at the beginning of the treatment trial was significantly associated with treatment gain. This is shown in Table 2. Although these associations are statistically significant, the scatter, expressed in the standard error of the estimate is large.

Thus, if we want to predict the response to treatment of a new patient on the basis of a pretreatment BUT, one in twenty times the prediction can be wrong 3.5 score points. This makes the pretreatment value of the BUT alone unsuitable for prediction in clinical practice.

The improvement of the Rb score under treatment and the treatment effect were statistically significantly associated. Also, the score in the Rb staining at the beginning of the treatment was significantly associated with the treatment effect, but again the scatter is large: i.e. 3.09. This is shown in Table 3.

Table 2. *Row 1:* The relation between the improvement of the break-up time (d. BUT) and the treatment gain (d. subj. sc.). *Row 2:* The relation between the break-up time at the beginning of the treatment trial (BUT 0) and the treatment gain (d. subj. sc.)

y = f(x)	r	t(33)	Sig.	2Sy
d (subj. sc.) * d(BUT)	0.33	2.02	P<0.06	3.63
d (subj. sc.) * BUT(0)	−0.42	2.64	P<0.02	3.50

Table 3. *Row 1:* The relation between the improvement of the Rose bengal score (d. Rb) and the treatment gain (d. subj. sc.). *Row 2:* The relation between the Rose bengal score at the beginning of the treatment trial (Rb 0) and the treatment gain (d. subj. sc.)

y = f(x)	r	t(33)	Sig.	2Sy
d (subj. sc.) * d(Rb)	−0.92	13.1	P<0.001	1.55
d (subj. sc.) * Rb(0)	0.60	4.27	P<0.001	3.09

So, it appeared that neither the BUT nor the Rb score at the beginning of the treatment, are of clinical value as predictors for treatment effect. Although the break-up time and the Rose bengal score are non-homogenous data, there is a good correlation between these two parameters: $r=-0.41$; $t(33)=3.73$, P <0.001. Therefore, a more reliable prediction can be made if both parameters are analyzed together as in a partial regression analysis. For any individual patient the predicted treatment effect, expressed in patient score can be calculated from the following formula:

$$Y(c) = \{0.45 * BUT(0)\} - \{0.12 * Rb(0)\} - 0.03$$

If this prediction would be of clinical value, than of course the observed treatment effect should be associated with the predicted treatment effect, and this we found: $r=0.60$, $t(33)=4,35$, P<0.001, 2 Sy=1.8. As the scatter, using both parameters, is small, the prediction has practical value: if the maximal treatment gain or loss is 5 score points the prediction is wrong 1.8 points once in twenty times.

Discussion

After 12 weeks of treatment the majority of our patients reported an improvement of their eye symptoms, but the amount of amelioration differed markedly between the patients. Laboratory tests for the diagnosis of KCS, such as the Schirmer test and tearfluid lysozyme concentration, reflect the acinar and tubular function of the teargland and have an excellent discriminatory ability, but they do not have an immediate relation to the degree of ocular discomfort. Therefore, it is not surprising that measurements of tearprotein concentrations and Schirmer values are not useful in predicting the effect of treatment.

On the other hand, the tear film break up time and the Rose bengal staining score have an association with superficial eye disease due to teargland deficiency, and therefore have a direct relation to ocular discomfort. In this model we demonstrated for one particular treatment the possibility to make an adequate prediction concerning treatment effect on the basis of both the break-up time and the Rose bengal score. An effort should be made to explore models for other artificial tears, which allows the physician not only to predict the treatment gain, but helps him to select the optimal treatment.

References

1. Schirmer O (1903) Studien zur Physiologie und Pathologie der Tränenabsonderung und Tränenabfuhr. Graefe's Arch Ophthalmol 56: 197–291
2. Marquardt R (1982) Der Schirmer-Test zur Prüfung der Tränensekretion. In: Marquardt R (ed) Chronische Conjunctivitis – Trockenes Auge. Springer, Wien New York, pp 136–138
3. van Bijsterveld OP (1969) Diagnostic tests in the sicca syndrome. Arch Ophthal 82: 10–14
4. van Bijsterveld OP (1974) Standardisation of the lysozyme test for a commercially available medium. Its use for the diagnosis of the sicca syndrome. Arch Ophthal 91: 432–434
5. Norn MS (1977) Outflow of tears and its influence on tear secretion and break up time. Acta Ophthalmol 55: 674–682

Corresponding Address

N. Klaassen-Broekema, M.D.
University Hospital Utrecht, Department of Ophthalmology, P.O. Box 85500,
NL-3508 G.A.-Utrecht, Niederlande

Behandlungsstrategien des trockenen Auges

R. Marquardt

Einleitung

Die Behandlung sogenannter „trockener Augen", d.h. Augen mit patholo-
gischer Zusammensetzung des Tränenfilms und/oder zu wenig Tränenflüssigkeit ist in den letzten Jahren immer bedeutungsvoller geworden. Dies zum
einen, weil die Zahl daran Erkrankter in den letzten Jahrzehnten immer mehr
zugenommen hat, zum anderen weil die Therapie eines Dryeye-Syndroms in
den meisten Fällen unbefriedigend ist, weil es bislang kein effizientes
Medikament gibt, das eine erloschene oder herabgesetzte Tränensekretion
befriedigend anfacht, und wir bislang in den meisten Fällen auf Substitutionspräparate angewiesen sind.

Ursachen des trockenen Auges

Das trockene Auge ist vielfach Teil- oder Endstadium zahlreicher, meistens
chronischer Augenkrankheiten. Kenntnis und Verlauf der verschiedenarti-
gen krankhaften Veränderungen, die ein trockenes Auge auslösen oder
unterhalten, sind daher Grundvoraussetzung sämtlicher Behandlungsstrate-
gien, denn gelingt es, die dem trockenen Auge zugrundeliegende Störung
auszuschalten oder das auslösende Grundleiden auszuheilen, so erspart man
sich die belastende Langzeittherapie mit Substitutionspräparaten.

Die Ursachen eines trockenen Auges sind vielartig. Das wichtigsten sind:

- Angeborener Mangel an Tränenflüssigkeit
- Erkrankungen oder Schädigungen, die zu Schrumpfungen oder Narben-
  bildungen der Bindehaut geführt haben
- Stellungsanomalien der Lider
- Lidschlußinsuffizienz
- Chronische Conjunctivitiden verschiedenster Genese
- Langzeiteinwirkung toxischer Substanzen
    berufliche Exposition
    Umweltverschmutzung
    Konservierungsmittel in Augenmedikamenten

Gramer/Kampik (Hrsg.) Pharmakotherapie am Auge
© Springer-Verlag Berlin Heidelberg 1992

- Senile Involution der tränenbildenden Drüsen
- Folgen von Allgemeinerkrankungen
- Nebenwirkungen von Medikamenten
- A-Avitaminose

Diese Vielzahl möglicher Ursachen eines trockenen Auges veranschaulicht wie wichtig es ist, stets mit einer gründlichen und gezielten Anamnese die Behandlung zu beginnen. Ebenso wichtig ist die Analyse möglicher Störfaktoren welche den Tränenfilm verändert haben. Hierzu verhelfen uns die zahlreichen diagnostischen Maßnahmen, die uns Prof. van Bijsterveld so anschaulich dargestellt hat.

Behandlung des Grundleidens

Die Behandlung des Grundleidens führt leider nicht immer zum gewünschten Erfolg. Ist die Ursache z.B. eine chronische allergische Erkrankung, so gelingt es gelegentlich mittels Testung das Allergen zu finden und zu eleminieren, beziehungsweise durch gezielte Hyposensibilisierung eine entscheidende Besserung herbeizuführen. Am Auge kommen als Allergene besonders Kosmetika, Reinigungsmittel von Contactlinsen, ebenso aber auch Konservierungsmittel in Augenmedikamenten in Frage. Handelt es sich andererseits um eine Medikamentennebenwirkung, so sollte in Zusammenarbeit mit dem behandelnden Arzt das auslösende Medikament durch ein anderes ersetzt werden. Ähnliches gilt für chemische Schadstoffe.

Der Tabelle 1 ist zu entnehmen, daß sich zahlreiche Ursachen operativ beseitigen lassen. Hierher gehören die Lidschlußinsuffizienz, zum einen infolge Facialisparese, zum anderen bedingt durch Stellungsanomalien oder Kolobome der Lider. Nicht selten führen auch Tumore, ebenso Narben an Lidern und Bindehaut zum trockenen Auge. Eine weite Lidspalte, ein seltener Lidschlag, eine Lidschlußinsuffizienz durch Exophthalmus bedingen bei fortgeschrittener Hyperthyreose eine vermehrte Austrocknung des praecornealen Tränenfilms. Letztlich seien die Trichiasis sowie Unregelmäßigkeiten der Hornhautoberfläche erwähnt.

Tabelle 1. Operativ beeinflußbare Ursachen des „trockenen" Auges

- Lidschlußinsuffizienz
- Stellungsanomalien der Lider
- Traumatische Kolobome der Lider
- Weite Lidspalte
- Tumoren der Lider
- Tumoren der Bindehaut
- Narbenbildungen der Bindehaut
- Trichiasis
- Unregelmäßigkeiten der Hornhautoberfläche

Tabelle 2. Willentlich beeinflußbare Ursachen des trockenen Auges (unvollständiger, seltener Lidschlag)

– Neuroparalytische Keratitis
– Schilddrüsenüberfunktion
– (Stellwag'sches Zeichen)
– Parkinsonismus
– Senile Demenz
– Stammhirnschädigungen
– (Exophthalmus)

Eine zweite kleine Gruppe (Tabelle 2) umfaßt die wenigen Erkrankungen, die zu einem unvollständigen und/oder seltenen Lidschlag führen und bei denen die Symptome des trockenen Auges zumindest teilweise durch kontrolliertes Blinken positiv beeinflußt werden können. Hierzu gehören in erster Linie die neuroparalytische Keratitis, bei der in Folge einer Störung der Neurotrophik der Abwehrblinkreflex weitgehend aufgehoben ist. Hierzu zählen auch die Basedow'sche Erkrankung (Stellwag'sches Zeichen), der Parkinsonismus, die senile Demenz, ferner Stammhirnschädigungen und zu einem gewissen Grad auch der Exophthalmus.

Beseitigung adjuvanter Störfaktoren

Als nächstes müssen Störfaktoren analysiert werden, die in der Regel ein trockenes Auge zwar nicht hervorrufen, wohl aber ein bestehendes richtungsweisend sowohl subjektiv als auch objektiv verschlechtern können.

Ganz allgemein sollten Patienten mit trockenem Auge möglichst im staubfreien Umfeld leben, weil sowohl Staub als auch Rauch insbesondere beim Fehlen der wäßrigen Kompomente des praecornealen Tränenfilms, den Ph-Wert am Auge so verändern, daß die Beschwerden ins Unerträgliche gesteigert werden. Dasselbe gilt, wenn die Luftfeuchtigkeit unter 50 % sinkt, was recht häufig in zentralgeheizten überhitzten Büros in den Wintermonaten gang und gäbe ist. Bedenkt man, daß schon der praecorneale Tränenfilm bei einem Gesunden bei geöffnetem Auge innerhalb von 10 Sekunden von 10 auf 4 μ abnimmt, so wird verständlich, wie sehr eine erheblich herabgesetzte Luftfeuchtigkeit einen Patienten mit einem trockenen Auge belastet. Abhilfe schaffen hier Luftbefeuchter, von denen es zahlreiche Modelle im Handel gibt. Nicht unerwähnt lassen möchte ich auch die Gebläseheizungen gewisser Kraftfahrzeuge die, wenn die Warmluft auf das Gesicht gerichtet ist, ebenfalls zu einer nicht unerheblichen Austrocknung des äußeren Auges führen.

Als nächstes sei die Astenopie erwähnt. Sei es nun eine Ametropie oder Phorie, die neben einem Druck- und Schweregefühl in der Regel Kopfschmerzen und Sehstörung bewirken, von denen letztere insbesondere im Laufe des Tages zunehmen. Wir wissen, daß derartige Störungen der beidäugigen Zusammenarbeit sich ebenfalls beim trockenen Auge negativ auswirken.

Erwähnen möchte ich ferner den negativen Einfluß aller Konservierungsmittel in Augenmedikamenten. Diese Problematik beschäftigt uns insbesondere in den letzten Jahren in zunehmendem Maße.

Gelingt uns die Elimination derartiger Störfaktoren, so ist damit einem Patienten mit einem trockenen Auge mitunter schon entscheidend geholfen.

Medikamentöse Therapie

Allgemein

Wenn es nicht gelingt, die Ursache einer Benetzungsstörung der Augen zu beseitigen, so muß medikamentös eingegriffen werden, was leider in den meisten Fällen von trockem Auge der Fall ist. Die zahlreichen unterschiedlichen Erkrankungsgruppen sind der Tabelle 3 zu entnehmen. Es handelt sich dabei um angeborene Störungen, Erkrankungen die zu Bindehautschrumpfungen geführt haben und schließlich auch um Symptome von Allgemeinerkrankungen. Besonders hervorzuheben sind langzeitige Einwirkungen toxischer Substanzen, die gerade in den letzten Jahren in Industrienationen zunehmend chronische Bindehautentzündugnen hervorrufen bzw. unterhalten. Hierher gehört auch unsere Umweltverschmutzung, besonders an dazu exponierten Orten, in zunehmendem Maße auch berufliche Exposition. Wir müssen auch daran denken, daß eine langzeitige Einnahme gewisser Medikamente zum trockenen Auge führen kann. Außerdem führen zahlreiche chronisch-allergische Erkrankungen zum trockenen·Auge. Gelegentlich kann dies schon durch die senile Involution der tränenbildenen Drüsen verursacht werden.

Um hiergegen einzugreifen stehen folgende medikamentöse Behandlungsprinzipien zur Verfügung:

1. Medikamentöse Stimulation der Tränenproduktion
2. Substitution
3. Protektion

Stimulation

In die Therapie des trockenen Auges haben zwei Substanzen, das Bromhexin und Eledoisin zur Anregung der Tränensekretion Eingang gefunden. Von vorneherein sei jedoch festgestellt, daß derartige, die Sekretion anregende Medikamente nur wirken können, wenn genügend funktionsfähiges Drüsengewebe vorhanden ist. Kein Medikament kann eine atrophierte Drüse wieder zur Sekretion anregen! Dies gilt auch für sogenannte Hausmittel wie das Zwiebelschneiden oder die Prise Schnupftabak.

Tabelle 3. Vorwiegend durch Substitution der Tränenflüssigkeit beeinflußbare Störungen, die zum trockenen Auge führten

1. Angeborene Erkrankungen
   Aplasie oder Hypoplasie der Tränendrüse
   (Riley-Day-Syndrom)

2. Erkrankungen die zu Bindehautschrumpfungen führten
   Erythema multiforme
   (Stevens-Johnson-Syndrom)
   Oculäres Pemphigoid
   Trachom
   Thermische, chemische, strahlenbedingte
   Schädigungen

3. Symptom einer Allgemeinerkrankung
   Rheumatische Arthritis
   Morbus Reiter
   (Sjögren-Syndrom)
   Sarkoidose
   Vitamin-A-Avitaminose (Xerophthalmie)
   Diabetes mellitus
   Sklerodermie

4. Langzeitige Einwirkung toxischer Substanzen
   Umweltverschmutzung
   Berufliche Exposition
   Medikamente
   Konservierungsmittel in Augentropfen
   Reinigungsmittel von Kontaktlinsen
   (Narkose)

5. Chronisch-allergisch
   Blepharoconjunctivitis (Rosazea)
   Frühjahrsconjunctivitis
   Chronische Ekzeme

6. Altersbedingt
   Senile Involution der tränenbildenden Drüsen und der Bindehaut

7. Chronische Conjunctivitis anderer Ätiologie
   bakteriell
   virusbedingt

8. Endokrine Dysfunktionen
   Klimakterium
   Ovulationshemmer

Bromhexin, das ursprünglich in der inneren Medizin systemisch zur Behandlung von Bronchialerkrankungen eingesetzt wurde, fand als 0,2 %ige wäßrige Lösung Eingang in die Behandlung des trockenen Auges. Die Behandlungsergebnisse über therapeutische Erfolge bei krankhaft verminderter Tränensekretion sind jedoch widersprüchlich. Hinzu kommt, daß das Medikament einerseits teuer ist, zum anderen bei Anwendung stark brennt. Dies dokumentiert, weshalb diese Substanz bislang keine breite Anwendung bei der Therapie des trockenen Auges finden konnte.

Eledoisin gehört zur Gruppe der Polypeptide. Diese Substanz wurde ursprünglich wegen ihrer Blutdrucksenkung durch periphere Vasodilatation bekannt. Eine dabei festgestellte gesteigerte Tränensekretion war zunächst ein lästiger Nebeneffekt. Rasch wurde jedoch erkannt, daß mit diesem Medikament insbesondere schwere Verlaufsformen des trockenen Auges günstig beeinflußt werden können. Zusammen mit den Augenkliniken Heidelberg und Köln haben wir an einer prospektiven randomisierten Studie teilgenommen um die Wirksamkeit dieser Substanz bei Keratokonjunktivitis sicca zu prüfen. Eine topische Anwendung von 3× tägl. 1 Tropfen brachte insbesondere bei schweren und hoffnungslosen Verlaufsformen, bei denen andere Medikamente versagten, gute Erfolge.

Substitution

Gelingt es nicht ein trockenes Auge durch Beseitigung der Ursachen bzw. Anregung der Sekretion positiv zu beeinflussen, so bleibt als nächste therapeutische Maßnahme die Substitution. Diese richtet sich danach, welche Bestandteile des Tränenfilms die Störung hervorgerufen haben. Beim trockenen Auge führen in der Regel entweder das Fehlen der wäßrigen und/oder mukösen Phase zum Zusammenbruch des praecornealen Tränenfilms zwischen den einzelnen Blinkintervallen. Liegt es an der mukösen Phase, so wird die hydrophobe Oberfläche der Hornhaut nicht mehr ausreichend von Mucinen, die die Hornhautoberfläche für die Tränenflüssigkeit erst benetzbar machen, bedeckt und geschützt. Die Folge ist, der Tränenfilm bricht auf, was die subjektiven Symptome des trockenen Auges hervorruft und erst ein erneutes Blinken vermag den Schaden vorübergehend zu beseitigen.

Fehlt es an der wäßrigen Komponente, so trocknet der Tränenfilm zu rasch aus, was letztlich zu derselben Symptomatik führt.

Entsprechend müssen wäßrige Lösungen visköser Substanzen dem pathologisch veränderten Tränenfilm zugeführt werden, um den gestörten physiologischen Tränenfilm auf der Hornhautoberfläche so gut als möglich zu normalisieren.

Das Hauptproblem, das auch bis heute noch nicht gelöst werden konnte ist, eine Substanz zu finden, die einerseits neben einer guten Verträglichkeit eine hohe Oberflächenstabilität und damit eine lange Verweildauer auf der Hornhaut hat, die andererseits aber wiederum nicht zu viskös sein darf, weil sonst die Sehschärfe negativ beeinflußt würde.

An ein ideales Tränenersatzmittel müssen folgende Anforderungen gestellt werden:

1. Es muß gut verträglich sein
2. Es darf nicht toxisch sein
3. Es muß beliebig häufig angewandt werden können
4. Es muß von der Hornhautoberfläche absorbiert werden um diese hydrophil zu machen

5. Es muß eine lange Verweildauer haben
6. Es darf die Optik des Auges nicht beeinflussen
7. Es darf die Tränensekretion, Schleimproduktion und Sekretion der Lidranddrüsen nicht behindern
8. Es darf keinen negativen Einfluß auf den Stoffwechsel der Hornhaut haben
9. Es darf die äußerste Lipidschicht des Tränenfilms nicht emulgieren
10. Es muß neutral sein
11. Es darf keine Fremdzusätze wie z.B. störende Konsiervierungsstoffe haben.

Substitutionstherapie durch Polymere. Wässrige Lösungen von Polymeren haben bisher am ehesten die Anforderungen, die an ein Netzmittel gestellt werden müssen, nämlich Hydrophilisierung der Hornhautoberfläche und vertretbare Verweildauer am Auge erfüllt. Es handelt sich um folgende Polymere:

1. Halbsynthetische Zellulosederivate als viskositätserhöhende Zusätze in 0,5 bis 1 %iger wäßriger Lösung
2. Polyvinylalkohol, Polyvinylpyrrolidon in 1,4 %iger wäßriger Lösung
3. Polyakrylsäureabkömmlinge als Tropfgele
4. Hyaluronsäure in 0,1 % bis 0,2 %iger wäßriger Lösung

Bei all diesen mehr oder weniger viskösen Lösungen muß stets bedacht werden, daß ihre Viskosität in Grenzen bleibt, weil sonst ab einer gewissen Konzentration die Sehfunktion negativ beeinflußt wird. Hieran kranken nahezu alle einschlägigen Präparate. Sie setzen zwar die Oberflächenspannung der Tränenflüssigkeit herab, verdicken und stabilisieren den Tränenfilm, haben wegen ihrer geringen Viskosität jedoch nur eine begrenzte Verweildauer am Auge. Dies wirkt sich besonders bei den Patienten negativ aus, die schwere und schwerste Benetzungsstörungen haben.

Einen gewissen Vorteil hiergegen bringen gelartige Tränenersatzmittel. Ein derartiges tropffähiges gelartiges Tränenersatzmittel, ein Akrylsäurepolymerisat, wurde von uns 1985 getestet. Neben einer guten Verträglichkeit und Verteilung auf Binde- und Hornhaut fanden wir eine um den Faktor 7 verlängerte Verweildauer am Auge gegenüber einem Tränenersatzmittel auf Polyvinylalkoholbasis. Damit ließ sich die Tropffrequenz insbesondere für Patienten mit schwereren Benutzungsstörungen auf eine 3, allenfalls 4-malige Anwendung in 24 Stunden reduzieren.

Als eine weitere Therapieform mit langer Verweildauer erwiesen sich sogen. *Inserte.* Es sind dies kleine solide, aber noch weiche Polymere, die in den Bindehautsack eingeführt werden und sich unter kontinuierlicher Befeuchtung durch die Resttränenflüssigkeit innerhalb von Stunden auflösen. Derartige Inserte, die insbesondere in den USA einen festen Platz in der Therapie gefunden haben, bei uns jedoch bislang nicht zugelassen sind, werden insbesondere von Patienten mit schwerergradiger Keratoconjunctivitis bevorzugt. Ein weiterer Vorteil der Inserte ist, daß sie kein Konservierungsmittel enthalten. Sie sind durch Bestrahlung keimfrei gemacht und einzeln verpackt.

Viskoelastische Substanzen. In diese Gruppe gehört die *Hyaluronsäure*, ein Glycosaminoglykan, eine organische Substanz, die nahezu in allen Geweben von Wirbeltieren vorkommt und kommerziell aus den Kämmen von Hähnen heute gewonnen wird. Diese viskoelastische Substanz, die chemisch inert und auch bei Langzeitanwendung nicht toxisch ist, wird heute weltweit in der Cataractchirurgie angewandt. In der Therapie des trockenen Auges fand eine 0,1 %ige wäßrige Lösung dieser Substanz Eingang. Leider erwies sich auch bei dieser Substanz die Verweildauer am Auge ähnlich derer anderer handelsüblicher Augentropfen, wobei der hohe Preis dieser Substanz bislang eine breite Anwendung verhinderte.

Ähnliche Ergebnisse erhielt man mit einer weiteren viskoelastischen Substanz, dem *Chontoitinsulfat*. Ich möchte diese Substanz nur erwähnen, bislang ist kein diesbezügliches Präparat in Handel.

Als weitere therapeutische Maßnahmen kommen in Frage:

Operative Maßnahmen

Verschluß der tränenableitenden Wege

Insbesondere in fortgeschrittenen Fällen von trockenem Auge kann durch vorübergehenden oder permanenten Verschluß der ableitenden Tränenwege der Tränenabfluß blockiert werden, was sowohl subjektiv als auch objektiv Besserung bringen kann. Dem stehen allerdings die Untersuchungsergebnisse von Norn entgegen, der fand, daß eine Behinderung des Tränenabflusses sich negativ auf die Tränensekretion auswirkt. Da diese Behandlungsmethode erfahrungsgemäß bislang nicht immer zum Erfolg führt, sollte zuerst durch einen vorübergehenden Verschluß mittels Kunststoffplomben die Wirksamkeit erprobt werden, ehe durch Elektrokoagulation, die derzeitige Methode der Wahl, eine verstümmelnde Maßnahme angewandt wird.

Transplantation des Parotisausführungsganges

Bei diesem Verfahren wird der Stenon'sche Gang der Glandula parotis in die untere Übergangsfalte der Bindehaut verpflanzt. Es liegen hierüber nur wenige Berichte vor, zumal dieses Verfahren allenfalls in verzweifelten Fällen Anwendung finden kann. Hier ist insbesondere zum Nachteil, daß diese Drüse etwa 1 l Speichel sezerniert und das Auge auch ständig agressiven Fermenten des Speichels ausgesetzt ist.

Tarsorrhaphie

Mit diesem einfachen Operationsverfahren wird die Lidspalte verkleinert und so die der Außenwelt ausgesetzte Tränenfläche verkleinert.

Anderweitige Hilfsmittel und Verfahren

Schutzgläser und feuchte Kammern

sind insbesondere als adjuvante Maßnahmen indiziert, wenn durch Substitutionspräparate alleinig keine Kompensation erreicht werden kann. Hierzu seien auch sogen. Infusionssysteme genannt, mit denen über eine kleine motorgetriebene Pumpe kontinuierlich Flüssigkeit, die im Bügel einer Brille enthalten ist, dem Auge zugeführt wird. Dieses Verfahren kann allenfalls in verzweifelten Fällen Linderung bringen, zumal ein solches Verfahren ein hohes Infektionsrisiko besitzt.

Kontaktlinsen

Nicht unerwähnt sollen *Kontaktlinsen* bleiben. Sie können am besten in Verbindung mit Tränenersatzflüssigkeit in ausgeprägten Fällen von trockenem Auge von Nutzen sein.

Legt man am Ende dieses Übersichtsreferates allem Erwähnten den aus der ärztlichen Erfahrung resultierenden Satz zugrunde: „Gibt es zur Behandlung eines Leidens 100 Behandlungsverfahren, so wirkt keines optimal", so müssen wir uns auch eingestehen, daß es bislang zur Behandlung des trockenen Auges keine optimale Therapie gibt, sondern das augenärztliche Wissen und die augenärztliche Erfahrung aus den gegebenen therapeutischen Möglichkeiten das für den Erkrankten optimale Behandlungsschema auszusuchen und zusammenstellen muß.

Zusammenfassung

Die Ursachen eines „Trockenen Auges" sind vielartig. Vor Beginn jedweder Therapie gegen dieses immer häufiger werdende Leiden muß mit einer gezielten Anamnese nach möglichen Ursachen gefahndet werden. Ist die Ursache allergischer oder toxischer Natur (z.B. Konservierungsmittel), so läßt sich durch Behandlung des Grundleidens oder Elimination des Schadstoffes mehr erreichen als mit einer rein symptomatischen Behandlung. Ebenso nötig ist die Beseitigung adjuvanter Störfaktoren.

Die medikamentöse Therapie gegen das trockene Auge ist vorwiegend symptomatisch und beruht, wenn eine Stimulation der tränenbildenden Gewebe versagt, auf der Substitution durch wäßrige Lösungen von Polymeren oder viskoelastischen Substanzen, deren Wirkung wegen der ungünstigen Relation von Viskosität zur Verweildauer begrenzt ist. Als weitere, oft adjuvante therapeutische Maßnahmen kommen ein Verschluß der tränenableitenden Wege, eine Tarsorrhaphie, die Transplantation des Parotisausführungsganges, Schutzgläser, feuchte Kammern und hochhydrophile Kontaktlinsen in Frage.

Literatur beim Verfasser

Korrespondenzadresse
Professor Dr. med. R. Marquardt
Direktor der Universitätsaugenklinik Ulm, Prittwitzstr. 43, D-7900 Ulm

Microbial Contamination of In-Use Ocular Medications

K.R. Kenyon, T. Starck, P.L. Hibberd, O.D. Schein,
and A.S. Baker

Abstract

Two hundred twenty in-use medications from 101 patients with non-microbial ocular surface disease were studied by sterile culture of the bottle caps, a drop produced by simple inversion, and the interior contents. Conjunctival cultures were taken from these patients and 50 aged-matched controls. Pathogenic organisms were harvested from conjunctivae significantly more frequently (p < 0.01) from cases (34%) than from controls (10%). Twenty-nine percent of medications had microorganisms cultured from at least one medication site. Gram negative organisms were significantly more likely (p < 0.00001) to be isolated from all medication sites than gram positive organisms. Forty-nine percent of the gram negatives, but none of the pathogenic gram positives (p < 0.01), isolated from the conjunctivae were also found in the drops of their associated medications. We conclude that this cycle of contamination between in-use medications and conjunctivae may represent an important risk factor for microbial keratitis in patients with ocular surface disease.

Introduction

Microbial keratitis, except in the specific setting of soft contact lens wear, is predominantly associated with gram positive organisms, principally staphylococci and streptococci that are prevalent on the eyelids and conjunctiva and that opportunistically invade the corneal stroma through breaks in the epithelium [1]. Yet, in a recent extensive review of microbial keratitis at the Massachusetts Eye & Ear Infirmary, among the corneal ulcers not related to contact lens wear, gram negative organisms accounted for one-third of cases [2]. The origin of these gram negative organisms was not usually evident. Moreover, Schein and associates have recently collected 7 cases of severe gram negative keratitis where the same organism was cultured from both the cornea and the topical ocular medications concurrently in use by these patients [3]. In all instances, antibiograms by Kirby-Bauer disc sensitivities were identical for the corneal and topical medication isolates. Importantly, 6 positive cultures were from timolol maleate and one from prednisone acetate.

Gramer/Kampik (Hrsg) Pharmakotherapie am Auge
© Springer-Verlag Berlin Heidelberg 1992

Examples from this case series include a 75 year-old woman with longstanding angle closure glaucoma and bullous keratopathy who developed *Pseudomonas* corneoscleritis eventually requiring enucleation, and a patient with aphakic bullous keratopathy who also developed *Pseudomonas* corneoscleritis resulting in light perception vision. Disasters such as these highlight *Pseudomonas aeruginosa* as a major contaminant of ocular medications.

Templeton reported 3 cases of *Serratia marcescens* keratitis in 1982, where the organism was recovered from either the inside of the eyedropper cap or from the grooves of the bottle top [4]. Solutions cultured directly from the medication bottles were sterile. Marion and Tapert uncovered significant growth of pathogens from the outside and inside of approximately one-third of timolol maleate bottles in a glaucoma clinic population [5].

The origin of these bacteria remains obscure. While it might be argued that it is actually the ocular surface which harbors the bacterial microorganisms and contaminates the eye drops, in fact pseudomonal colonization of the conjunctiva is infrequent (1 % or less) and *Serratia* and *Proteus* are even more unusual in this setting [6, 7]. *Pseudomonas* and *Serratia* do not normally inhabit the skin. However both are commonly found in foodstuffs and in kitchens [8, 9]. *Pseudomonas* in particular has a predilection for moist environments like kitchens and bathrooms and has been cultured repeatedly from water supplies and faucets [10]. Hence it is perhaps not surprising that medications and contact lens solutions kept weeks at a time in a bathroom environment become contaminated with *Pseudomonas*.

The foregoing experiences heightened our concern about the source of these virulent gram negative organisms. Therefore we performed a prospective study to examine the bacteriology of the conjunctiva of patients using topical medications in comparison with controls using no medications in order: (1) to investigate the bacteriology and rate of contamination of in-use medications obtained from these patients, and (2) to determine the risk factors for contamination of topical medications.

Materials and Methods

The study involved 101 patients with noninfectious ocular surface diseases (49 unilateral, 52 bilateral) who had used topical medications for more than 2 months. Control subjects comprised 50 age-matched individuals not using medication. Conjunctival cultures were obtained from the retracted lower lid with a moistened cotton swab. The medications were cultured as follows: (1) a swab of the inside surface of the cap, (2) one drop from the bottle allowed to fall on the culture media, and (3) contents withdrawn sterilely with a syringe. Multiple media were used for each culture and growth on one or more solid media (except for anaerobes) was required for a culture to be considered positive. Concordance was defined as the same organisms being isolated from the conjunctiva and from the medications applied to that conjunctiva.

Risk factors for contamination and the use of medications were evaluated by observations of the patient during medication administration, by interview, and by chart review. The data analysis was assessed for continuous variables using an unpaired two sample t-test or analysis of variance, and for proportions, the chi square and Fisher exact tests.

Results

These 101 patients with ocular surface disease demonstrated the following active diagnoses: post-corneal transplant surgery 64 %, lid disease 19 %, dry eye 13 %, corneal edema 8 %, and other corneal epithelial disease 12 %. (Note that several patients had more than one active ocular surface disease.) A total of 220 medications were cultured, a mean of 2.2 per patient with a range of 1 to 6. Eye drops accounted for 71 % of the sample and ointments for 29 %. These specifically comprised steroids 34 %, antibiotics 29 %, lubricants 17 %, beta-blockers 14 %, and others 10 %.

The results of conjunctival cultures were noteworthy in disclosing that 60–75 % of the subjects had positive conjunctival cultures with no statistically significant difference between the in-use medication and the control groups (Table 1). However control eyes only rarely demonstrated a gram negative

Table 1. Conjunctival microbiology

	Patients with ocular surface disease (n=101)	Controls (n=50)
Gram positive		
Coagulase negative Staphylococci	51	21
Diphtheroids	15	17
S. aureus	14	1
Propionobacterium spp	3	–
Streptococcus spp	9	–
Gram negative		
Pseudomonas spp	3	2
Proteus spp	3	1
Klebsiella spp	1	–
Serratia spp	2	–
Enterobacter spp	1	–
Citrobacter spp	1	–
Acinetobacter	1	–
H. parainfluenza	1	–
Unidentified nonenteric Gram negative rods	2	–
Fungi		
Yeast	2	
Filamentous		1

[Total > 101 because more than one organism was cultured from the conjunctiva of 7 patients.]

organism on the conjunctiva, and importantly, once coagulase negative staphylocci and diptheroids were excluded, control eyes had significantly fewer positive conjunctival cultures than in-use medication eyes ($\sim 10\%$ vs. $\sim 34\%$; $p < 0.01$). Overall, medication cultures disclosed that 29% had at least one culture positive site, and caps were the most frequent site growing almost exclusively skin flora (Table 2). Nevertheless, despite excluding skin flora, the contribution of gram negative contamination to drops and/or contents was relatively large ($\sim 10\%$). Ocular lubricants, beta blockers and steroid drops exhibited the highest rate of contamination (Table 3).

We further examined the concordance of microorganisms cultured from the conjunctiva and from the medications. Forty-two patients (42%) had at least one medication which was contaminated, and of these, 28 (60%) had the same organism on the conjunctiva to which the contaminated medication was applied. Twenty-eight pathogenic organisms were isolated from the medications of 19 patients. Among these, 68% of the gram negative organisms but none of the gram positive organisms or fungi isolated from the medication contents were also found on the conjunctiva to which that medication was applied ($p < 0.01$). From the opposite perspective, 50 potential pathogens were isolated from the conjunctiva of 34 patients using ocular medications. Forty-eight percent of the gram negative organisms but none of the pathogenic gram positive or fungi isolated from the conjunctiva were also found in the medications which had been applied to these conjunctivas ($p < 0.001$).

Based on the observed application of drops and/or ointments, the patient interview and the chart review, the following were identified as risk factors for contamination at any site ($p < 0.05$): older age, increasing number of medications, ocular cicatricial disease, observed dropper contact with eye, eyelid or facial skin, observed spoilage of medication, and observed tremor. If

Table 2. Contamination of medications

	Drops $n=156$			Ointments $n=64$	
Any growth	45(29%)			17(27%)	
	Cap	Drop	Content	Cap	Content
Any growth	42(27%)	20(13%)	21(14%)	17(27%)	3(5%)
Coagulase negative staphylococci and diphtheroids	21(13%)	5 (3%)	2 (1%)	13(20%)	–
Other gram positive	5 (3%)	1(0.6%)	1(0.6%)	1(1.5%)	–
Gram negative	18(12%)	16 (10%)	18 (12%)	2 (3%)	1(1.5%)
Fungi	7 (5%)	4 (7%)	5 (3%)	6 (9%)	3 (5%)

Coagulase negative staphylococci and diphtheroids.

[Totals > 100% because multiple organisms were cultured from 8 medications and 26 medications had more than one site culture positive.]

Table 3. Medications with contaminated drops or contents

	Drops	*Ointments*
Steroids	8/73 (11%)	0/1 (0%)
Lubricants	7/24 (29%)	1/14 (7%)
Antibiotics	1/21 (5%)	2/43 (5%)
β Blockers	5/30 (17%)	–
Other*	2/18 (11%)	1/4 (25%)

[Total > 100% because 8 medications were combinations of steroid and antibiotic.]
* Miotics, mydriatics, vasoconstrictors, cromolyn-sodium, and vitamin A preparations.

one only considered contamination of bottle, drops and contents, observation of the dropper contact with eyelid, eye or face remained a significant association. The following potential risk factors were not associated with contamination: handwashing prior to administration of medication, location of medication storage, location where medication applied, duration of medication use, drops vs. ointments, and visual acuity.

Conclusions

The present study suggests a high rate of contamination of in-use ocular medications. There are several potential reservoirs of contamination, and bottled drops and contents may be the more importent sites. Importantly as gram negative organisms account for much of this contamination, the question of preservative efficacy must be considered. The ocular surface is likely to be colonized with the same gram negative organisms as are found in the contaminated medication. The dropper mechanism actually touching the eye, eyelid or face is a major risk factor for contamination. Such contamination by gram negative organisms may additionally comprise a significant risk factor for the development of microbial keratitis among patients with ocular surface diseases who are known to be at increased risk of infection.

What can be done to lessen contamination? Among the possible avenues which are probably best approached in combination, technologic modifications such as the use of pipette dispensers or unit dose administration and/or improved preservatives may prove important. Observation of patient habits and education of patients to avoid dropper contact with eye or periocular sites is seemingly straightforward. In patients who are at highest risk of microbial keratitis, such as those with ocular surface disease, possibly the periodic culture of medications, conjunctiva, and solutions on a surveillance basis is indicated. Such medical interventions and possibly the use of prophylactic antibiotics are worthy of consideration. Finally, in a patient who presents with suspected microbial keratitis, we strongly recommend that all topical medications and contact lens solutions be cultured. These measures may be helpful beyond the stage of initial diagnosis and treatment, as they may uncover inadequacies in medication delivery technique and/or contaminated solutions that place such patients at ongoing risk. Clearly the high prevalence of medication contamination, especially with virulent gram negative organisms, should increasingly prioritize such considerations by both physician providers and pharmaceutical manufacturers.

Acknowledgement. This work was supported by a research grant from Allergan pharmaceuticals, Irvine, CA, USA.

References

1. Fahmy JA, Moller S, Bentzon MW (1974) Bacterial flora of the normal conjunctiva I. Topographical distribution. Acta Ophthalmol 52: 786–800
2. Schein OD, Ormerod LD, Barraquer E et al (1989) Microbiology of contact lens-related keratitis. Cornea 8 (4): 281–285
3. Schein OD, Wasson PJ, Boruchorff SA, et al (1988) Microbial keratitis associated with ontaminated ocular medications. Am J Ophthalmol 105: 361–365
4. Templeton WC, Eiferman RA, SnyderJW, et al (1982) Serratia keratitis transmitted by contaminated eyedroppers. Am J Ophthalmol 93: 723–726
5. Marion AD, Tapert MJ (1986) Bacterial contamination of timolol in use by a non-selected clinic population. ARVO Abstracts. Invest Ophthalmol Vis Sci 26: 3
6. Hovding G (1981) The conjunctival and contact lens bacterial flora during lens wear, Acta Ophthalmol 59: 387
7. Rauschl RT, Rogers JJ (1978) The effect of hydrophilic contact lens wear on the bacterial flora of the human conjunctiva. Int Contact Lens Clin 5: 37
8. Remington JS, Schimpff SC (1981) Please don't eat salads. N Engl J Med 304: 433
9. Dainty RH (1985) Bacterial growth in food, a nutritionally rich environment. In: Fletcher MM, Floodgate GD (eds) Bacteria in their natural environment. Academic Press, Orlando, pp 171–188
10. Hoadley AW (1977) Potential health hazards with Pseudomonas aeruginosa. In: Hoadley AW, Dutka BJ (eds) Bacterial indicators-health hazards associated with water. ASTM STP 635. American Society for Testing and Materials, Philadelphia, pp 80–114

Corresponding Address
Professor K. R. Kenyon, M.D., FACS
Cornea Consultant, 100 Charles River Plaza, Boston, MA 02114, USA

Retina

Therapie der Endophthalmitis

H.-P. Heidenkummer und A. Kampik

Einleitung

Eine postoperative, posttraumatische oder endogene Endophthalmitis stellt trotz moderner Antibiotika eine gefürchtete ophthalmologische Komplikation dar. Nur rasches und gezieltes Handeln kann den Verlust der Funktion oder gar des Organs vermeiden. Unter Berücksichtigung weniger Grundsätze ist es jedoch möglich, die Diagnose klinisch zu stellen, die Ätiologie zu klären und die notwendigen therapeutischen Maßnahmen rechtzeitig in die Wege zu leiten. Da zwischen dem klinisch erkennbaren Krankheitsbeginn und einer noch erfolgversprechenden Therapie oftmals nur eine Zeitspanne von 24 h liegt, erfordert die diagnostische und therapeutische Strategie klare und schnelle Entscheidungen. Vor nur etwas mehr als einem Jahrzehnt war mit der Diagnose einer Endophthalmitis das Schicksal des Auges besiegelt. Entweder zwang eine Panophthalmie oder eine sich entwickelnde Phthisis bulbi schließlich zur Enukleation des Auges. Die rechzeitige intravitreale Applikation von Antibiotika in Kombination mit einer pars-plana-Vitrektomie hat die Prognose dieser oftmals foudroyant verlaufenden Erkrankung entscheidend verbessert (Chen, 1983; Davidson, 1985; Ficker et al., 1988; Kampik et al., 1986; Kroll et al., 1981; Laatikainen et al., 1987; Lund et al., 1983; Majerovics et al., 1984; Talley, 1987; Vastine DW et al., 1979; Verbraeken et al., 1985 und 1988).

Pathogenetische Faktoren und Erreger

Häufigste Erreger einer akuten Endophthalmitis sind Bakterien, die über eine operative oder traumatische Bulbuseröffnung in das Auge gelangen. Nach intraokularen Eingriffen liegt die Inzidenz einer bakteriellen Endophthalmitis bei 0,02 bis 0,5 % (Allen et al., 1964 und 1974; Bohigian et al., 1986; Christy et al., 1973; Francois et al., 1980; Lund et al., 1983). Häufigste Ursache einer Endophthalmitis ist, bedingt durch die hohe Operationsfrequenz, eine Kataraktoperation, wobei Wundprobleme prädestinierend wirken können (Driebe et al., 1986). Das Erregerspektrum umfaßt in diesen Fällen meist koagulase-negative Staphylokokken, gefolgt von Staphylokokkus aureus, Streptokokken, gram-negativen Erregern, anaeroben Bakterien

Gramer/Kampik (Hrsg.) Pharmakotherapie am Auge
© Springer-Verlag Berlin Heidelberg 1992

und Pilzen. Ein besonders virulenter Erreger ist Bazillus cereus. Während der Erkrankungsbeginn nach einer Kataraktoperation typischerweise in den ersten 3-5 postoperativen Tagen liegt, kann nach fistulierenden Glaukomoperationen die intraokulare Infektion über eine lokale Filterkisseninfektion noch Jahre nach der Erstoperation erfolgen (Wilson, 1986). Bei extrakapsulärer Kataraktextraktion scheint die intakte hintere Linsenkapsel eine Barrierefunktion gegen das Vordringen von Bakterien in den Glaskörperraum zu haben. Untersuchungen an Primaten zeigten, daß bei Implantation von 10 000 Staphylokokkus aureus in die Vorderkammer vorher operierter Augen, die intakte hintere Linsenkapsel eine Endophthalmitis verhindern konnte (Beyer et al., 1984).

Bakterielle Infektionserreger können aber auch auf hämatogenem Weg bei einer Septikopyämie oder über infizierte Injektionskanülen z. B. bei Drogenabhängigen in das intraokulare Milieu gelangen. Seit Mitte der siebziger Jahre ist Bacillus cereus häufigster Erreger einer hämatogen gestreuten Endophthalmitis und löste damit Meningokokken als dominierende Erreger ab (Greenwald et al., 1986).

Pilze sind vor allem bei penetrierenden Bulbusverletzungen mit pflanzlichen Fremdkörpern Erreger einer mykotischen Endophthalmitis, können aber auch durch jede andere traumatische oder operative Bulbuseröffnung in das Auge gelangen. Im Rahmen einer langdauernden Antibiotikatherapie, bei erworbener Immunschwäche, nach schweren Traumata, bei Diabetes mellitus oder Leukämie oder nach multiplen intraabdominellen Eingriffen können jedoch normalerweise saprophytär lebende Pilze auch hämatogen meist über eine vorausgehende fokale Chorioretinitis den Glaskörperraum infiltrieren. Der Augenhintergrundsuntersuchung kommt bei derartig gefährdeten Patienten deshalb für die Früherkennung eine entscheidende Bedeutung zu. Pilze verursachen ca. 13 % aller Endophthalmitiden (Forster et al., 1980).

Viren (Yanoff et al., 1977) und Parasiten wie Toxocara (Rodriguez, 1986) spielen in ihrer Häufigkeit eine nur untergeordnete Rolle.

Klinisches Bild

Klinisch ist eine bakterielle Endophthalmitis durch eine rasch zunehmende intraokulare Entzündung mit gemischter konjunktivaler Injektion, Chemose der Bindehaut, evtl. Lidödem, zunehmendem Hypopyon, subjektiven Schmerzen, deutlicher Visusabnahme einhergehend mit zunehmender entzündlicher Trübung des Glaskörpers gekennzeichnet (siehe auch Abb. 1). Als Frühzeichen kann in manchen Fällen eine retinale Periphlebitis beobachtet werden, deren morphologisches Korrelat perivaskuläre Infiltrate von polymorphkernigen Leukozyten sind (Packer et al., 1983).

Hypopyon und Fibrin in der Vorderkammer, Glaskörperinfiltration und Schmerzen sind klinisch alarmierende Zeichen, die unbedingt engmaschige Verlaufskontrollen in 4 bis 6-stündigem Abstand erforderlich machen. Bei

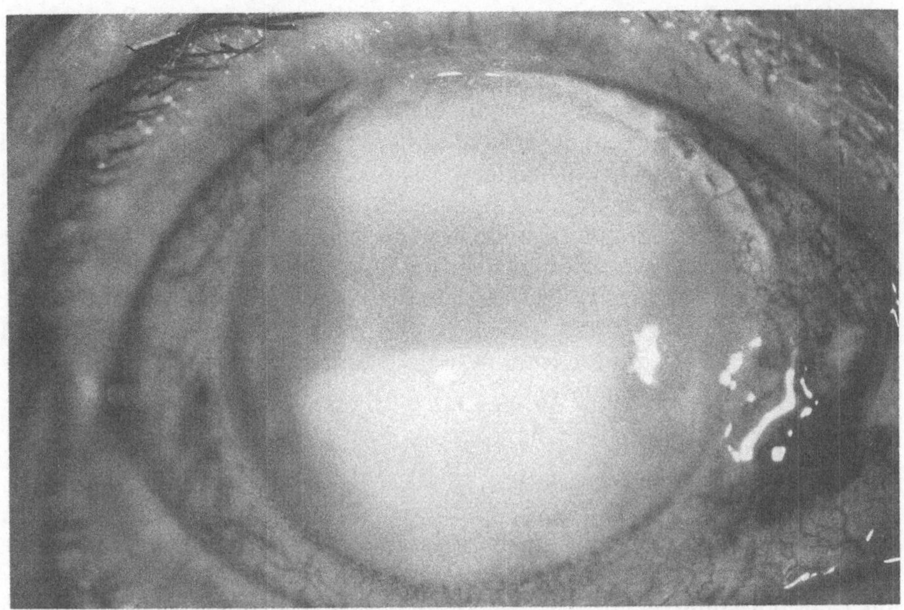

Abb. 1. Akute bakterielle Endophthalmitis nach Kataraktextraktion mit großem Hypopyon und diffuser Hornhauttrübung

rascher Zunahme dieser Symptomatik, spätestens aber beim Verlust des Fundusreflexes ist der Zeitpunkt für eine operative Intervention gekommen. Der klinische Verlauf kann in Abhängigkeit von der Art des Erregers variieren (Ficker et al., 1986).

Staphylokokkus aureus oder gramnegative Keime verursachen eine sich innerhalb von Stunden entwickelnde Endophthalmitis (Rowsey et al., 1982), während z. B. Staphylokokkus epidermidis erst relativ spät zum Vollbild einer Endophthalmitis führt und sich der klinische Verlauf subakut über Tage erstrecken kann. U. U. kompliziert eine ausgeprägte korneale Trübung durch Endotheldekompensation oder stromale Infiltration von Entzündungszellen die Beurteilung der tieferen Bulbusabschnitte. Ultrasonographische Zusatzbefunde zur Verifizierung vitrealer Infiltrate oder einer Verdickung der Aderhaut evtl. mit uvealer Effusion können in diesen Fällen die klinische Diagnose erhärten (Wilson, 1986).

Die Häufigkeit einer Endophthalmitis nach einer Vitrektomie ist zwar sehr niedrig, jedoch kann insbesondere bei diabetischen Patienten das klinische Bild durchaus üblichen und weitaus weniger bedrohlichen postoperativen Verläufen ähneln. Nicht immer lassen sich abakterielle fibrinöse Entzündungsreaktionen oder intravitreale Hämorrhagien klinisch sofort von bakteriell bedingten Entzündungen unterscheiden. Die Diagnose kann sich dadurch in dieser Patientengruppe zeitlich verzögern. Daraus erklärt sich eine möglicherweise ungünstigere Prognose für diese Patientengruppe (Ho et al., 1984).

Mykotische Endophthalmitiden sind in ihrer klinischen Progression wesentlich langsamer als bakterielle Formen der Endophthalmitis und zeigen einen eher subakut bis chronischen Verlauf. Die endogenen Formen der mykotischen Endophthalmitis beginnen mit einem chorioretinalen Infiltrat, aus dem sich die Pilze schließlich in den Glaskörper ausbreiten können und dort umschriebene, schneeballartige Glaskörperverdichtungen verursachen. Bereits im Stadium der chorioretinalen Infiltrate kann die typische Anamnese die Verdachtsdiagnose andeuten und ein erhöhter Antikörpertiter z. B. gegen Candida albicans die Diagnose untermauern. Die Notwendigkeit eines operativen Eingreifens bei einer mykotischen Endophthalmitis steht bei weitem nicht unter dem gleichen Zeitdruck wie bei einer batkeriell verursachten intraokularen Infektion und kann dementsprechend elektiv geplant werden (Barrie, 1987).

Morphologische Befunde

Nach kurzer Zeit sich entwickelnde irreparable intraokulare Gewebszerstörungen erfordern eine rasche und effektive Therapie einer akuten bakteriellen Endophthalmitis. Die Erreger breiten sich nicht nur in den vorderen Augenabschnitten aus, sondern vermehren sich auch im Glaskörperraum, der schließlich Hauptfokus der Infektion wird. In den Anfangsstadien des

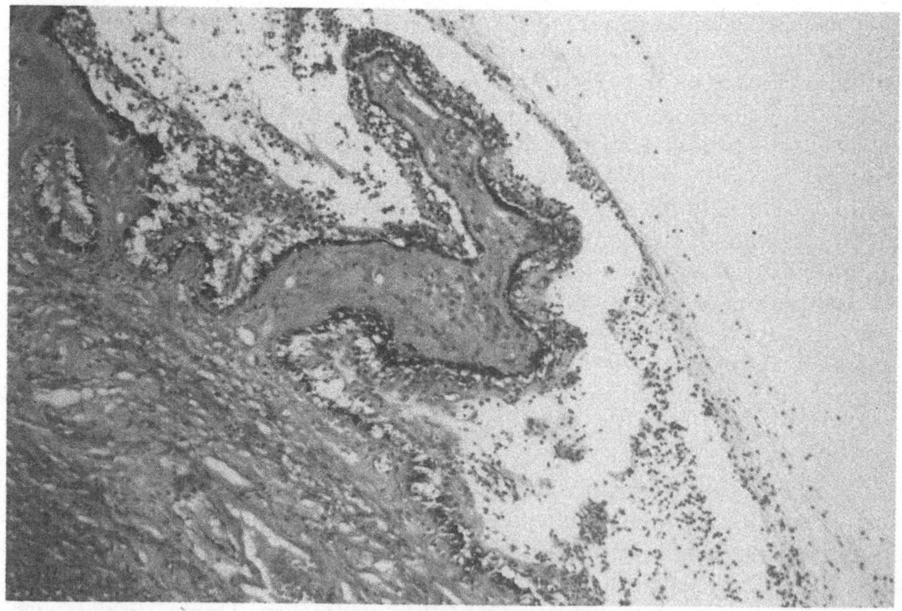

Abb. 2. Akute bakterielle Endophthalmitis mit Leukozyteninfiltraten im Bereich des Ziliarkörpers. Lichtmikroskopischer Befund, HE, Original 200x

Entzündungsprozesses dringen polymorphkernige Granulozyten über die pars plana des Ziliarkörpers in den Glaskörperraum ein (siehe Abb. 2). Nach kurzer Zeit ist die Glaskörperbasis dicht von Leukozyten infiltriert, wie dies in Abb. 3 bei einer hämatogenen Endophthalmitis dargestellt ist, die auch durch choroidale septikopyämische Herde gekennzeichnet ist.

Entzündliche Gewebsnekrosen intraokularer Sturkturen führen schließlich zu irreversiblen Gewebsschäden. Zerstörungen großer Anteile des Ziliarkörpers sind möglicher Wegbereiter einer Phthisis bulbi. Die gefürchteten Nekrosen der Retina limitieren das postentzündliche funktionelle Ergebnis (siehe Abb. 4). Die intraokulären Gewebszerstörungen sind ausgeprägter bei Infektionen mit Streptokokken oder gramnegativen Bakterien wie z. B. Pseudomonas aeruginosa. Abb. 5 zeigt einen derartigen Befund mit ausgedehnten hämorrhagischen Nekrosen und völliger Destruktion der intraokularen Gewebsstrukturen. Schließlich kann die Entzündung auf alle okulären Schichten übergreifen und zu einer Panophthalmie führen. Sind zusätzlich, z. B. bei einem penetrierenden Bulbustrauma, Linsenpartikel im Auge verblieben, verschlechtert die dadurch provozierte phakogene Entzündung die Prognose. Wie in Abb. 6 ersichtlich ist, richten sich die zellulären Entzündungsreaktionen aggressiv gegen die Linsenanteile und komplizieren zusätzlich den Verlauf der Infektion.

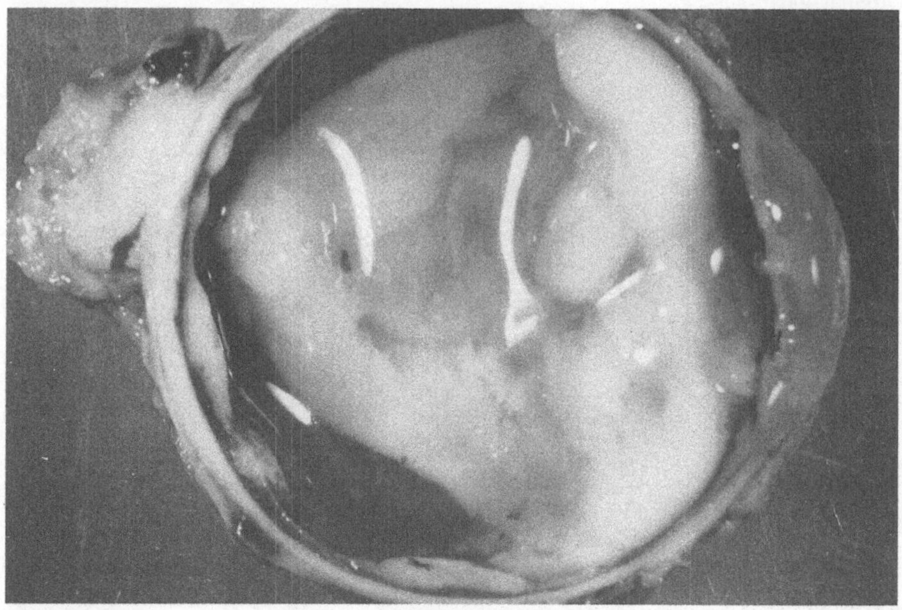

Abb. 3. Endogene bakterielle Endophthalmitis bei Septikopyämie. Multiple konfluierende choroidale Abszesse. Infiltration des Glaskörpers mit starken Verdichtungen an der Glaskörperbasis. Hintere Glaskörperabhebung. Keine Infiltrate im subhyaloidalen Raum

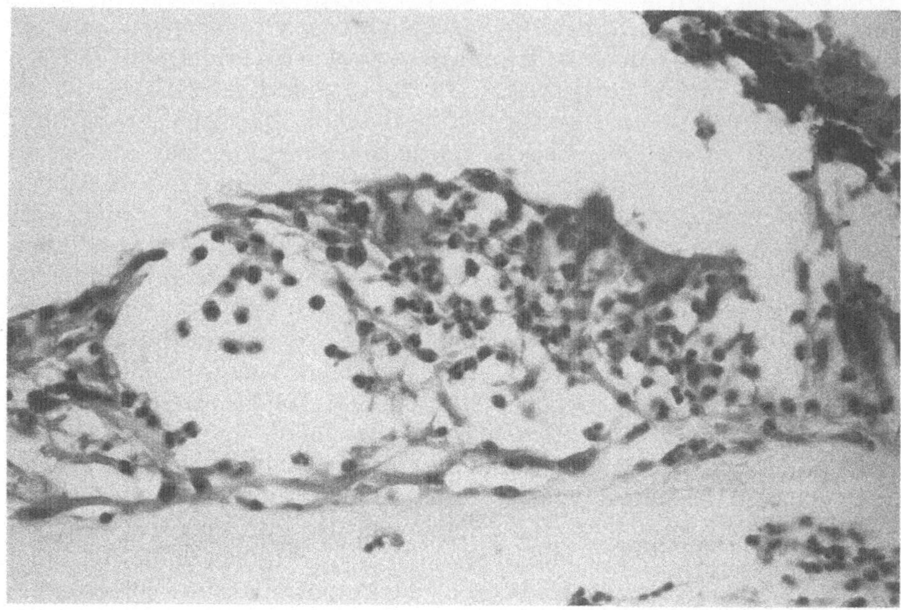

Abb. 4. Intraretinaler Abszeß mit polymorphkernigen Leukozyten bei bakterieller Endophthalmitis. Destruktion aller retinalen Schichten. Lichtmikroskopischer Befund, HE, Original 400x

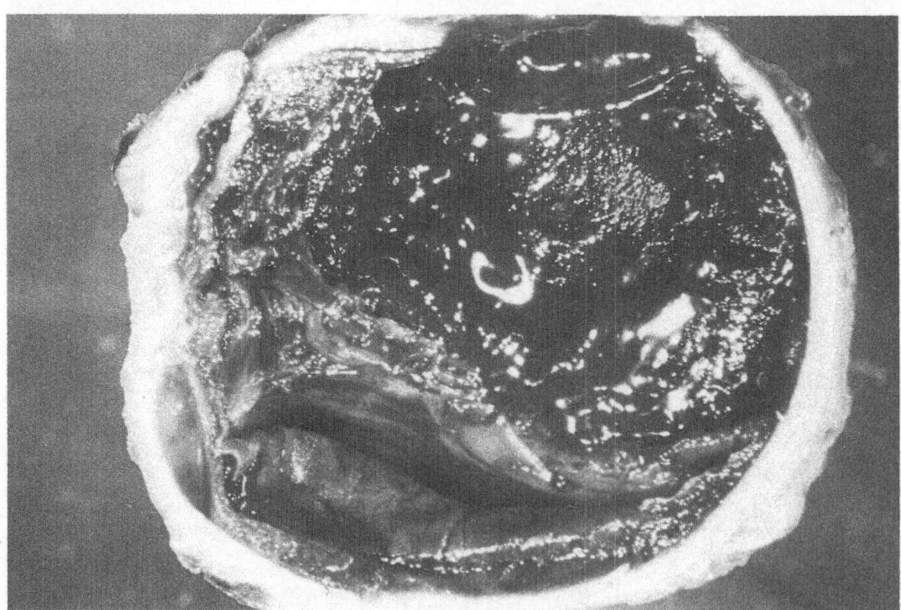

Abb. 5. Bulbus mit total destruiertem intraokulärem Gewebe. Große hämorrhagische Nekrosen bei endogener Endophthalmitis durch Pseudomonas aeruginosa

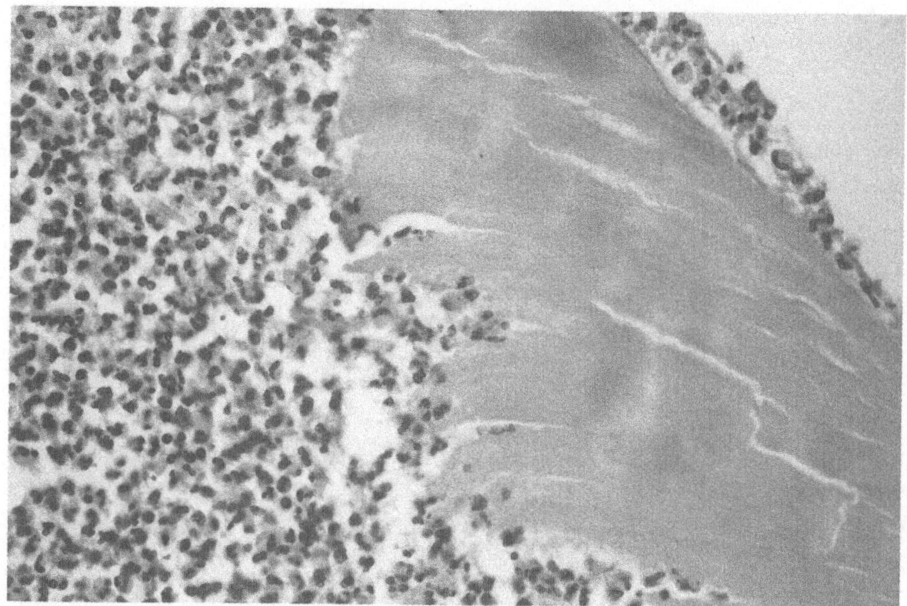

Abb. 6. Posttraumatische bakterielle Endophthalmitis mit zusätzlicher phakogener Entzündung. Dichte leukozytäre Reaktion um Linsenpartikel. Lichtmikroskopischer Befund, HE, Original 400x

Pharmakokinetische Aspekte

Ziel jeder Therapie einer Endophthalmitis ist deshalb die Elimination des infektiösen Agens und die Prävention sekundärer Gewebszerstörungen mit ihren schwerwiegenden funktionellen Folgen. Antibiotika, Kortikosteroide und im Fall einer Pilzinfektion Antimykotika sind die Medikamentengruppe der Wahl. Vor allem im Glaskörperraum müssen hohe Medikamentenkonzentrationen erreicht werden, wobei bei der Auswahl von Pharmaka die Wirksamkeit, die Pharmakokinetik und die retinale Toxizität zu beachten sind. Eine exakte Dosierung (Angaben siehe Tabelle 1) intravitreal applizierter Medikamente ist jedoch unbedingt erforderlich, um retinale Schäden zu vermeiden. So sind bei zu hoher Dosierung insbesondere makuläre Infarkte beschrieben worden (Conway et al., 1986).

Der Transport von Pharmaka in das Auge wird an drei anatomischen Barrieren funktionell gehemmt (Barza, 1989). Das Hornhautepithel hemmt durch seine „tight junctions" den Durchtritt hydrophiler Substanzen. Nur lipidlösliche Pharmaka können ein intaktes Hornhautepithel überwinden. Im Gegensatz zum Hornhautepithel stellt das Hornhautstroma eine Diffusionsbarriere für hydrophobe Substanzen dar. Der Übertritt lipophiler Substanzen aus dem retinalen Gefäßsystem in die Netzhaut und den Glaskörperraum wird durch die nicht fenestrierten retinalen Kapillaren

Tabelle 1. Empfehlungen für die Dosierung intravitrealer antimikrobieller Pharmaka. (Nach Kattan und Pflugfelder 1989)

	Dosis (mg/0,1 ml)
Antibiotika	
Aminoglykoside	
Gentamycin	0,10
Tobramycin	0,10
Amikacin	0,40
Netilmicin	0,10
Kanamycin	0,40
Cephalosporine	
Cefazolin	2,25
Cephalotin	2,0
Cephaloridin	0,25
Vancomycin	1,0
Clindamycin	0,45 – 1,0
Penicilline	
Methicillin	2,0
Oxacillin	0,50
Carbenicillin	2,0
Ampicillin	5,0
Erythromycin	0,50
Lincomycin	1,5
Imipenem	0,50
Antimykotika	
Amphotericin B	0,005 – 0,010
Miconazol	0,025 – 0,040
Fluconezol	0,10

gehemmt. Das retinale Pigmentepithel hemmt wegen seiner interzelluären „tight junctions" ebenfalls die Passage hydrophiler Pharmaka.

Bei topischer, subkonjunktivaler, parabulbärer und systemischer Medikamentenapplikation müßten diese Diffusionsbarrieren überwunden werden, um hohe intravitreale Wirkspiegel zu erreichen. Dies gelingt mit vorhersagbarer Sicherheit jedoch nur durch eine direkte intravitreale Medikamenteninstillation. Bereits in den vierziger Jahren leisteten von Sallman et al. (1944), Leopold (1945), Duguid et al. (1947) und Sorsby et al. (1948) Pionierarbeiten in der Behandlung der bakteriellen Endophthalmitis durch intravitreale Penicillininjektionen. 1974 berichteten dann Peyman et al. über die intravitreale Injektion von Gentamycin und Dexamethason in ein menschliches Auge über den pars plana und den translimbalen Zugang.

Intravitreal applizierte Pharmaka werden über zwei Wege wieder aus dem Auge eliminiert (Maurice, 1976). Über den anterioren Weg verlassen

Pharmaka über die Vorderkammer und Schlemm'schen Kanal den intraokulären Raum. Die intraokuläre Halbwertszeit für Aminoglycoside oder Vancomycin, die über diese engen Kanäle aus dem Auge eliminiert werden, ist am nicht entzündeten Kaninchenauge mit 20 bis 30 Stunden deshalb relativ lange. Sie dürfte am menschlichen Auge doppelt so lange sein (Barza, 1989), bei Entzündungszuständen ist sie jedoch möglicherweise verkürzt.

Der posteriore Weg besteht aus einem aktiven Transportmechanismus durch die retinalen Kapillaren oder durch das retinale Pigmentepithel. Auf diesem Wege werden z. B. β-Lactam-Antibiotika und Clindamycin eliminiert. Die intravitreale Halbwertszeit derartig eliminierter Pharmaka liegt oft nur im Bereich von drei bis sechs Stunden. Dieser posteriore Eliminationsweg zeigt eine Sättigungskinetik und kann im Falle von β-Lactam-Antibiotika durch Substanzen der gleichen Klasse kompetitiv gehemmt werden. Eine Hemmung ist jedoch auch mit systemisch appliziertem Probenecid möglich (Barza et al., 1982).

Die Clearancerate intravitreal applizierter Medikamente ändert sich nach einer vorher durchgeführten Vitrektomie und ist z. B. in vitrektomierten Kaninchenaugen für Amphotericin B im Vergleich zu nicht vitrektomierten Augen deutlich erhöht (Doft et al., 1985). Dies kann auch in der klinischen Behandlung relevant sein und eine wiederholte intravitreale Applikation antimikrobieller Substanzen erforderlich machen.

Experimentelle Untersuchungen an Kaninchen zeigten, daß zwischen der intravitrealen Antibiotikakonzentration und der Abnahme der Bakterienkonzentration eine lineare Beziehung besteht. Bemerkenswert ist dabei das Fehlen einer maximalen Effektkonzentration, oberhalb derer eine weitere Erhöhung der Medikamentenkonzentration ohne Einfluß auf die weitere Abnahme der Bakterienkonzentration bleibt (Davey et al., 1987). Folglich sollten die höchstmöglichen intravitrealen Antibiotikakonzentrationen, die noch ohne retinotoxische Wirkung sind, in der Behandlung einer Endophthalmitis erreicht werden. Experimentell bestätigt sich auch die Wichtigkeit des Zeitfaktors, da im Falle einer Infektion mit Pseudomonas aeruginosa bei einer zeitlichen Verzögerung des Behandlungsbeginns von mehr als 24 Stunden die untersuchten Antibiotika die Bakterienkonzentrationen nicht mehr reduzieren konnten.

Therapeutische Maßnahmen und mikrobiologische Diagnostik

Die intravitreale Medikamentenapplikation allein ist für eine effiziente Therapie einer Endophthalmitis jedoch nicht ausreichend, beinhaltet aber die Gefahr der Symptomverschleierung und gibt dadurch dem Therapeuten möglicherweise eine falsche Sicherheit. Erst in Kombination mit einer pars-plana-Vitrektomie kann der gewünschte Behandlungserfolg erreicht werden. Die Prognose einer Endophthalmitis, die bis zum Jahre 1980 für das Organ noch infaust war (Kampik et al., 1986), konnte durch dieses rechzeitig eingesetzte Verfahren – wobei die Zeit der wichtigste prognostische Faktor ist – so verbessert werden, daß in 80 % der Fälle eine Sehfunktion erhalten werden kann (Buhl et al., 1991). Das zur Verfügung stehende Zeitintervall, in dem ein therapeutisch erfolgreiches Eingreifen noch möglich ist, kann bei foudroyantem Verlauf im Bereich von nur wenigen Stunden liegen.

Die Indikation zum operativen Vorgehen richtet sich in erster Linie nach dem klinischen Bild. Ist bei kurzfristiger Kontrolle des Patienten eine schnelle Zunahme der intraokularen Entzündung vor allem mit Hypopyon und Fibrin in der Vorderkammer und Mitbeteiligung des Glaskörpers erkennbar, duldet der notwendige operative Eingriff keine weitere Aufschiebung mehr. Die Vitrektomie führt zu einer sofortigen Reduzierung der intravitrealen Bakterienkonzentration und einer dadurch günstigeren Dosis-Bakterien-Relation. Mit der Entferung des Glaskörpers wird auch ein für das Bakterienwachstum förderliches biologisches Kulturmedium (Maylath et al., 1955) entfernt zusammen mit bakteriellen Enzymen, Toxinen und einer Diffusionsbarriere für die intravitreal gegebenen Pharmaka.

Der Versuch, die Diagnose durch eine Glaskörperpunktion präoperativ zu sichern, bleibt ein unsicheres Unterfangen. Bei noch nicht verflüssigtem Glaskörper ist eine ausreichende Probenentnahme mit dünner Kanüle aufgrund der Glaskörperkonsistenz oftmals nicht möglich. Auch die Gefahr eines iatrogenen Netzhautforamens durch Aspirationszug an der Glaskörperbasis sollte nicht unberücksichtigt bleiben. Ein negatives Ausstrichergebnis schließt jedoch eine bakterielle Komponente nicht aus, ein Kulturergebnis kann nicht abgewartet werden und ein positiver Ausstrich würde schließlich die Operationsindikation nur bestätigen. Trotzdem bleibt die mikrobiologische Diagnostik ein wichtiger Stützpfeiler für klinische Entscheidungen. Sie kann aber besser im Zusammenhang mit einer Vitrektomie durchgeführt werden.

Mit Beginn des glaskörperchirurgischen Eingriffes werden je drei Ausstrichpräparate aus Vorderkammer und Glaskörper angefertigt. Intraoperativ ist es somit möglich durch eine leicht durchführbare Gramfärbung die Unterscheidung zwischen einer bakteriellen und mykotischen Endophthalmitis zu treffen und innerhalb der Bakterienarten grampositive von den gefürchteten gramnegativen Bakterien zu unterscheiden. Eine derartige Diagnostik kann auch im Notdienst durch einen Assistenten erfolgen. Typischerweise finden sich polymorphkernige Granulozyten und intrazytoplasmatisch gelegene Bakterien (siehe Abb. 7). Zur zytologischen Diagnostik kann spätestens am nächsten Tag noch jeweils eine Giemsa-Färbung und zur besseren Diagnostik von Pilzen eine PAS-Färbung durchgeführt werden.

Eine wichtige Ergänzung zur sofortigen Ausstrichdiagnostik sind mikrobiologische Kulturuntersuchungen der entnommenen Proben vor allem zur Resistenzbestimmung gegenüber Antibiotika. Kulturuntersuchungen ergeben jedoch nur in etwa 50 % der Fälle ein positives Ergebnis. Dies unterstreicht umsomehr die Wichtigkeit einer sofortigen intraoperativen Diagnostik.

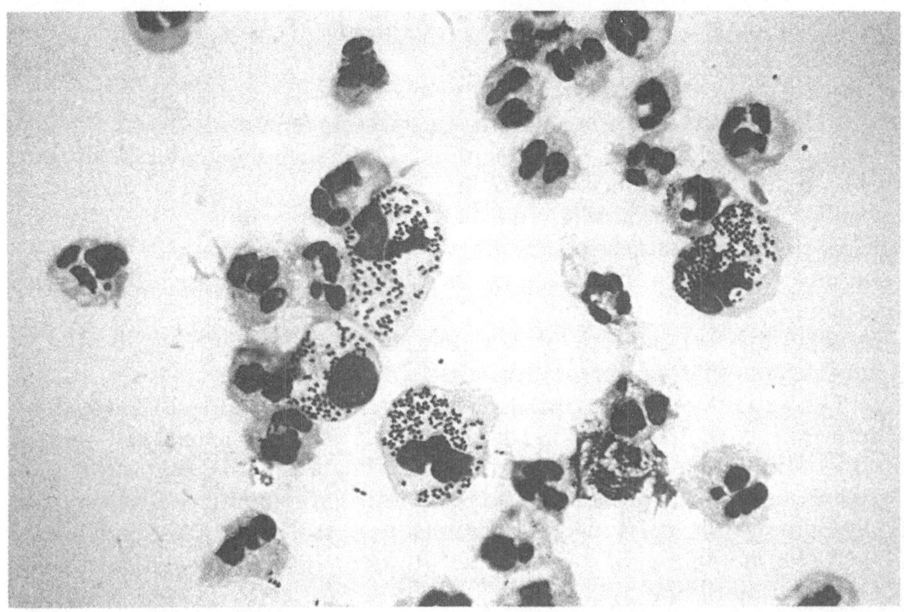

Abb. 7. Gramfärbung eines Glaskörperausstrichpräparates bei bakterieller Endophthalmitis. Polymorphkernige Leukozyten mit intrazellulären grampositiven Bakterien. Lichtmikroskopischer Befund, Original 1000x

Vitrektomie und intravitreale Medikamentenapplikation

Vor Beginn des eigentlichen glaskörperchirurgischen Eingriffes müssen häufig Fibrin- und Eitermembranen aus der Vorderkammer entfernt werden, da sie die Sicht auf die tieferen Bulbusabschnitte deutlich einschränken können. Intraokularlinsen werden in der Regel belassen, doch sollte die hintere Linsenkapsel zur besseren Reinigung des Kaspelsackes und zur besseren Diffusion intravitrealer Medikamente eröffnet werden. Bei penetrierenden Verletzungen mit noch vorhandenen Linsenpartikeln müssen diese zur Verhinderung einer phakogenen Reaktion entfernt werden. Der Glaskörper wird dann so gründlich wie möglich entfernt unter besonderer Einbeziehung auch der Glaskörperbasis, die fast immer dicht leukozytär infiltriert ist. Membranös verdichtete Leukozytenbeläge der Netzhaut können vorsichtig abgesaugt werden. Manipulationen in der Nähe der Netzhaut erfordern jedoch große Vorsicht, da entzündliche intraretinale Infiltrate zu iatrogenen Netzhautläsionen prädestinieren.

Mit Beendigung des glaskörperchirurgischen Eingriffes erfolgt eine intravitreale Medikamentenapplikation. Für die Antibiotikaauswahl sind ein optimales Spektrum hinsichtlich des vermuteten Erregers und eine potentielle toxische Wirkung vor allem auf Netzhaut und Linse zu beachten. Verwendbare Antibiotika und ihre jeweilige Dosierung sind in Tabelle 1 nach den Empfehlungen von Kattan und Pflugfelder (1989) aufgeführt. Bei bakterieller Endophthalmitis hat sich die zusätzliche intravitreale Gabe von Kortikosteroiden als sehr vorteilhaft erwiesen, um die intraokuläre Entzündungsreaktion mit ihren negativen Auswirkungen auf das intraokuläre Gewebe zu hemmen. Tierexperimentelle Untersuchungen mit positivem Effekt auf den Verlauf einer bakteriellen Endophthalmitis bei kombinierter Anwendung von Antibiotika und Dexamethason waren in den frühen siebziger Jahren bereits durchgeführt worden (Graham et al., 1974).

Aus unserer eigenen Erfahrung hat sich folgendes medikamentöse Therapieschema in Kombination mit einer Vitrektomie bewährt:

Intraoperativ bei bakterieler Endophthalmitis: Intravitreal 20 Mikrogramm Dexamethason-Azetat pro ml BSS-Spülflüssigkeit.

Mit Operationsende intravitreale Eingabe einer Gesamtdosis von 0,1 mg Gentamycin gelöst in 0,1 ml BSS (dies enspricht einer 40-fachen Verdünnung von 1 Ampulle Gentamycin mit einer ursprünglichen Konzentration von 40 mg/ml) und 1 mg Dexamethason-Azetat. Parabulbäre Injektion von 40 mg Gentamycin und 4 mg Dexamethason-Azetat.

Die Lokaltherapie wird perioperativ über ca. 10 Tage mit einem Breitspektrumantibiotikum ergänzt.

Bei mykotischer Endophthalmitis werden intravitreale Antibiotika und Kortikosteroide ersetzt durch die intravitreale Injektion von Amphotericin B in einer Gesamtdosis von 0,005-0,010 mg in 0,1 ml BSS in Ergänzung mit systemisch verabreichten Antimykotika. Amphotericin B hat sich als das Mittel der Wahl bei mykotischer Endophthalmitis bewährt (Pflugfelder et al., 1988; Wilmarth et al., 1983).

Die akute Endophthalmitis gefährdet wie kaum ein anderer Notfall in der Augenheilkunde das gesamte Organ. Die Hauptgründe für ein Versagen aller therapeutischen Anstrengungen liegen meist in einer Verzögerung des Behandlungsbeginns, im Verzicht auf eine intravitreale Medikamentenapplikation, in einer inadäquaten Medikamentendosierung und nicht zuletzt auch an der Virulenz des Infektionserregers. Für den Erfolg der Therapie ist auch eine enge Kooperation zwischen dem erstuntersuchenden Ophthalmologen und dem vitreoretinalen Chirurgen erforderlich. Im heutigen Trend zum ambulanten Operieren muß auch der Patient über Frühsymptome informiert sein, und es muß, auch außerhalb einer stationären Beobachtung, eine kontinuierliche Patientenüberwachung gewährleistet sein. Bei rechtzeitiger kombinierter medikamentöser und operativer Therapie kann diese potentiell so gefährliche Erkrankung heutzutage in den meisten Fällen erfolgreich behandelt und dem Patienten eine noch brauchbare Sehfunktion erhalten werden.

Literatur

Allen HF, Mangiaracine AB (1964) Bacterial endophthalmitis after cataract extraction: A study of 22 infections in 20 000 operations. Arch Ophthalmol 72:454

Allen HF, Mangiaracine AB (1974) Bacterial endophthalmitis after cataract extraction. Arch Ophthalmol 91:3

Barrie T (1987) The place of elective vitrectomy in the management of patients with candida endophthalmitis. Graefe's Arch Exp Clin Ophthalmol 225:107

Barza M (1989) Antibacterial agents in the treatment of ocular infections. Infect Dis Clin North Am 3 (3):533

Barza M, Kane A, Baum J (1982) The effects of infection and probenecid on the transport of carbenicillin from the rabbit vitreous humor. Invest Ophthalmol Vis Sci 22:720

Beyer TL, Vogler G, Sharma D, O'Donnel FE jr (1984) Protective barrier effect ot the posterior lens capsule in exogenous bacterial endophthalmitis – an experimental study. Invest Ophthalmol Vis Sci 25:108

Bohigian GM, Olk RJ (1986) Factors associated with a poor visual result in endophthalmitis. Am J Ophthalmol 101:332

Buhl M, Heidenkummer H-P, Schönfeld K, Kampik A (1991) Klinische Ergebnisse nach Endophthalmitis. Jahrestagung der Bayerischen Augenärzte, Würzburg, 14./15. 06. 91

Chen CJ (1983) Management of infectious endophthalmitis by combined vitrectomy and intraocular injection. Ann Ophthalmol 15:968

Christy NE, Lall P (1973) Postoperative endophthalmitis following cataract surgery. Arch Ophthalmol 90:361

Conway BP, Campochiaro PA (1986) Macular infarction after endophthalmitis treated with vitrectomy and intravitreal gentamicin. Arch Ophthalmol 104:367

Davey PG, Barza M, Stuart M (1987) Dose response of experimental Pseudomonas endophthalmitis to ciprofloxacin, gentamicin, and imipenem: Evidence for resistance to "late" treatment of infections. J Infect Dis 155:518

Davidson SI (1985) Post-operative bacterial endophthalmitis. Trans ophthalmol Soc UK 104:278

Doft BH, Weiskopf J, Nilsson-Ehle I, Wingard LB (1985) Amphotericin clearance in vitrectomized versus nonvitrectomized eyes. Ophthalmology 92:1601

Driebe WT jr, Mandelbaum S, Forster RK, Schwartz LK, Culbertson WW (1986) Pseudophakic endophthalmitis. Diagnosis and management. Ophthalmology 93:442

Duguid JP, Ginsberg M, Fraser IC,m Macasakill J, Michaelson IC, Robson JM (1947) Experimental observation on the intravitreal use of penicillin and other drugs. Br J Ophthalmol 31:193

Ficker L, Peacock J (1986) Infectious endophthalmitis. Trans Ophthalmol Soc UK 105:319

Ficker LA, Meredith TA, Wilson LA, Kaplan HJ (1988) Role of vitrectomy in staphylococcus epidermidis endophthalmitis. Br J Ophthalmol 72:386

Forster RK, Abbott RL, Gelender H (1980) Management of endophthalmitits. Ophthalmology 87:813

Francois J, Verbraeken H (1980) Complications in 1000 consecutive intracapsular cataract extractions. Ophthalmologica 180:121

Graham RO, Peyman GA (1974) Intravitreal injection of dexamethasone. Treatment of experimentally induced endophthalmitis. Arch Ophthalmol 92:149

Greenwald MJ, Wohl LG, Sell CH (1986) Metastatic bacterial endophthalmitis: A contemporary reappraisal. Surv Ophthalmol 31:81

Ho PC, Tolentino FI (1984) Bacterial endophthalmitis after closed vitrectomy. Arch Ophthalmol 102:207

Kampik A, Dabov B (1986) Aktue Endophthalmitis. In: Lund O-E, Waubke TN (Hrsg) Akute Augenerkrankungen – Akute Symptome. Bücherei des Augenarztes, Bd 109. Enke, Stuttgart, S 177-193

Kattan P, Pflugfelder SC (1989) Complications of intraocular microbial agents. Int Ophthalmol Clin 29:188

Kroll P, Busse H (1981) Ergebnisse der Vitrektomie bei akuter und chronischer Endophthalmitis. Klin Mbl Augenheilk 179:514

Laatikainen L, Tarkanen A (1987) Early vitrectomy in the treatment of post-operative purulent endophthalmitis. Acta ophthalmol 65:455

Leopold IH (1945) Intravitreal penetration of penicillin and penicillin therapy of infections of the vitreous. Arch Ophthalmol 33:211

Lund O-E, Kampik A (1983) Vitrektomie bei Endophthalmitis. Klin Mbl Augenheilk 182:30

Majerovics A, Tanenbaum HL (1984) Endophthalmitis and pars plana vitrectomy. Can J Ophthalmol 19:25

Maurice DM (1976) Injection of drugs into the vitreous body. In: Leopold IH, Burns RP (eds) Symposium on Ocular Therapy, vol 9. Wiley, New York, 59

Maylath FR, Leopold FH (1955) Study of experimental intraocular infection. Am J Ophthalmol 40:86

Packer AJ, Weingeist TA, Abrams GW (1983) Retinal periphlebitis as an early sign of bacterial endophthalmitis. Am J Ophthalmol 96:66

Peyman GA, Herbst R (1974) Bacterial endophthalmitis. Arch Ophthalmol 91:416

Pflugfelder SC, Flynn HW, Zwickey TA, Forster RK, Tsiligianni A, Culbertson WW, Mandelbaum S (1988) Exogenous fungal endophthalmitis. Ophthalmology 95:19

Rodriguez A (1986) Early pars plana vitrectomy in chronic endophthalmitis of toxocariasis. Graefe's Arch Clin Exp Ophthalmol 224:218-220

Rowsey JJ, Newsome DL, Sexton DJ, Harms WK (1982) Endophthalmitis. Current approaches. Ophthalmology 89:1055

von Sallmann L, Meyer K, DiGrandi J (1944) Experimental study on penicillin treatment of exogenous infection of vitreous. Arch Ophthalmol 32:179

Sorsby A, Ungar J (1948) Intravitreal injection of penicillin. Study of the levels of concentration reached and therapeutic efficacy. Br J Ophthalmol 32:857

Talley AR, D'Amico DJ, Talamo JH, Casey V-NJ, Kenyon KR (1987) The role of vitrectomy in the treatment of postoperative bacterial endophthalmitis. Arch Ophthalmol 105:1699

Vastine DW, Peyman GA, Guth SB (1979) Visual prognosis in bacterial endophthalmitis treated with intravitreal antibiotics. Ophthalmic Surgery 10:76

Verbraeken H, van Laethem J (1985) Treatment of endophthalmitis with and without pars plana vitrectomy. Ophthalmologica Basel 191:1

Verbraeken H, Geeroms B, Karemera A (1988) Treatment of endophthalmitis by pars plana vitrectomy. Ophthalmologica Basel 197:19

Wilmarth SS, May DR, Roth AM, Cole RJ, Nolan S, Goldstein E (1983) Aspergillus endophthalmitits in an intravenous drug user. Ann Ophthalmol 15:470

Wilson LA (1986) Acute bacterial infection of the eye: Bacterial keratitis and endophthalmitis. Trans ophthalmol Soc UK 105:43

Yanoff M, Allman MI, Fine BS (1977) Congenital herpes simplex virus, type 2, bilateral endophthalmitis. Trans Am Ophthalmol Soc 75:325

Korrespondenzadresse

Dr. med. H.-P. Heidenkummer

Universitätsaugenklinik Würzburg, Josef-Schneider-Straße 11, D-8700 Würzburg

Experimental Intravitreal Drug Delivery for Retinal Disease

W.R. Freeman, C.A. Wiley, K. Assil, R. Gariano, A. Listhaus,
D. Munguia, T. Schneiderman, and P. Svendson

Abstract

Infectious retinitis and proliferative vitreo-retinopathy (PVR) are two disorders in which there is a need for antiviral and antiproliferative drugs to be delivered to the retina giving therapeutic levels over intervals of weeks to months. Currently, intravitreal ganciclovir is given to AIDS patients with cytomegalvirus rentinitis who are intolerant or unwilling to take ganciclovir intravenously. Antimetabolites capable of inhibiting PVR would be an important therapeutic modality; treatment trails with intraocular irrigation of daunorubicin are currently underway. We have explored the intraocular toxicity of polar anti-CMV drugs and anti-proliferative agents which we have previously shown can be incorporated into a multivesicular liposome system. We have shown that these drugs are not toxic at concentrations many times above those necessary for therapeutic effect when injected intravitreally. We will review electrophysiologic and morphologic data on the toxicity of both the drugs and their liposome preparations injected intravitreally. Our laboratory studies suggest that certain polar antiviral and antimetabolite drugs can be delivered at efficacious concentrations without evidence of toxicity in animal models.

Introduction

Intravitreal drug therapy for retinal disease has been considered and used in several types of retinal disorders which can be broadly classified into infectious and proliferative disorders. Degenerative diseases and other disorders may be amenable to such local therapy however, and all retinal diseases should be considered as potential candidates for local intravitreal drug delivery. The advantage of this type of delivery is the accessability of the retina to intravitreal therapy and the potential for accumulating prolonged and high concentrations of a variety of therapeutic compounds in the region of the retina. Local therapy may also avoid systemic toxicity of potent drugs thus allowing the delivery of therapeutic agents to the retina in concentrations which, if delivered systemically, would be otherwise toxic (Freeman 1989). This manuscript will focus on therapy of viral infections of the retina and therapy of proliferative vitreo-retinopathy.

Gramer/Kampik (Hrsg.) Pharmakotherapie am Auge
© Springer-Verlag Berlin Heidelberg 1992

Viral Retinitis

Viral retinitis has become a more common problem in recent years. Both Herpes Zoster and Simplex infections of the retina occur and cause the syndrome of acute retinal necrosis. In addition, in immunosuppressed patients, cytomegalovirus retinitis has become a major problem, particularly as the worldwide incidence of AIDS has grown. In the latter disease it is important to realize that CMV retinitis occurs in up to 40 % of patients with the acquired immunodeficiency syndrome and that as new therapies prolong life in these patients, CMV retinitis will be seen with ever increasing frequency (Jabs 1989).

The acute retinal necrosis syndrome (ARN) is classically described as a fulminant retinitis accompanied by moderate to severe uveitis that generally occurs in otherwise healthy patients, but on occasion has been observed in milder forms and in immunocompromised hosts (Culbertson 1986).The ARN patient typically presents with progressive visual blurring in one or both eyes occurring over days to weeks. Examination reveals a prominent anterior uveitis which may be granulomatous or non-granulomatous in nature. The diffuse vitritis may make the view of the retina difficult, and may contribute to the high degree of delayed and/or misdiagnosis which occurs in the early stages of the disease. Days to weeks after onset of the infection, the discrete peripheral lesions typically coalesce into a white or yellow ring of infected retina, and the associated vasculature is obliterated. Necrotic retina desquamates into the vitreous resulting in vitreous "sheets". Eventually, seventy-five percent of all untreated eyes can be expected to develop retinal detachment due to development of multiple full thickness retinal breaks accompanied by traction. Both Herpes simplex type 1 and Herpes simplex type 2 (HSV-1, HSV-2) may cause ARN. In a single report, Cytomegalovirus (CMV) particles were identified in and cultured from the retina of an enucleated eye of a non-immunosuppressed patient suffering from bilateral ARN (Rungger-Brandle 1984). Varicella zoster virus (VZV), has been reported most frequently as the viral etiologic agent of ARN.We have demonstrated herpes family viral particles in endoretinal biopsy specimens taken from patients in the active stage of the disease showing an enormous viral load (Freeman 1986).These studies, combined with the failure of many enucleated eyes with ARN to demonstrate evidence of viral particles, indicate that the virus is present only in the active stages of the disease and that gliotic retina will not demonstrate the etiologic agent.

Some strains of Herpes viruses known to have caused ARN syndrome are inhibited only by acyclovir concentrations greater than the achievable aqueous concentrations after oral administration (400 mg five times per day) of acyclovir. Intravenous therapy with 1500 mg per square meter per day in three divided doses achieves peak plasma levels of 30-40 uM without significant toxicity to the patient and is therefore the recommended regimen (Blumenkranz 1986). Aqueous acyclovir levels of 8.7 to 11.2 uM are achievable using intravenous acyclovir (1500 m,g per square meter per day), and these levels are sufficient to treat most cases of ARN. Because of the high doses of acyclovir necessary to inhibit certain strains of Varicella Zoster virus some investigators have suggested that intravitreal acyclovir be used, particularly at the time of vitrectomy in these patients (Peyman 1984). These investigators have suggested either the use of acyclovir in the infusion fluid or direct intravitreal injections (Pulido 1985). Because the disease may proceed with a rapid tempo, it has been argued that high dose intravitreal therapy may be more efficacious in halting replication of the virus than the relatively lower intraocular levels attained by intravenous or oral therapy with acyclovir. In addition, it should be realized that resistance of Herpes Simplex and Varicella Zoster virus to acyclovir has been reported and that such resistant strains may be more susceptible to the very high levels attainable with intravitreal therapy.

Despite a high prevalence of antibody positivity in the population, clinical ocular disease secondary to CMV infection in adults is rare or nonexistent in the absence of immunosuppression due to malignancies, autoimmune disease, AIDS or therapeutic intervention. CMV retinitis occurs in 15 to 40 % of AIDS patients (Henderly 1987) and, in contrast to the non-infectious lesions of AIDS, demands aggressive treatment to prevent severe visual loss. Progression of the retinitis generally occure with a leading edge of active retinitis and a trailing region of thin gliotic retina. This pattern indicates cell to cell transmission of the virus. CMV is a slowly progressive necrotizing retinitis that may affect the posterior pole, the peripheral retina, or both and may be unilateral or bilateral. Involved areas appear as white intraretinal lesions, areas of infiltrate and often necrosis, along the vascular arcades in the posterior pole. In addition, prominent retinal hemorrhages are often seen within the necrotic area or along its leading edge. Ganciclovir, also known as DHPG (tradename Cytovene), a hydroxylated derivative of acyclovir, was licensed for use in the United States in 1989. Treatment with ganciclovir is usually successful at controlling CMV infection, but is difficult and requires a multidisciplinary team approach. Oral bioavailability of ganciclovir is low and inconsistent; therefore, the drug is available only intravenously although trails of oral ganciclovir are planed. Intravenous ganciclovir has a short half-life (3.6 hours), and must be given on a once or twice daily basis intravenously (Henderly 1987). Side effects are numerous with myelosuppression and life threatening neutropenia being the most difficult to manage. In many patients, concurrent treatment with AZT, which has been shown to prolong life in HIV infected individuals, is often not possible.

The only other drug used to treat CMV is foscarnet. This drug also has significant systemic toxicity and, like ganciclovir, is poorly water soluble at neutral pH. Foscarnet (trisodium phosphonoformate hexahydrate) is a potent virustatic agent with in vitro antiviral activity against HIV and Herpesviruses. It inhibits RNA and DNA virus polymerases and has been found and reversible anemia noted in 30 % in one series (Walmsley et al. 1988). Tremor, nausea, serum calcium and/or phosphorous changes have also been noted in association with Foscarnet treatment. Virtually all patients placed on foscarnet have shown improvement of CMV retinitis with partial or complete resolution of retinitis. The recurrence rate is equal to that seen with ganciclovir (Lehoang et al. 1989). Response to foscarnet has been described in patients who have retinitis unresponsive to ganciclovir (Walmsley et al. 1988). It is clear that administration of either ganciclovir or foscarnet systemically will be associated with significant toxicity particularly in ill patients. For this reason, recent attention has been focused on the administration of ganciclovir intravitreally.

In rabbitis, intravitreal ganciclovir injections of up to 400 micrograms produced no ophthalmoscopic, histologic, or electroretinographic changes. Multiple intraocular injections of ganciclovir have been successful in controlling CMV retinitis in at least one patient who was treated over three months with a total of 28 intravitreal injections of 200 micrograms each (Henry et al. 1987). No evidence of retinal toxicity was noted and the estimated half life of the drug in the human vitreous was thirteen hours.

Several investigators have found intravitreal injection to be efficacious in controlling CMV retinitis (Cantrill 1989; Heinemann 1989; Henry 1987; Ussery 1988). The usual dose is 200µg in 0.1 cc intravitreally. Injections have been performed in the out patient setting under retrobulbar or local (4 % xylocaine injection or 4 % cocaine hydrochloride topically) anesthesia both in the clinic and under sterile conditions in the operating room. Those injections performed in the clinic have used topical gentamicin drops the night before the injection. However, sterilization of the conjunctiva with povidone-iodine is perferable. The complications of intraocular injections are well known and must be considered carefully (Freeman 1989). Review of the literature shown that intravitreal injection of ganciclovir is controversial. Between 1 and 58 injections per patient have been administered. Of 463 intravitreal injections in 30 patients two cases of endophthalmitis (Staphylococcus aureus and Staphylococcus epidermidis) and one retinal detachment have been described.

Proliferative Vitreoretinopathy

Proliferative vitreopretinopathy (PVR) is a complication that occurs in 5-19 % of patients with retinal detachment. Membranes grow on the surface of the retina and occasionally beneath the retina causing recurrent traction and redetachment of the retina (Steinberg 1986). A variety of surgical techniques are used to remove the tractional forces from the retina and internal tamponade is used in combination with retinopexy to assure reattachment. Silicone oil has been used in the eye in the repair of retinal detachments for over 20 years. Initially, silicone oil was used for retinal detachments complicated by proliferative vitreo-retinopathy in whom scleral buckling had failed. It was used prior to the advent of vitrectomy surgery and was initially injected in the vitreous cavity and sometimes under epiretinal membranes in order to disect them from the surface of the retina. This technique was an extremely difficult one and required the use of indirect ophthalmoscopy at the time of silicone oil injection. Poor results were reported utilizing these techniques.

With the advent of modern pars plana vitrectomy techniques, silicone oil is used quite differently. The major goals of retinal detachment repair including identification of all breaks and relieving of all traction still hold and must be fulfilled. In particular, intraocular surgery with vitrectomy instrumentation must be utilized to remove all traction. Silicone oil is most helpful in the repair of complicated retinal detachments in eyes whom have failed previous attempts with long acting gases. In general, such failures are often due to recurrent re-proliferation which often takes place inferiorly. The surface tension of silicone oil is significantly less than that of intraocular gases; thus, it will easily extrude through retinal breaks and enter the subretinal space if any residual traction remains. The major advantage of silicone appears to be the fact that it may be used as a permanent or semi-permanent tampanode. Recurrent traction inferiorly with or without new break formation may result in inferior retinal detachment.

Intraocular corticosteroids at high doses have been evaluated in animal models (Tano, 1980). Such studies show that there may be some decrease in the incidence of redetachment utilizing such intraocular therapy. Other investigators have evaluated antiproliferative agents to prevent redetachement of the retina (Weideman, 1987). Weideman and associates have pioneered the use of intraocular doxorubricin which appears to be taken up by retinal and glial elements and which may have a relatively long lasting effect. This compound can be used at the time of vitrectomy by exposing the retina to the drug for a relatively brief period of time and then washing the drug from the eye. Results in animal models of PVR have been encouraging. We have pursued another approach, the use of liposomes to encapsulate drug for sustained release in the vitreous cavity. Based on work indicating that the polar congener of 5 fluorouracil, 5-FUMP may be a useful antimetabolite, we have encapsulated the drug in large liposomes and have evaluated its toxicity in the vitreous cavity. Preliminary results show that at levels which have previously been shown to inhibit PVR in a rabbit model, the drug is not toxic to the retina. The major problems encountered in evaluating intraocular therapy for patients with PVR include the aphakic status of many of the eyes. Aphakia causes exit of intravitreal drug to occur more rapidly and studies with smaller liposomes have suggested that in aphakic eyes, liposomes may leave the anterior segment relatively rapidly. The second problem encountered in intravitreal anti-PVR therapy is the fact that eyes which have developed full blown PVR and redetachment of the retina commonly have intraocular gas or silicone oil filling the vitreous cavity. In such cases, placement of a drug within the eye will cause the drug to achieve extremely high concentration in the portion of the eye which is filled with aqueous fluid. This is likely to cause toxicity although it would place a very high concentration of the drug on the surface of the inferior retina where re-proliferation is most likely to occur. Certainly a number of eyes with PVR may be phakic however and such therapy may have a role, particularly in preventing early reproliferation in eyes which are developing PVR and in whom intraocular tamponade is not present. It is even possible that antiproliferative therapy will be eventually used in high risk eyes prior to the development of PVR if such therapy can be shown to reliably reduce the incidence of PVR and be non-toxic to the retina and other intraocular structures.

Materials and Methods

All injections of medication into the vitreous cavity were carried out under sterile conditions. New Zealand white rabbits were anesthetized with an intramuscular injection of ketamine and xylazine. All animal experimentation was done in strict accordance with the guidelines of the UCSD office of veterinary affairs. Pupils were dilated with topical cyclogyl and phenylephrine. Injections were given through a 25 gauge needle placed 1 mm posterior to the limbus and injected posteriorly into the vitreous cavity. In all cases a total of 0.1 cc of drugs or control solution was injected. After the injections and aqueous paracentesis was performed utilizing a 30 gauge needle which was left open to air. This caused normalization of the intraocular pressure. For subtenon injections, a volume of 0,5 ml was injected into the posterior subtenon space standard techniques.

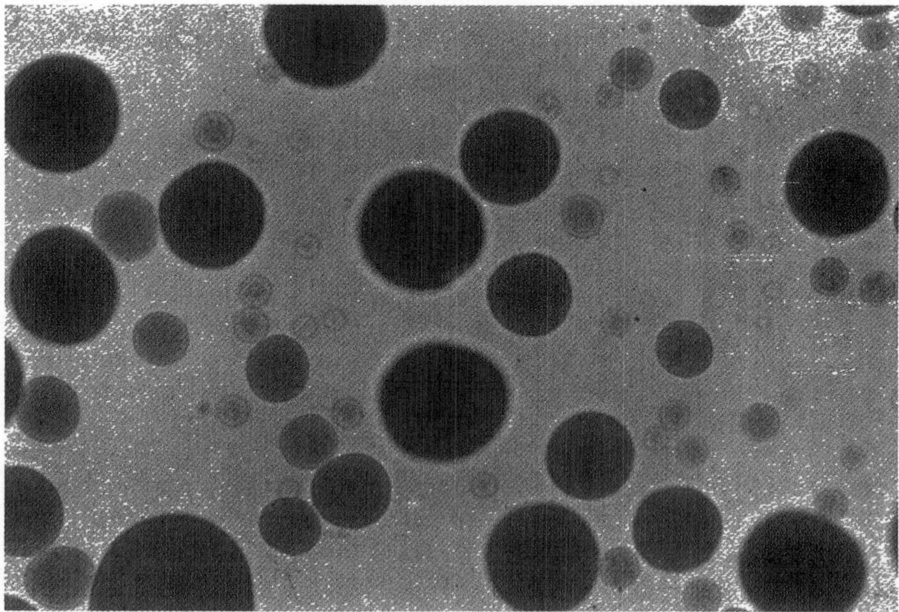

Fig. 1. Photograph of multivesicular liposomes containing red dye. Multiple lipid lamellae are present in each liposome causing drug to be retained in the aqueous interior.

The liposomes which we utilize, we refer to as multivesicular liposomes and they have previously been described in detail (Assil 1987; Kraim 1983). The antivirals thus far evaluated inculde ganciclovir (DHPG), Trifluorothymidine (TFT) and a phosphorylated derivative of ganciclovir. The molecular weight of ganciclovir is 255.23 mg per mole and solubility in water at 25°C is 50 mg/ml (5). The phosphorylated derivative of ganciclovir has a molecular weight of 340 and is water soluble up to concentrations of 100 mg per ml (Fig. 1).

In carrying out the pharmacokinetic studies, 1 cc of multivesicular liposome encapsulated drug is suspended in each of three 20 cc syringes containing phosphate buffered saline. These are then incubated at 37 degress, mounted on a LabQauke revolving rotor (Labindustries Clinical and Research Instruments, Berkeley, California) at 20 revolutions per minute. At set time intervals, 1 ml aliquots are removed from each syringe and centrifuged at 400 g for ten minutes. The resultant liposomal pellet is then isolated. Next, the liposomes are disrupted by resuspension in 1 cc of distilled and deionized water. HPLC determination of drug concentration is then carried out. Drug amount remaining within the liposomal compartment is thus determined and averaged for all three samples at each time point. A standard curve was generated with the percent of drug retained within the liposomes on the abscissa and time on the ordinant. Utilizing this technique, half-life for drug release (hours) with standard deviation are determined.

Clinical examinations were performed with the animals awake or under Ketamine/Xylazine anesthesia after delation the pupils with cyclopentoate 1 % and phenylephrine 2.5 %. In all cases an external ocular examination was performed in conjunction with indirect ophthalmoscopy and examination of the anterior segment with the indirect ophthalmoscope or operating microscope.

Electrophysiologic studies were performed under Ketamine/Xylazine anesthesia. In all cases five to ten bright flash ERG's which gave good signal tracings were performed and then signal averaged to obtain one tracing. Silver wire electrodes were placed on both corneas after topical anesthetic instillation. A Grass stimulator was used at a distance of fourteen inches from the eyes and signals were amplified and fed to a 286 based personal computer. In all animals, electrophysiologic studies were carried out in both eyes. Baseline (preinjection) studies were carried out in all animals. Other control data included ERG amplitude and latencies on fellow eyes and a databank of normal ERG amplitudes and latencies in New Zealand White rabbits corrected for age and weight of the animals. Post-operative studies were performed at various intervals between one day and three months after injection of drug.

Animals were sacrificed utilizing an overdose of pentobarbitol. In all cases in which drug toxicology studies were performed, the animals were perfusion fixed via trans-aortic-perfusion of buffered 2 % gluteraldehyde and 2 % buffered paraformaldahyde while the animal was under deep anesthesia. After removal of the eyes, a small incision was placed at the limbus and the eyes were allowed to soak for up to 24 hours in fixative. The eyes were then placed in a buffer prior to sectioning. In general, one half of the globe was prepared for thin plastic light microscopy and the other half was prepared for electron microscopy.

For phosphorylated 5-Fluoruracil studies, 20 New Zealand White animals were used. Eyes were injected in duplicate with saline, dextrose containing liposomes and drug at 50, and 100 micrograms per 0.1 cc of liposome solution. Animals were sacrificed at 1 week, 2 weeks, 8 weeks, and 12 weeks after injection. Electroretinography and clinical examinations were performed prior to sacrifice and at all of the aforementioned time intervals.

Results

Injection of multivesicular liposomes containing dextrose and saline controls showed no evidence of alteration in the ERG after the one week time point post injection. In addition, at all time points morphologic studies by both light and electron microscopy revealed no evidence of morphologic changes. A standard curve was generated with the percent of drug retained within the liposomes on the abscissa and time on the ordinant. Utilizing this technique, half-life for drug release (hours) with standard deviation are as follows: 13±3.5 (DHPG), 68±6.7 (TFT) and 1000±84 (phosphorylated ganciclovir) (Fig. 2).

Studies of injection of repository preparations of ganciclovir injected in the subtenon space at doses up to 70 mg (preparation kindly provided by Syntex Corp., Palo Alto) revealed a level of 3.85 micrograms per milliliter however not detectable ganciclovir was present at day seven.

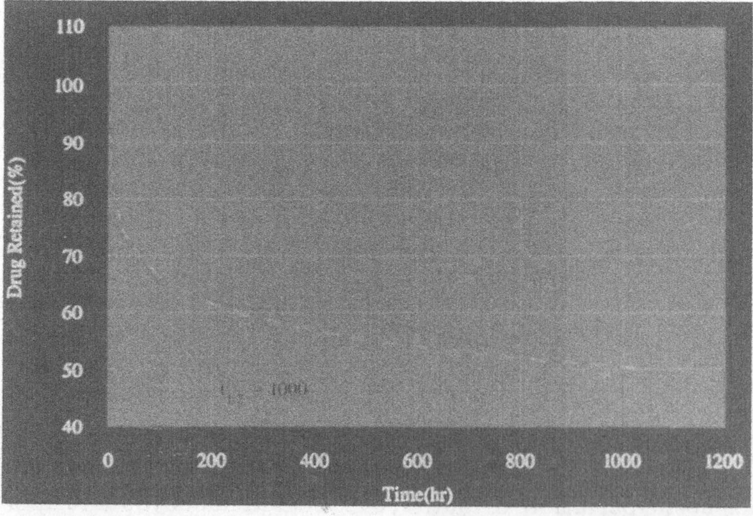

Fig. 2. In vitro dialysis study showing elimination of antiviral drugs from multivesicular liposomes

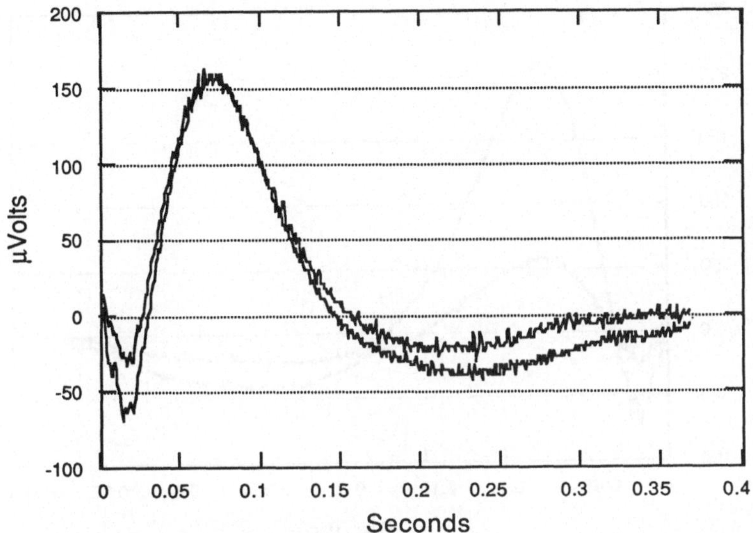

Fig. 3. Electroretinogram of rabbit two weeks after injection of a non-toxuc dose of antiviral drug. The post-injection tracing is normal

Injection of a phosphorylated congener of ganciclovir revealed slight depression of the electroretinogram at doses of 20 micrograms which returned to normal within weeks (Fig. 3). Injection of drug at higher doses (over 50 micrograms) revealed severe depression of the electroretinogram (Fig. 4) which did not return to normal with time. Morphologic changes were determined by thin section (2 micron) light microscopy of methacrylate embedded tissue. At doses over 50 micrograms, irreversible changes and degeneration of the middle and outer nuclear layers were seen (Fig. 5). Infiltration of the outer with phagocytic cells was also documented. Calculations show that this drug therefore appears to have a therapeutic index in the 10-20 range when injected in the free form.

Injection of a liposome encapsulated phosphorylated derivative of 5-FU failed to reveal significant retinal toxicity at doses up to 100 micrograms. An initial slight depression of the ERG and subtle morphologic changes normalized within three weeks at this dose. This dose has been shown in other studies to inhibit proliferative vitreoretinopathy in animal models. These studies also showed that control liposome (filled with dextrose) did not cause changes in the electroretinogram.

Discussion

Review of the current therapy of viral retinitis and proliferative vitreoreti- nopathy revels the need for development of local therapy to inhibit virus replication and intraocular proliferation. Our studies of subtenon ganciclovir in both soluble and repository forms reveal that this route of injection doses not lead to significant levels of the antiviral drug ganciclovir in the eye.

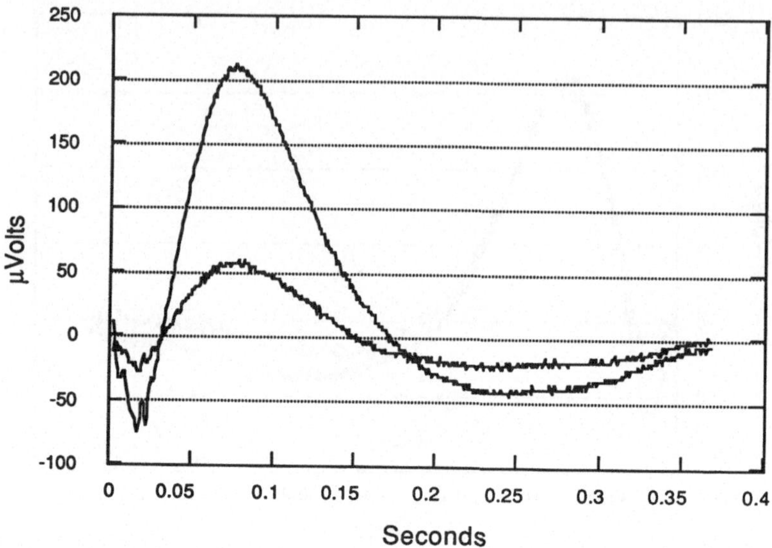

Fig. 4. Electroretinogram of rabbit before one and two weeks after injection of a toxic dose of antiviral drug. Note abnormal waves from and significant loss of amplitude seen at two weeks (lower cure) post injection

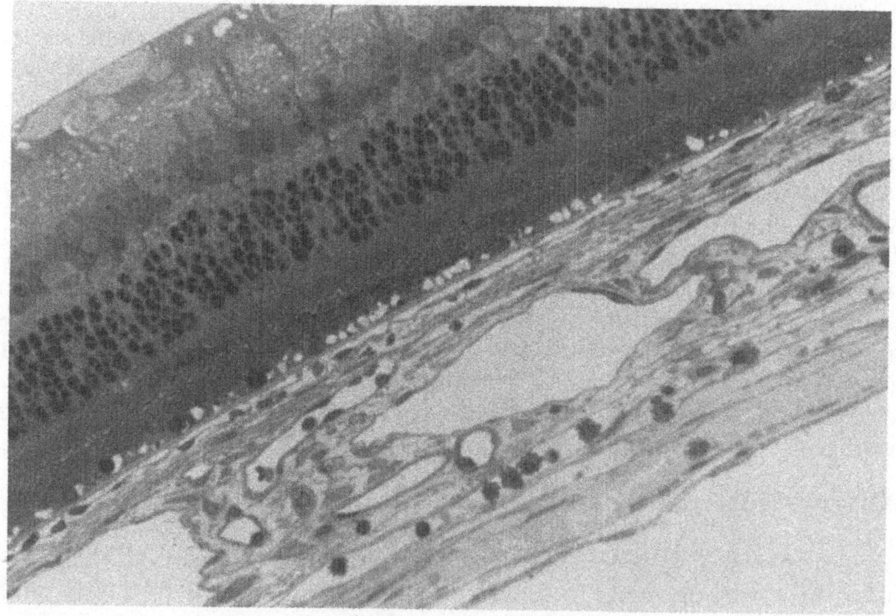

Fig. 5. Thin section light micrograph (400x) of perfusion fixed rabbit after toxic dose of phosphorylated ganciclovir. Note vacuoles in outersegment layer of retina

Our studies do indicate that the multi-vesicular liposome system is not toxic to the rabbit retina. Morphologic studies utilizing toluidine blue stained 2 micron sections and electron microscopic studies of perfusion fixed rabbit retina reveal no evidence of morphologic abnormalities up to one month after empty liposome injection into the vitreous cavity. Electroretinographic studies revealed normal ERG latencies and amplitudes two weeks and later post injection. Our electrophysiologic studies indicate nonspecific changes in the electroretinogram both in the injected eye and in the fellow eye of all animals within the first week post-injection. Performance of electroretinography within one week of injection of any substance within the vitreous cavity will lead to nonspecific ERG changes. For this reason, elecroretinography cannot be relied upon as a sensitive indicator of drug toxicity within the first week of injection. Studies of toxicity with a variety of drugs after this time period however, do reveal that changes in electroretinogram parallels the severity of changes seen morphologically. Our studies cannot discriminate as to which of the techniques are more sensitive to drug toxicity.

As expected, molecular weight and water solubility of antiviral and related drugs are significant in determining the rate of release from liposomes. Ganciclovir, which is the least polar and of lowest molecular weight is released most rapidly by the liposomes; while a phosphorylated derivative of ganciclovir, which is the most water soluble and of highest molecular weight, enjoys the slowest rate of release. Since drug must traverse numerous lipid bilayers prior to release from the multivesicular liposomes, it is reasonable that larger and less lipid soluble drugs would require a longer transit time. Furthermore, in evaluating the therapeutic indices of these drugs in HCMV infected mammalian cell lines, TFT has the lowest therapeutic index at 3.5, with DHPG intermediate at 8.0 and the phosphorylated derivative of ganciclovir, the greatest at 20. It thus appears that the in-vitro dialysis system, coupled with knowledge of a drug's toxicity and efficacy can help to reselect liposomal encapsulated antivirals for local treatment of viral retinitis.

Work with polar derivatives of anti-metabolites and antiviral drugs reveal that concentrations of drugs many times above those required to inhibit virus or intraocular proliferation can be safly achieved within the rabbit eye. Polar derivatives of medications are highly water soluble and therefore are well retained within most liposome system. These results, in combination with the encouraging negative toxicologic studies utilizing a multi-vesicular liposome system, would indicate that injection of polar drugs which have been encapsulated within the aqueous phase of liposomes may be a promising therapeutic modality. Further studies which need to be performed include studies of the pharmacokinetics of both free and liposome encapsulated drugs as well as determining the most efficacious method to retain therapeutic drug levels in the eyes of vitrectomized and/or lensectomized animals.

References

Assil K., Weinreb RN. (1987) Multivesicular liposomes: sustained release of the antimetabolite cytosine arabinoside in the eye. Arch Ophthal 105:400

Blumenkranz MS, Culbertson WW, Clarkson JG et al. (1986) Treatment of the acute retinal necrosis syndrome with acyclorvir. Ophthalmology 93:296-300

Cantrill HL, Henry K, Melroe H, Knobloch WH, Ramsay RC, Balfour HH (1989) Treatment of cytomegalovirus retinitis with intravitreal ganciclovir. Ophthalology 96:367-374

Culbertson W, Blumenkran MS, Pepose JS, et al. (1986) Varicella zoster virus is a cause of the acute retinal necrosis syndrome Ophthalmology 93:559-569

Freeman WR (1989) Intraocular antiviral therapy. Ach Ophth 107:1737-1739

Freeman WR, Thomas EL, Rao NA et al. (1986) Demonstration of herpes group virus in acute retinal necrosis syndrome. Am J Ophthalmol 102:701-9

Gariano R, Assil K, Svendsen P, Munguia D, Bergeron-Lynn G, Heckenlively J, Weinreb RN, Freeman WR (1990) Retinal toxicity of intravitreal injection of FUMP using multivesicular liposomes. Investigative Ophthalmology Visual Science (suppl) 31:306

Heinemann MH (1989) Long term intravitreal ganciclovir therapy for cytomegalovirus retinopathy. Arch Ophth 107:1767-1772

Henderly DE, Freemanm WR, Causey DM et al (1987) Cytomegalovirus retinitis and response to therapy with ganciclovir. Ophthalmology 425-34

Henry K, Cantrill H, Fletcher C, et al. (1987) Use of ganciclovir (dihydroxy propoxymethyl guanine) for cytomegalovirus retinitis in a patient with AIDS. Am J Ophthalmol 103:17-23

Jabs DA, Enger C, Bartlett JG (1989) Cytomegalovirus retinitis and acquired immunodeficiency syndrome. Arch Ophthalmol 107:75-80

Kimm S, Turker, MS, Chi EY, Shifa S, Martin GM (1983) Preparation of multivesicular liposomes. Bioch Bioph Acta 728:339-398

Lehoang P, Girard B, Robinet P et al. (1989) Foscarnet in the treatment of cytomegalovirus retinitis in acquired immune deficiency syndrome. Ophthalmology 96:865-873

Peyman GA, Goldberg MF, Uninsky E et al. (1984) Vitrectomy and intravitreal antiviral drug therapy in acute retinal necrosis syndrome. Arch Ophthalmol 102:1618-1621

Pulido J, Peyman GA, Lesar T, Vernot J (1985) Intravitreal toxicity of hydroxyacyclovir (BW-B759U), a new antiviral agent. Arch Ophthalmol 103:840-841

Rungger-Brandle E, Roux L, Leuenberger PM (1984) Bilateral acute retinal necrosis (BARN); identification of the presumed infectious agent. Ophthalmology 91:1648-58

Soushi S, Ozawa H, Matsuhashi M et al. (1988) Demonstration of varicella-zoster virus antigens in the vitreous aspirates of patients with acute retinal necrosis syndrome. Ophthalmology 95:1394-98

Steinberg RH (1986) Research update: Report from a workshop on cell biology of retinal detachment. Exp Eye Res 43:695-706

Tano Y, Chandler D, Machemer R (1980) Inhibition of intraocular proliferation with intraviteal injection of triamcinilone acetonide. Am J Ophthalmol 90:810-816

Ussery FM, Gibson SR, Conklin RH, Piot DF, Stool EW, Conklin AJ (1988) Intravitreal ganciclovir in the treatment of AIDS-associated cytomegalovirus retinitis. Ophthalmology 95:640-648

Walmsley SL, Chew E, Read SE, Vellend H, Salit L, Rachlis A, Fanning MM (1988) Treatment of cytomegalovirus retinitis with trisodium phosphoformate hexahydrate (foscarnet). J Infectious Dis 157:569-572

Wiedemann P, Heimann K (1987) Proliferative vitreoretinopathy. Pathogenesis and possibilities for treatment with cytostatic drugs. Am J Ophthal 104(1):10-14

Wiedemann P, Lemmen K, Schmiedl R, Heimann K (1987) Intraocular daunorubicin for the treatment and prophylaxis of traumatic proliferative vitreoretinopathy. Am J Ophthal 104:10-14

Corresponding Address
Professor W. R. Freeman, M.D.
University of California, UCSD Eye Center, Department of Ophthalmology,
9500 Gilman Drive, La Jolla, San Diego, California 92093-0618, USA

Medikamentöse Therapie der proliferativen Vitreoretinopathie (PVR)

P. Wiedemann

Einleitung

Jedes Auge mit einer Netzhautablösung entwickelt eine PVR, wenn auch in verschiedenem Ausmaß und Grad. Als PVR oder proliferative Vitreoretinopathie bezeichnet man die narbige Organisation von Glaskörper und Retina durch opake, kontraktile Zellmembranen zu beiden Seiten der Retina. Die Vernarbung im Glaskörperraum ist der häufigste Grund für einen Mißerfolg der Netzhautchirurgie. Voraussetzung für Beginn und Fortschreiten des Krankheitsprozesses ist ein *Zusammenspiel von natürlichen und iatrogenen Ursachen: Art* (z. B. Entscheidung zur primären Vitrektomie) und *Intensität* der Behandlung (ausgedehnte Kryopexie oder Laserkoagulation) spielen ebenso eine Rolle wie die initiale *Schädigung der Netzhaut* (Größe und Ausmaß von Hufeisenforamina mit großflächiger Exposition des Pigmentepithels) und der *Zusammenbruch der Blut-Retinaschranke* (Glaskörperblutung) (Bonnet, 1989; Cowley et al., 1989). Wenn das feine Gleichgewicht zwischen *Zellen* und *extrazellulären modulierenden Faktoren* gestört ist, kommt es durch unkontrollierte Zellproliferation (Hiscott et al., 1985) zur Narbenbildung der PVR. Im Verlauf der Krankheit können wir eine zelluläre *Aktivierungsphase* von einer *Proliferationsphase* und einer *Kontraktionsphase* unterscheiden: Dem entspricht bei der Wundheilung das Stadium der Entzündung, Proliferation und Narbenschrumpfung (Weller et al., 1990; Widemann und Weller, 1988).

Ziel einer medikamentösen Behandlung ist die Unterbrechung der Ereignisfolge, die zur Proliferation und Kontraktion periretinaler Membranen und damit zur Traktionsamotio führt.

Zellen und extrazelluläre modulierende Faktoren

Zellen

Mit licht- und elektronenmikrokopischen sowie immunologischen Techniken lassen sich vier verschiedene Zelltypen in den Traktionsmembranen nachweisen. *Pigmentepithelzellen* werden zum Zeitpunkt der Netzhautablösung als Tabakstaub in den Glaskörperraum ausgestreut, siedeln sich der Schwer-

Gramer/Kampik (Hrsg.) Pharmakotherapie am Auge
© Springer-Verlag Berlin Heidelberg 1992

kraft folgend meist in der unteren Fundushälfte an – die PVR ist eine Erkrankung der unteren Fundushälfte – und können sich metaplastisch in Fibroblasten umwandeln (Vidaurri-Leal et al., 1984) und Traktion ausüben (Glaser et al., 1987).

Monozyten sind in besonderer Weise zur Aktivierung anderer Zellen befähigt, denn sie sezernieren verschiedene lösliche Faktoren, die chemotaktisch und proliferationsfördernd auf andere Zellen wirken. Sie sind daher in der Initialphase der Erkrankung von äußerster Bedeutung, spielen aber auch eine wichtige Rolle bei der Fibrosierung einer Narbe (Weller et al., 1988).

Gliazellen dienen als Gerüst und Ankerpunkt für die Proliferation und Kontraktion anderer Zellen (Hiscott et al., 1984). Stoffwechselprodukte von Gliazellen fördern die Proliferation von Pigmentepithelzellen und Fibroblasten (Burke und Foster, 1985). Gliazellen können auch Traktionskräfte ausüben (Hui et al., 1987).

Fibroblasten bilden die extrazelluären fibrösen und amorphen Komponenten der Membranen. Sie finden sich in der PVR-Membran, jedoch ist die genaue Herkunft dieser Zellen nicht geklärt. Fibroblasten können sich in Myofibroblasten umwandeln und kontrahieren.

Extrazelluläre modulierende Faktoren

Für die Zellen gilt: "The milieu is the message". Das Milieu wird in den frühen Phasen der Erkrankung durch den Zusammenbruch der Blut-Retina-Schranke entscheidend verändert, später kommt es durch Kontakt des Immunsystems mit retinalen Antigenen eventuell zu einer chronischen autoimmunbedingten Entzündung (Broekhuyse et al., 1990; Grisanti et al., 1990). Bei den extrazellulären Faktoren müssen wir trennen und unterscheiden zwischen im Auge vorhandenen, aus dem Plasma stammenden und im Verlauf der Krankheit von den an der Membranbildung beteiligten Zellen erzeugten Faktoren. Der meist diskutierte Faktor ist der *Transforming growth factor-beta (TGF-ß)*, der die Proliferation, vor allem aber die Kontraktion und Fibrose fördert (Raymond und Thompson, 1990). Bei einer PVR ist TGF-ß entsprechend dem Schweregrad der Erkrankung erhöht (Glaser, 1988; Gaudric et al., 1989). Viele andere Faktoren wurden im Auge nachgewiesen: aber nicht ein einzelner Wachstumsfaktor ist "der" PVR-Faktor, sondern unterschiedliche Kombinationen von Faktoren bewirken eine verschieden starke Proliferation (Burke, 1989). Die verschiedenen Faktoren sind sozusagen Buchstaben in einem Alphabet, mit dem man verschieden starke Proliferationsbefehle schreiben kann.

Pharmakologische Therapie der PVR

Begründung einer medikamentösen PVR-Therapie

Warum brauchen wir überhaupt eine medikamentöse Behandlung der PVR?
Die Verbesserung der mikrochirurgischen Techniken, die erleichterte intraoperative Manipulation mit Perfluorocarbonflüssigkeit sowie die Tamponade
der Netzhaut mit langdauerndem Gas oder Silikonöl bewirken einen
anhaltenden Erfolg bei ca 60-70 % der operierten Augen. Umgekehrt kann
man sagen: *bei etwa einem Drittel der Patienten mit PVR reicht die einmalige
chirurgische Behandlung allein nicht aus.* Diese Patienten benötigen einen
neuen, einen pharmakologischen Therapieansatz. Denn die Chirurgie hat die
meisten technischen Probleme der Behandlung der komplizierten Traktionsamotio gelöst, aber das *biologische Problem der Reproliferation* kann nur
pharmakologisch angegangen werden.

Ziele der medikamentösen PVR-Therapie

Die Ziele der pharmakologischen Therapie der PVR sind offensichtlich:

- *Rezidivprophylaxe*, d. h. Verhinderung von Reamotio und Reoperation
  durch Verhinderung der Reproliferation, da bekanntlich jede Operation
  das PVR-Risiko steigert, und
- *Funktionsstabilisierung* und gegebenenfalls *-verbesserung*.

Es handelt sich bei der medikamentösen PVR-Therapie um eine *tertiäre
Prävention*, d. h. eine Verhinderung von Rückfällen. Eine sekundäre Prävention, d. h. Krankheiten so rechtzeitig zu erkennen, daß sie mit sicherem
Erfolg behandelt werden können, oder eine primäre Prävention, d. h.
Erkennung von Risikoaugen, ist bisher in der Praxis nur ansatzweise
möglich. Die klinisch zur Behandlung eingesetzten Medikamente greifen in
der inflammatorischen Aktivierungs- bzw. chronischen Entzündungsphase,
der proliferativ-synthetischen Phase und der Kontraktionsphase der PVR an.
Obowhl diese Prozeße nicht streng getrennt ablaufen, hält man einen
möglichst *frühzeitigen Eingriff in die Ereignisfolge* für sinnvoll, da dann ja
auch die späteren Schritte gehemmt werden.

Viele Medikamente greifen in mehreren Phasen der PVR-Entwicklung an,
aber meistens läßt sich eine Hauptwirkung (s. Tabelle 1) benennen. Die
folgenden Medikamente werden vorgestellt, weil sie experimentell und/oder
klinisch eine deutliche Wirkung haben und eine erträgliche Toxizität
zeigen.

Kriterien zur Auswahl eines Medikaments

Medikamente werden nach drei Kriterien beurteilt:

Tabelle 1. Hauptwirkung verschiedener Medikamente bei der PVR-Behandlung

Medikament	Entzündung	Matrix-adhäsion	Prolifera-tion	Matrix-synthese	Kontraktion
Steroide	+		+		
Heparin		+	+		+
Daunomycin	+		+		+
Fluoropyrimidin			+		+
Colchicin			+	+	+
Penicillamin				+	

Die pharmakodynamischen Eigenschaften. Die Wirksamkeit hängt ab von der Wirkstärke, einem Maß für die Dosis, die zur Erzielung einer bestimmten gewünschten Wirkung erforderlich ist, und von der Wirkaktivität (intrinsic activity), also dem in einem biologischen System erreichbaren Maximaleffekt, der mit der Empfindlichkeit des biologischen Substrats korreliert.

Die pharmakokinetischen Eigenschaften. Natürlich hängt die Wirkung ab von der erreichbaren Expositionszeit. Die pharmakokinetischen Eigenschaften des Medikaments sind von entscheidender Bedeutung für die kontrollierte und für den Patienten erträgliche Zufuhr des Medikaments und für die Verteilung des Medikaments im Auge und Körper. Man darf bei systemischer Therapie nie vergessen, daß das Auge und insbesondere der Glaskörperraum nur ein sehr kleiner, für Medikamente schlecht zugänglicher Teil des Körpers ist.

Die toxikologischen Eigenschaften. Die Sicherheit des Medikaments hängt von der Toxizität ab und von der Selektivität mit der das Medikament schädliche Prozesse verhindert und normale Funktionen des Auges unbeeinflußt läßt. Die meisten der zur PVR-Behandlung verwendeten Medikamente haben nur ein kleines therapeutisches Fenster. Es gilt also sicher der Satz von G. Kuschinsky: „Wenn behauptet wird, daß eine Substanz keine Nebenwirkung zeigt, so besteht der dringende Verdacht, daß sie auch keine Hauptwirkung hat" (Kuschinsky, 1980).

Antiproliferativ wirkende Medikamente

Die proliferative Phase gab der Krankheit ihren Namen. Wir wenden uns daher zunächst antiproliferativen Medikamenten zu: diese Therapie scheint relativ spezifisch, denn die ortsständigen Netzhautzellen (Pigmentepithel, Rezeptoren, Ganglienzellen) teilen sich unter normalen Umständen nicht und sollten daher weniger empfindlich gegenüber den Medikamenten sein.

Colchicin. In erster Linie wirkt Colchicin als Zytostatikum. Colchicin ist ein Mitosehemmstoff, der während des Kernteilungvorgangs die Ausbildung der Teilungsspindel verhindert und zu polyploiden Kernen führt. In vitro wirkt Colchicin auch antikontraktil, hemmt die Makrophageninvasion und die Kollagensekretion. Im Tierversuch senkt Colchicin bei oraler Gabe die Amotiorate von 78 % auf 30 % (Lemor et al., 1986). Das z. Z. erprobte Therapieschema sieht die mehrwöchige orale Gabe hoher Dosen vor, die Dosierung beträgt etwa 1.2 mg viermal täglich für 6 Wochen oral (Glaser, 1988). Patienten mit einem Riesenriß, also Patienten mit hohem Risiko eine PVR zu entwickeln, bekamen unter Colchicin seltener eine PVR als eine kleine Kontrollgruppe. Das Medikament war also scheinbar prophylaktisch wirksam. In einer randomisierten Studie fand sich bei mit Colchicin behandelten Patienten eine geringere Notwendigkeit zur Reoperation als bei Kontrollaugen (Glaser, 1988). Eine andere Arbeitsgruppe fand dagegen bei unterschiedlichem Protokoll das Medikament unwirksam (Berman und Gombos, 1989). Colchicin wird wegen seiner geringen therapeutischen Breite in der Krebstherapie nicht mehr eingesetzt. Es erstaunt daher nicht, daß Colchicin in der verwendeten Dosierung toxisch für den Sehnerv ist.

Fluoropyrimidine. Die Fluoropyrimidine – die am häufigsten eingesetzten Vertreter sind Fluorouracil, Fluorouridin und Fluoroorotat – sind die Zytostatika, über die bisher im Zusammenhang mit der PVR-Behandlung am meisten publiziert wurde. Sie wirken entweder wie Fluorouracil hauptsächlich auf die DNA-Synthesephase oder beeinflussen über die RNA auch den Proteinstoffwechsel wie die beiden letztgenannten effektiveren Vertreter. Über den Metabolismus zu Fluorouridin-Monophosphat werden sie in die RNA eingebaut und stören damit die Funktion von ribosomaler und Boten-RNA. Auch die Hemmung der Glykosilierung von Membranproteinen (Heath et al., 1990) soll von therapeutischer Bedeutung sein. Fluoropyrimidine werden intravitreal oder subkonjunktival appliziert oder in Liposomen verpackt.

Wie alle Zytostatika sind die Fluoropyrimidine bei höherer Dosierung toxisch für Retina und Sehnerv, bei subkonjunktivaler Gabe treten schwer heilende Hornhautulcera auf. In einer nicht randomisierten Studie mit Fluorouracil war Blumenkranz bei 60 % seiner PVR-Patienten erfolgreich (Blumenkranz et al., 1984). Tavakolian und Wollensak berichteten über ermutigende Resultate (Tavakolian and Wollensak, 1985).

Daunomycin. Wir selbst haben zur Behandlung der PVR Daunomycin eingesetzt. Daunomycin hemmt die Zellproliferation sehr effektiv, aber auch die Zellmigration, allerdings nicht die Kollagensekretion. Bei proliferationshemmender Dosierung wird auch die Kontraktion gehemmt (Heath et al., 1990). Wir spülen mit 7.5 mg/l die vitrektomierte Glaskörperhöhle für 10 min. (Wiedemann et al., 1987). Damit ist eine exakte Dosierung und Verteilung des Medikaments im periretinalen Raum gewährleistet. Daunomycin wirkt besonders starkt in der S-Phase des Zellzyklus, greift aber auch an anderen

Stellen, z. B. durch Schädigung der Zellmembranen, in den Zellstoffwechsel ein und ist deshalb in seiner Wirkung weitgehend *unabhängig vom Zellzyklus*. Damit – und das ist in der Praxis sehr vorteilhaft – genügen *kurze Expositionszeiten*.

In einer prospektiven randomisierten Studie zur Behandlung der idiopathischen PVR mit Daunomycin konnten wir zeigen, daß die Zahl der periretinalen Proliferationen von 78 % auf 24 % gesenkt werden konnte und die Zahl der notwendig erachteten Reoperationen von 44 % auf 15 %. Dabei ist auch der funktionelle Erfolg zufriedenstellend (Wiedemann et al., 1988). Die Langzeitergebnisse wurden in einer retrospektiven Studie ermittelt. Nach 18 Monaten lag bei 73 % der Augen mit 1.1 Operationen die Netzhaut an, 89 % hatten eine Sehschärfe größer 1/50. Diese Ergebnisse sind günstiger als die früherer Studien (Wiedemann et al., 1991). Der Wert des Medikaments soll in einer multizentrischen von der DFG unterstützen Studie überprüft werden.

Andere zur PVR-Behandlung eingesetzte Medikamente

Steroide. Steroide waren die ersten Medikamente, die zur Behandlung der PVR eingesetzt wurden (Machemer et al., 1979): Prednison, Prednisolon, Methylprednisolon, Triamcinolon und Dexamethason wurden experimentell oder klinisch erprobt (cf. Wiedemann, 1988). Steroide stabilisieren die Blut-Retina-Schranke und hemmen die Makrophageninvasion. Außerdem hemmen sie die Fibroblastenbildung und damit die Kollagensynthese. Schließlich wirken sie immunsuppressiv und verhindern damit die chronische autoimmun bedingte Entzündungsphase. Sie werden systemisch oder intravitreal appliziert, ihre intraokulare Toxizität ist minimal. Machemer fand beim Kaninchen und beim Affen keine Nebenwirkungen. Deshalb gibt Machemer bei ausgewählten Patienten 2 mg Triamcinolon intravitreal. Eine randomisierte Studie (Körner et al., 1982) belegte den Wert systemischer Prednisolongaben, denn es konnte bei diesen Patienten eine deutliche Reduktion der frühen Zeichen der PVR gefunden werden.

Machemers Gruppe konnte auch zeigen, daß die Vorbehandlung mit Steroiden im Tiermodell zu einer deutlichen Verminderung der PVR-Rate führt (Chandler et al., 1987). Dies betont die Bedeutung der Hemmung der entzündlichen Aktivierungsphase, in der die antiphlogistische Wirkung der Steroide voll zur Geltung kommt.

Pharmakologische Interaktion mit der Matrix. Nach dem Therapieziel Abdichtung der Blut-Retina-Schranke wenden wir uns nun einem anderen wesentlichen Punkt in der Pathogenese der PVR zu: Anheftung der Zellen an der extrazellulären Matrix und Interaktion mit den Matrixproteinen, die über den Fibronexus die Zellmorphologie, Permeabilität und Kontraktion, aber auch das Proliferationsverhalten beeinflussen. Die Anheftung ist eine unbedingte Voraussetzung für das Wachstum der Zellen und damit für alle folgenden Schritte der PVR-Pathogenese. Für den therapeutischen Einsatz in der Initialphase der PVR diskutiert man Heparin (Johnson und Blankenship, 1988; Alvira et al., 1989). Fibrin, das Endprodukt der Koagulationskaskade fördert die Membranbildung (Murray et al., 1990), Heparin hemmt die Fibrinbildung. Auf der anderen Seite erhöht Heparin die intraokulare Blutungsneigung und fördert damit die Entstehung der PVR. Heparin ist ein Glykosaminoglykan sehr heterogener Zusammensetzung, das hydriert ein großes Volumen einnimmt. Es wirkt antikoagulativ, bindet Wachstumsfaktoren und hemmt die Kontraktion in vitro. Die sogenannten niedermolekularen Heparine sollen die Koagulationskaskade ohne verstärkte Blutungsneigung hemmen (Hirsh et al., 1985) und man kann damit in Zukunft vielleicht die positiven Eigenschaften der Heparine zur vollen Geltung bringen. Die Hoffnungen, die auf diese Medikamente gesetzt werden, beruhen großenteils auf in vitro Versuchen, die exakte therapeutische Wertigkeit ist noch nicht abgeklärt, trotz Anwendung bei Patienten.

RGDS-Peptide, so benannt nach ihrer Aminosäuresequenz (Avery and Glaser, 1986) hemmen in vitro die Bindung von Fibronektin an die Strukturproteine (Kollagen) und reduzieren daher die Fähigkeit der Zellen zur hypozellularen Gelkontraktion. Darunter verseht man die Kontraktion eines Kollagengels durch wenige nicht im Zusammenhang stehende Zellen, im Gegensatz zur syncytialen Kontraktion der myofibroblastenartigen Zellen.

Als Beispiel eines Medikaments, das die Kollagensynthese hemmt, sei das Penicillamin genannt, das aber keine größere Bedeutung bei der Behandlung der experimentellen PVR erlangte. Medikamente, die selektiv die kontraktile Phase beeinflussen, sind bisher nicht bekannt.

Neue Applikationsformen

Das Hauptproblem der medikamentösen PVR-Therapie scheint nicht ein pharmakodynamisches zu sein sondern eher ein pharmakokinetisches: Um eine Wirkung zu erzielen, muß ein Medikament mit den Zielzellen für eine kritische minimale Zeit in Kontakt kommen; die typische Halbwertszeit eines Medikaments im Glaskörper beträgt 2-4 Stunden, nach der Vitrektomie verringert sich diese Zeit um den Faktor 2.5. Wie kann man nun therapeutische Spiegel erreichen und erhalten?

Experimentelle Ansatzpunkte liegen in der Applikation in Liposomen (Joondeph, Peyman et al., 1988), dem Einbringen im Plombenmaterial (Snady-McCoy et al., 1988), Targeting mit Antikörpern (Anti-Transferrin-Rezeptor (Weller et al., 1989)) und insbesondere Lösung der Medikamente im Silikonöl, z. B. Carmustin (Tolentino et al., 1988) oder Retinol (Campochiaro et al., 1990). Silikonöl wird bei schwierigen Netzhautablösungen häufig verwendet, denn es verhindert Blutungen, schwächt die Wirkung kontraktiler Membranen und hemmt intraokulare Flüssigkeitsströmungen. Aber bedingt durch die Emulsifikation des Öls, toxische niedermolukulare Anteile und die Konzentration von Zellen und Wachstumsfaktoren im ölfreien Raum in der unteren Fundushälfte werden immer wieder Beobachtungen publiziert, die dem Öl eine ursächliche Rolle bei der Reproliferation zusprechen.

Die einfachste Methode der Wirkungsteigerung liegt wohl in der *Kombination verschiedener Arzneimittel:* Die Kombination von Heparin mit Fluorouracil verstärkt die proliferationshemmende Wirkung.

Das Kölner Therapie-Schema

Das derzeitige *Kölner Schema* sieht die perioperative Gabe von 100 mg Ultralan bei Amotio und Trauma vor, sowie die intraoperative Daunomycinspülung bei Patienten mit offensichtlicher PVR, bzw. prophylaktisch bei Patienten mit hohem PVR-Risiko, z. B. bei Riesenrissen.

Zusammenfassung

Alle bisher eingesetzten Medikamente waren keine Wundermittel, die auf einem Schlag das Problem der Reproliferation in den Griff bekamen. Mit der Kombination verschiedener Medikamente sollte es aber in Zukunft möglich sein, den Patienten mehrfache Operationen zu ersparen und für einige Jahre zu orientierendem Sehen zu verhelfen.

Literatur

Alvira G, Hartzer M, Blumenkranz M, Camacho H (1989) Heparin, a possible new approach to the treatment of proliferative vitreoretinopathy. In: Heimann K, Wiedemann P (Hrsg) *Proliferative Vitreoretinopathy.* Kaden, Heidelberg, S 268-271
Avery R, Glaser B (1986) Inhibition of retinal pigment epithelial cell attachment by a synthetic peptide drived from the cell binding domain of fibronectin. Arch Opthalmol 104:1220-1222
Berman DH, Gombos GM (1989) Proliferative vitreoretinopathy: does oral low-dose colchicine have an inhibitory effect? A controlled study in humans. Ophthalmic Surg 20:268-72
Blumenkranz M, Hernandez E, Ophir A und Norton EW (1984). "5-fluorouracil: new applications in complicated retinal detachment for an established antimetabolite." Ophthalmoloogy. 921(2):122-30
Bonnet M (1989). Clinical findings associated with the development of postoperative PVR in primary rhegmatogenous retinal detachment. In Heimann K, Wiedemann P (Hrsg) *Proliferative Vitreoretinopathy.* Kaden, Heidelberg, S 18-20
Broekhuyse R, Rademakers A, Vugt Van A und Winkens H (1990). "Autoimmune responsiveness to retinal IRBP, S-antigen and Opsin in proliferative vitreoretinopathy." Exp Eye Res. 50:197-202
Burke J (1989). Cell interactions in proliferative vitreoretinopathy: do growth factors play a role? In Heimann K, Wiedemann P (Hrsg) *Proliferative Vitreoretinopathy. Kaden, Heidelberg, S 80-87*

Burke J und Foster S (1985). "Induction of DNA-synthesis by coculture of retinal glia and pigment epithelium." Invest Ophthalmol Vis Sci. 26:636-642

Campochiaro P, Hackett S und Conway B (1990). "Retinoic acid promotes a differentiated morphology and density-dependent growth arrest in human retinal pigment epithelial cells." Invest Ophthalmol Vis Sci. 31:69

Chandler DB, Hida T, Sheta S, Proia AD und Machemer R (1987). "Improvement in efficacy of corticosteroid therapy in an animal model of proliferative vitreoretinopathy by pretreatment." Graefes Arch Clin Exp Ophthalmol. 225:259-65

Cowley M, C.B.P., Campochiaro PA, Kaiser D und Gaskin H (1989). "Clinical risk factors for proliferative vitreoretinopathy." Arch Ophthalmol. 107:1147-51

Gaudric A, Glacet-Bernard A, Falquerho L, Barritault D und Coscas G (1989). Transforming growth factor beta in vitreous from patients with epiretinal proliferation. In Heimann K, Wiedemann P (Hrsg) Proliferative Vitreoretinopathy. Kaden, Heidelberg, S 118-119

Glaser B, Cardin A und Biscoe B (1987). "Proliferative vitreoretinopathy. The mechanism of development of vitreoretinal traction." Ophthalmol. 94:327-332

Glaser BM (1988). Pathobiology of PVR. In Freeman HM, Tolentino FI (Hrsg) Proliferative Vitreoretinopathy (PVR), Springer-Verlag New York, S 12-21

Grisanti S, Esser P, Weller M, Heimann K und Wiedemann P (1990). Zur Bedeutung des Komplementsystems bei der proliferativen Vitreoretinopathie. DOG, Baden-Baden

Heath T, Brown C und Stern W (1990). "Ocular Cicatricial Disease. Drug Effects in Vitro on Cell Proliferation, Contraction, and Viability." Invest Ophthalmol Vis Sci. 31:1245-1251

Hirsh J, Ofosu F und Buchanan M (1985). "Rationale behind the development of low molecular weight heparin derivatives." Sem Throm Hemostasis. 11:13-16

Hiscott P, Grierson I, Trombetta C, Rahi A, Marshall J und McLeod D (1984). "Retinal and epiretinal glia – an immunohistochemical study." Br J Ophthalmol. 68:698-707

Hiscott P, Grierson I und McLeod D (1985). "Natural history of fibrocellular epiretinal membranes. A quantitative, autoradiographic and immunohistochemical study." Br J Ophthalmol. 69:810-823

Hui Y, Goodnight R, Sorgente N und Ryan S (1987). "Glial epiretinal membranes: do they contract." Invest Ophthalmol Vis Sci. 28:207

Johnson R und Blankenship G (1988). "A prospective, randomized clinical trial of heparin therapy for postoperative intraocular fibrin." Ophthalmology. 95:312-317

Joondeph B, Peyman G und Khoobehi B (1988). Liposome-Encapsulated 5-Fluorouracil: A New Approach to PVR. In Freeman HM, Tolentino FI (Hrsg) Proliferative Vitreoretinopathy (PVR), Springer-Verlag, New York, S 130-133

Körner F, Merz A, Gloor B und Wagner E (1982) "Postoperative retinal fibrosis – a controlled clinical study of systemic steroid therapy." Graefe's Arch Clin Exp Ophthalmol 219:268-271

Kuschinsky G (1980). Taschenbuch der modernen Arzneibehandlung. Georg Thieme Verlag, Stuttgart New York, S 715

Lemor M, Yeo JH und Glaser BM (1986). "Oral colchicine for the treatment of experimental traction retinal detachment." Arch Ophthalmol. 104:1226-9

Machemer R, Sugita G und Tano Y (1979). "Treatment of intraocular proliferation with intravitreal steroids." Trans Am Ophthalmol Soc. 77:171-178

Murray T, Stern W, Chin D und MacGowan-Smith E (1990). "-Collagen Shield heparin delivery for prevention of postoperative fibrin." 108:104-106

Raymond MC und Thompson JT (1990). "RPE-mediated collagen gel contraction. Inhibition by colchicine and stimulation by TGF-beta." Invest Ophthalmol Vis Sci. 31:1070-1096

Snady-McCoy L, Buzney S, Bishara S und Gaynon M (1988). Five Fluorouracil Buckles and Retinal Pigment Epithelium (RPE) Proliferation in Situ. In Freeman HM, Tolentino FI (Hrsg) Proliferative Vitreoretinopathy (PVR), Springer-Verlag, New York, S 134-139

Tavakolian U und Wollensak J (1985). "Ergebnisse von Silikonölinjektionen in verschiedenen Stadien der proliferativen Vitreoretinopathie." Klin Monatsbl Augenheilkd. 186:268-271

Tolentino F, Cajita V, Chung H, Ueno N und Refojo M (1968). Carmustine (BCNU) in Silicone Oil prevents proliferation of cultured cells. In Freeman HM, Tolentino FI (Hrsg) Proliferative Vitreoretinopathy (PVR), Springer-Verlag, New York, S 162-165

Vidaurri-Leal J, Hohmann R und Glaser B (1984). "Effect of vitreous on morphologic characteristics of retinal pigment epithelial cells: A new approach to the study of proliferative vitreoretinopathy." Arch Ophthalmol. 102:1220-1223

Weller M, Heimann K und Wiedemann P (1988). "Role of macrophages and fibronectin in vitreoretinal proliferation." J Fr Ophtalmol. 11(3):243-7

Weller M, Wiedemann P, MH und K Heimann (1989). "Transferrin and transferrin receptor expression in intraocular proliferative disease. APAAP-immunolabeling of retinal membranes and ELISA for vitreal transferrin." Graefes Arch Clin Exp Ophthalmol. 227(3):281-6

Weller M, Heimann K und Wiedemann P (1990). "Proliferative Vitreoretinopathy – Is it Anything More than Wound Healing at the Wrong Place?" Int Ophthalmol. 14:105-117

Wiedemann P (1988). Die medikamentöse Behandlung der proliferativen Vitreoretinopathie unter besonderer Berüchsichtigung des Zytostatikums Daunomycin. Enke, Stuttgart

Wiedemann P und Weller M (1988). "The pathophysiology of proliferative vitreoretinopathy." Acta Ophthalmol Suppl (Copenh). 189:3-15

Wiedemann P, Lemmen K, Schmiedl R und Heimann (1987). "Intraocular daunorubicin for the treatment and prophylaxis of traumatic proliferative vitreoretinopathy." Am J Ophthalmol. 104:10-14

Wiedemann P, Lemmen KD, Wiedemann R, Moter H und Heimann K (1988). "A randomized, prospectice study of the treatment of proliferative vitreoretinopathy with daunomycin." Fortschr Ophthalmol. 85:503-4

Wiedemann P, Leinung C, Hilgers RD und Heimann K (1991). "Daunomycin and silicone oil for the treatment of proliferative vitreoretinopathy." Graefe's Arch Clin Exp Ophthalmol. 229:150–152

Korrespondenzadresse

Professor Dr. med. P. Wiedemann
Universitätsaugenklinik Köln, Josef-Stelzmannstr. 9, D-5000 Köln 41

Infektionsprophylaxe

V. Klauß

Infektionsprohphylaxe ist in der Ophthalmologie seit Jahrzehnten Anliegen von Ärzten, Sprechstundenhilfen sowie Ambulanz- und Operationsschwestern in Kliniken. Anlaß für infektionsprohylaktische Maßnahmen war die Erkenntnis, daß Augenerkrankungen von Auge zu Auge übertragen werden können und daß jeder intraokulare Eingriff mit dem Risiko einer Endophthalmitis verbunden ist.

Mit Einführung des routinemäßigen Gebrauchs von Antibiotika in der Ophthalmologie sind einige bewährte Grundregeln der Infektionsprophylaxe in den Hintergrund getreten, da Antibiotika scheinbar alle Probleme lösen konnten. Dies gilt jedoch nicht für Viren und Pilze, die in der Augenheilkunde eine große Rolle spielen sowie die zunehmende Resistenzentwicklung von Bakterien gegen Antibiotika. Speziell die perioperative Infektionsprophylaxe zur Reduzierung des Endophthalmitisrisikos hat große Bedeutung erlangt, auch in Zusammenhang mit gestiegenen Cataractoperationszahlen und mit Einführung des ambulanten Operierens. Schmierinfektionen und geeignete Desinfektion sind Mitte der 80er Jahre in Zusammenhang mit der erworbenen Immunschwäche AIDS heftig und kontrovers diskutiert worden. Es stellte sich die Frage, ob das HIV-Virus über Tonometerköpfe, Kontaktgläser, Ultraschallköpfe oder Untersucherhände übertragen werden kann. Auch die Frage nach dem Infektionsrisiko medizinischen Personals bei Behandlung von HIV-Positiven erlangte großes Interesse.

Übertragbare Erkrankungen

Erreger gelangen exogen oder hämatogen an das Auge wobei die Mehrzahl der Keime von der Haut des Patienten selbst (Saprophyten), von den Schleimhäuten des Patienten (Gonokokken, Chlamydien, Herpes simplex) oder über Schmierinfektion oder Vektoren von Infizierten in den Bindehautsack oder auf die Hornhaut gelangen (Abb. 1). Endogene Infektionen stellen eine Ausnahme dar. Ein gesundes Auge ist gegen die Mehrzahl möglicher Krankheitserreger gut geschützt: unspezifische und spezifische Abwehrmechanismen des äußeren Auges reduzieren das Infektionsrisiko. Zu den unspezifischen Abwehrfunktionen gehören Lidschluß, Tränenfluß, intaktes Bindehaut- und Hornhautepithel, epitheliale Desquamation, epitheliale

Gramer/Kampik (Hrsg.) Pharmakotherapie am Auge
© Springer-Verlag Berlin Heidelberg 1992

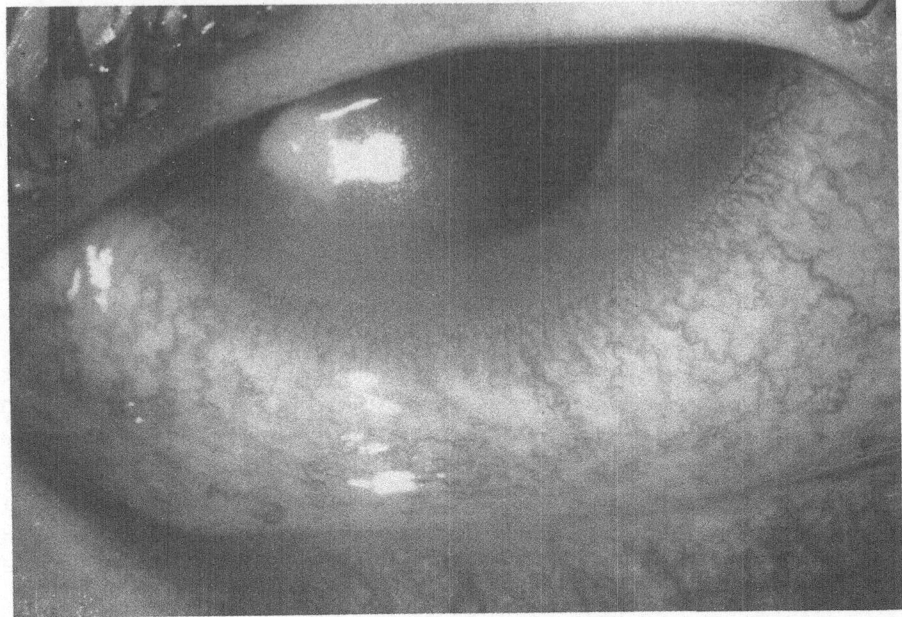

Abb. 1. Hornhautulcus nach Tragen von weichen Kontaktlinsen. Erreger: Pseudomonas aeruginosa

Phagozytose und niedrige Oberflächentemperatur. Lysozym, Mucin und Lactoferrin in der Tränenflüssigkeit wirken bakteriolytisch oder bateriostatisch. Die spezifischen Abwehrfunktionen laufen als zelluläre oder humorale Abwehr über die Bindehaut ab.

Nicht jedes Auge bzw. jeder Patient ist gleich infektionsgefährdet. Entscheidend für das Auftreten einer Infektion nach Kontakt mit infektiösem Material ist einerseits die Zahl der Keime, die mit dem Auge in Berührung kommen auf der anderen Seite Faktoren, die das Infektionsrisiko des einzelnen Patienten erhöhen. Hierzu gehören:

– Sicca-Syndrom
– Tragen von – speziell weichen – Kontaktlinsen
– Anwendung von Antibiotika und Kortikosteroiden über längere Zeit
– Diabetes mellitus
– Immunsuppression (Tabelle 1)

Die angegebenen Schutzmechanismen reichen speziell bei Viruserkrankungen nicht aus, das Auge oder den Menschen vor einer Infektion zu bewahren.

Schleimhäute stellen die wichtigste Eintrittspforte für Viren in den Körper dar. Die intakte Epidermis ist für Viren nur durch Verletzung oder Insektenstiche überwindbar.

Tabelle 1. Voraussetzungen für eine Infektionsauslösung

Infektion abhängig von
- Erreger
- Keimzahl
- Risikofaktoren
  - Sicca Syndrom
  - Kontaktlinsen
  - Antibiotikaanwendung
  - Cortisonanwendung
  - Diabetes mellitus
  - Immunsuppression

Für alle Viren gilt, daß die Organschädigung primär degenerativ und sekundär entzündlich erfolgt. Damit erfolgt die Virusproduktion und auch die Ausscheidung – womit die Kontagiosität verbunden ist – vor Krankheitsausbruch.

Dies gilt insbesondere für die *Keratoconjunctivitis epidemica (KCE)*. Die KCE wird durch Adenovirus 8 und 19 hervorgerufen. Adenoviren können generell zu lokalisierten Schleimhautinfektionen des Auges, der Luftwege oder des Intestinaltrakts führen. Kombinierte Infektionen von mehreren Organen sind außerordentlich selten. Die Immunität ist typenspezifisch und wenig fundiert. Antikörper lassen sich bei 5 % der Bevölkerung in den USA nachweisen. Eine Viruskultur aus dem Bindehautabstrich ist möglich. Die Infektion beginnt einseitig als akute follikuläre Conjunctivitis. Das akute Stadium dauert ein bis zwei Wochen, das zweite Auge wird nach einem unterschiedlich großen Zeitintervall zumeist weniger intensiv mitbefallen. Zu Beginn der Erkrankung zeigen die Patienten grippeähnliche Allgemeinsymptome, dann auf der betroffenen Seite eine präaurikuläre Lymphknotenschwellung. Die Hornhaut ist in der ersten Erkrankungswoche in Form einer diffusen oberflächlichen epithelialen Keratitis mitbeteiligt, die übergeht in eine fokale fluoreszeinpositive epitheliale Keratitis, nach ca. 2 Wochen sind subepitheliale Trübungen erkennbar, die über lange Zeit persistieren oder auch rezidivierend auftreten können. Bei zentralem Befall resultiert eine Visusherabsetzung verbunden mit Photophobie. An der Bindehaut kann es zu einer Membranbildung kommen, eine Vernarbung der Bindehaut ist möglich. Im Gegensatz zur Lungeninfektion mit Adenoviren handelt es sich am Auge nicht um eine Tröpfchen- sondern um eine Schmierinfektion. Epidemien ausgehend von Augenarztpraxen und Augenkliniken sind seit langem bekannt, auch ein saisonales Auftreten wurde beschrieben. Aus der Infektiosität und den beobachteten und beschriebenen Epidemien läßt sich ableiten, daß es sich bei der KCE um eine Erkrankung handelt, die auch über kleinste Mengen infektiösen Materials übertragen werden kann. Dies trifft sicher für die Übertragung durch Tonometerköpfe, Dreispiegelkontaktgläser und Untersucherhände zu.

Es liegen keine gesicherten Berichte über die Übertragung von *Herpes simplex Virus* durch den Augenarzt vor. Da es sich auch hier um eine

Schmierinfektion handelt, ist die Möglichkeit einer Übertragung gegeben. Die Primärinfektion zum Auge erfolgt häufig bereits im Kindesalter bei oral okulärem Kontakt. Es ist darauf zu achten, bei einer Herpesinfektion der Lippen Hautkontake zu vermeiden. Die Primärinfektion am Auge äußert sich in einer unspezifischen Conjunctivitis verbunden mit einzelnen oder zahlreichen Herpesbläschen an der Lidhaut. Die Rezidive werden durch Fieber, Trauma, Erschöpfung oder auch psychischen Streß induziert. Die Rezidivhäufigkeit kann durch gezielte Ausschaltung der Provokationsfaktoren verringert werden. Um eine Übertragung des genitalen HIV Typs II zu vermeiden, ist bei bekannter aktiver Infektion der Mutter ein Kaiserschnitt zur Entbindung angezeigt. Das *Varicella Zoster Virus* wird aerogen übertragen, die Durchseuchung beträgt 100 %. Hyperimmunglobuline können bei Patienten mit Immunsuppression einer Infektion vorbeugen.

Es gibt keine gesicherten Berichte über eine Übertragung des *Hepatitis B Virus* in der augenärztlichen Praxis. Da immer multiple Risiken vorliegen, wäre der anamnestische Hinweis auf einen Augenarztbesuch ungewöhnlich. Vom Verhalten des Virus kann jedoch die Möglichkeit einer Übertragung durch den Augenarzt nicht ausgeschlossen werden.

Enterovirus 70 ist der Erreger der *akuten epidemischen hämorrhagischen Conjunctivitis,* auch Apolloconjunctivitis genannt. Diese tritt vor allem in große Bevölkerungszahlen betreffenden Epidemien in feuchtheißen Küstengebieten der Tropen auf, wird durch internationalen Reiseverkehr bei Ausländern und deutschen Touristen jedoch auch bei uns zunehmend häufiger gesehen. Das Bild ähnelt dem der KCE, auffällig sind jedoch die zusätzlich auftretenden flächenhaften Bindehautblutungen. Die Inkubationszeit beträgt nur wenige Stunden, was die schnelle Ausbreitung begünstigt (Abb. 2)

Seltenere aber auch potentiell von Auge zu Auge übertragbare Viruserkrankungen sind hervorgerufen durch *Molluscum contagiosum* und das humane *Papilloma Virus.*

Die *HIV-Infektion* hat den Ophthalmologen mit einer Reihe von neuen Problemen konfrontiert: es stellt sich die Frage, ob eine Übertragung des HIV-Virus von Auge zu Auge oder von Patient zu Mediziner möglich ist. Weiterhin werden bisher außerordentlich seltene klinische Bilder bei AIDS-Patienten häufiger beobachtet. Dies betrifft im wesentlichen die opportunistischen Infektionen.

Die Infektionswege einer HIV-Infektion sind heute bekannt, dementsprechend ist es möglich, das Infektionsrisiko auszuschalten. Eine Übertragung erfolgt

- auf sexuellem Wege
- durch infizierte Injektionsnadeln (vor allem bei Drogenabhängigen)
- durch Blut und Blutprodukte
- von der Mutter auf das Kind intrauterin oder über die Muttermilch

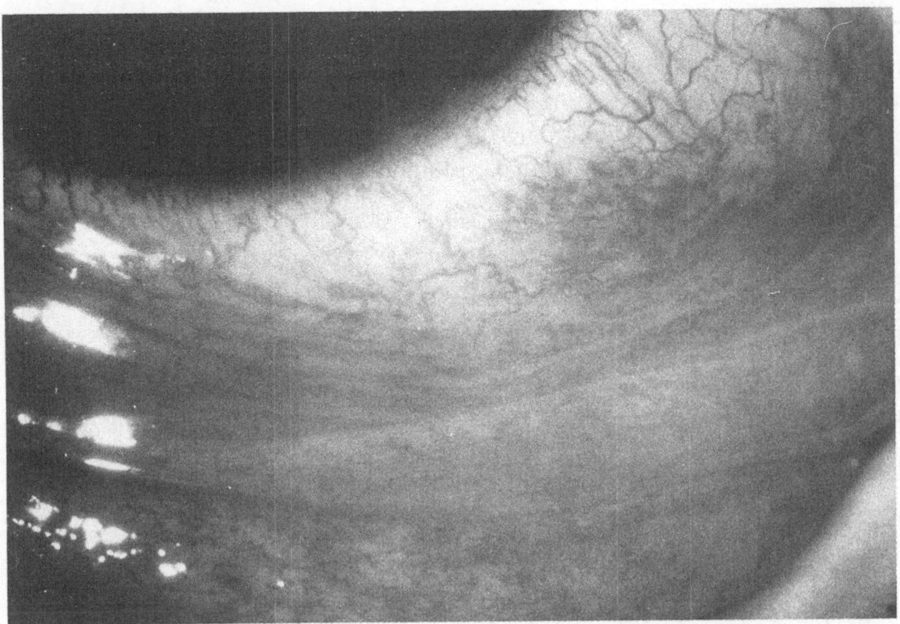

Abb. 2. Akute epidemische hämorrhagische Conjunctivitis: petechiale Blutungen in der Conjunctiva bulbi und Conjunctiva tarsi

In der augenärztlichen Praxis und Klinik sind alle Maßnahmen zu treffen, um eine Virusübertragung von Patient zu Patient oder von Patient zu Mitarbeiter auszuschalten. Das Virus wurde am Auge in der Tränenflüssigkeit, in der Bindehaut und in der Retina nachgewiesen. Es muß damit gerechnet werden, daß das Virus auch über Blutzellen in der Hornhaut vorkommen kann. Deshalb ist der HIV-Test vor Keratoplastik angezeigt.

Dem Augenarzt kommt eine wesentliche Bedeutung bei der Diagnose einer HIV-Infektion bzw. Diagnose und Therapie opportunistischer Infektion zu. Da heute alle das Auge befallenden opportunistischen Infektionen therapierbar sind, kann durch frühe Diagnostik und adäquate Therapie einer vorzeitigen Erblindung vorgebeugt werden. In den vergangenen Jahren ist es in der Bundesrepublik Deutschland weltweit zu einer jährlichen Verdopplung der Erkrankungszahlen gekommen. Die Erkrankungszahlen sind von bedingter Aussagekraft, da bei einer mittleren Inkubationszeit von 8,5 Jahren die heutigen Erkrankungen auf eine Infektion am Anfang der 80er Jahre zurückgehen, als prophylaktische Maßnahmen noch nicht üblich waren.

Bei einer geschätzten Zahl von 50 000 Infizierten in der Bundesrepublik Deutschland muß der Augenarzt damit rechnen, daß infizierte Patienten in seine Praxis kommen, die häufig während der langen symptomfreien Inkubationszeit noch nicht von ihrer Infektion wissen oder eine bekannte Infektion verschweigen.

Hieraus ergeben sich zwei Konsequenzen:

1. Alle Maßnahmen zur Ausschaltung einer Infektionsübertragung in der augenärztlichen Praxis müssen ergriffen werden.
2. DerAugenarzt sollte mit den typischen okulären Zeichen einer HIV-Infektion vertraut sein, da er, wenn auch selten, als erster die Diagnose stellen kann.

Das klinische Bild der okulären Beteiligung bei HIV-Infektion und AIDS

70 % der AIDS-Kranken entwickeln okuläre Komplikationen im Spätstadium der Erkrankung. Eine frühe okuläre Symptomatik ist nur in Einzelfällen mitgeteilt worden. Am häufigsten finden sich Cotton-wool-Herde der Netzhaut (70 %) und Zytomegalievirusretinitis (22 bis 30 %).

Die okulären Veränderungen bei HIV-Infizierten lassen sich in vier Gruppen einteilen:

1. Mikroangiopathiesyndrom
2. Tumoren
3. opportunistische Infektionen
4. neurologische Veränderungen

Mikroangiopathiesyndrom

Zu den Gefäßveränderungen bei AIDS gehören vor allem Cotton-wool-Exsudate der Netzhaut aber auch Netzhautblutungen und Mikroaneurysmen. Cotton-wool-Herde treten typischerweise multipel im Zentrum der Netzhaut und in der mittleren Peripherie auf. Sie können sich spontan zurückbilden, die Zahl variiert stark im Lauf der Erkrankung.

Tumoren

Unter Tumoren, die die Augenregion mitbetreffen, sind vor allem das Kaposi-Sarkom von Lid- und Bindehaut sowie Orbitalymphome, speziell das Burkitt-Lymphom zu erwähnen. Der Befall von Lidern und Bindehaut tritt im Rahmen eines disseminierten Kaposi-Sarkoms auf.

Opportunistische Infektionen

Eine große Zahl von Krankheitserregern, vor allem Viren und Parasiten, die vor Auftreten der erworbenen Immunschwäche nur ausnahmsweise gesehen und beschrieben wurden, verursachen bei AIDS-Patienten okuläre Infektionen, die rasch zur Erblindung führen können. Früherkennung, Diagnose und adäquate Therapie der Infektion können dem Patienten die Sehkraft für den Rest seines Lebens erhalten. Folgende Keime sind als Erreger von Infektionen am Auge identifiziert worden: Cytomegalievirus, Herpes simplex Virus, Varicella Zoster Virus, Cryptokokkus neoformans, Mycobacterium avium intracellulare, Toxoplasma gondii, Candida albicans, Histoplasma capsulatum, Pneumozystis carnii, Treponema pallidum.

Die klinischen Bilder opportunistischer Infektionen am Auge, speziell der Retinitiden, können sich sehr ähneln. Typisch für die häufigste opportunistische Infektion, die Cytomegalieretinitis, sind das Fortschreiten entlang den Gefäßen, das multifokale Auftreten, die geringe Glaskörperreaktion und die rasche Ausbreitung. Neben Entzündungsarealen werden Blutungen, Nekrosen und spontane Vernarbung beobachtet (Abb. 3). Die Differentialdiagnose ist anhand des klinischen Bildes, durch Erregernachweis und Serologie möglich. Besonders zu erwähnen ist ein Präparat zur Behandlung einer Cytomegalievirusinfektion, das Dihydroxipropoximethyl-Guanin (DHPG). Das Medikament wird täglich intravenös über eine Kurzinfusion appliziert. Die Suppressionstherapie wird zeitlebens fortgesetzt. Die Entzündungsareale hinterlassen Netzhautnarben mit vollständigem Funktionsausfall. Aus diesem Grund ist eine schnelle Diagnose und früheinsetzende Therapie erforderlich.

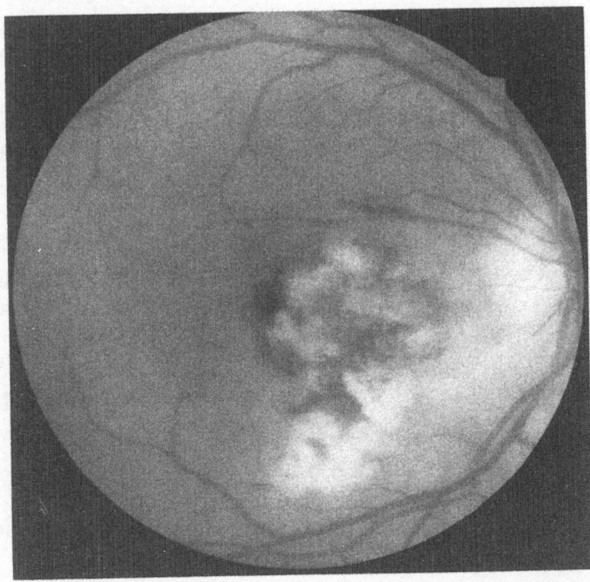

Abb. 3. Zentraler Cytomegalievirus-Retinitis-Herd bei einem AIDS-Patienten: gelb-weißliches Entzündungsareal mit aufgelagerten Blutungen

Neurologische Veränderungen

Neurologische Störungen im Augenbereich sind meistens Ausdruck einer zerebralen Erkrankung, z. B. einer Toxoplasmose. Neben Motilitätsstörungen bei Hirnnervenschädigung kommt es zu Gesichtsfeldausfällen, Stauungspapille, Neuritis nervi optici und Sehnervenatrophie.

Eine enge Zusammenarbeit zwischen Ophthalmologen und Ärzten anderer Fachrichtungen ist erforderlich. Der Ophthalmologe kann, wenn er mit dem klinischen Bild der okulären Veränderung bei HIV-Infektion vertraut ist, als erster eine HIV-Infektion diagnostizieren. Er kann auch einen wertvollen Beitrag zu Diagnose und Differentialdiagnose opportunistischer Infektion leisten. Es ist empfohlen, jeden HIV-Patienten einmal jährlich, jeden AIDS-Kranken einmal vierteljährlich und bei Auftreten von Augenkomplikationen entsprechend häufiger ophthalmologisch zu untersuchen.

Eigenen Untersuchungen zur Infektiosität der Tränenflüssigkeit haben bei 19 Patienten in der Viruskultur negative Ergebnisse erbracht. Hieraus läßt sich schließen, daß die Infektiosität von Tränen als sehr gering oder sogar negativ eingestuft werden muß. Jedoch sollten auch bei extrem geringem Infektionsrisiko alle erforderlichen Maßnahmen einer Infektionsprophylaxe ergriffen werden.

Infektionsprophylaxe in der Praxis/Ambulanz

Die Summe von Einzelmaßnahmen zur Infektionsprophylaxe kann die Übertragung von Keimen von Auge zu Auge nahezu 100 %ig ausschließen.

Händedesinfektion. Vor Untersuchung eines Patienten müssen die Hände desinfiziert werden. Hierfür reicht Händewaschen allein nicht aus, sondern ein Desinfektionsmittel ist erforderlich. Werden die Lider bei der Untersuchung an der Spaltlampe, bei der Tonometrie, usw. mit den Fingern geöffnet, ist die Kontamination der Finger unausweichlich. Es ist deshalb ratsam, die Lider unter Zuhilfenahme von Watteträgern zu öffnen (Abb. 4).

Verwendung von Einzeldosisbehältnissen in Diagnostik und Therapie. Besonders die Kappen von Tropfflaschen stellen ein bekanntes Risiko als potentielle Keimträger dar, insbesondere für Feuchtkeime wie Pseudomonas aeruginosa. Auch Fluopreszeinlösungen stellen ein gutes Kulturmedium für Feuchtkeime dar. Auge oder Lider können mit der Tropfflasche sehr leicht in Berührung kommen, vor allem wenn die Tropfen nicht vom Augenarzt selbst appliziert werden. Die Applikation aus Einzeldosisbehältnissen für Oberflächenanaesthetika, Fluoreszein, Mydriatika, Zycloplegika und Therapeutika, letzteres speziell im Op-Bereich, helfen nosokomiale Infektionen zu vermeiden.

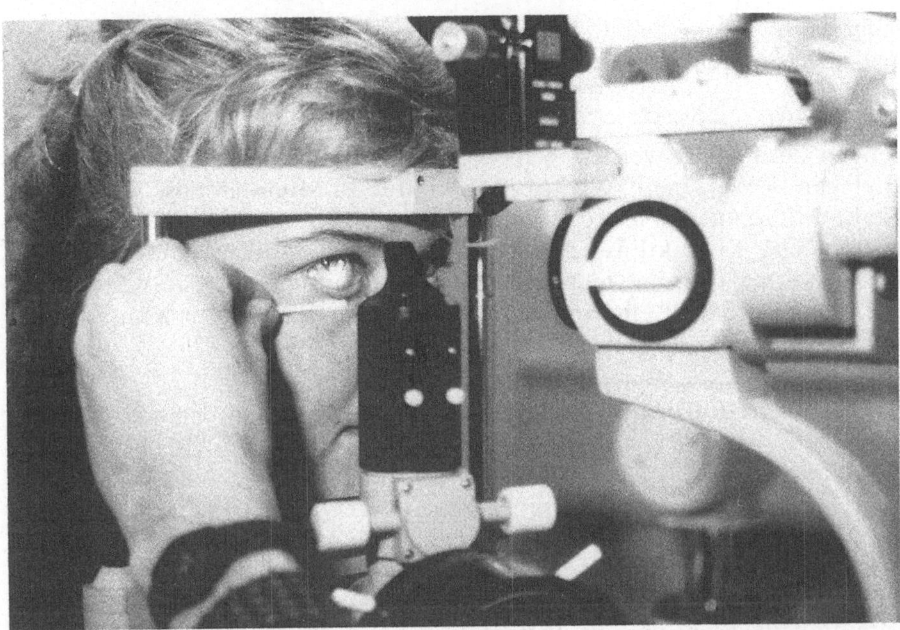

Abb. 4. Spaltlampenuntersuchung und Tonometrie mit Hilfe eines Watteträgers ohne Kontakt der Finger mit Lidern oder Tränenflüssigkeit

Desinfektion von Tonometerköpfen, Kontaktgläsern, Ultraschallköpfen usw. Alle Instrumente, die direkt mit dem Patientenauge in Berührung kommen, müssen sorgfältig desinfiziert werden. Speziell Tonometerköpfe sollten in der Praxis mehrfach vorhanden sein, um sie in einem Rotationsverfahren desinfizieren zu können. Als Maßnahmen kommen infrage:

- zunächst mechanische Reinigung mit einem Tupfer/Watte
- Einlegen in eine Gigasept/Pantasept 2 % Lösung für mindestens 10 Minuten
- oder Abwischen mit 70 % Isopropylalkohol
- oder Sterilisation durch Formaldehyddampf über 6 Stunden
- oder UV-Bestrahlung

Als Gefäße für die Gigasept-/Pantaseptlösungen können von der Industrie angebotene Behälter, in die die Tonometerköpfe eingehängt werden bzw. Petrischalen verwendet werden. Die Desinfektionslösung muß einmal wöchentlich erneuert werden. Bei der UV-Bestrahlung ist darauf zu achten, daß die angegebene Zeit nicht überschritten wird, da hierdurch die Instrumente leiden können. Weiterhin darf nicht nur die Kontaktfläche mit dem Auge, sondern es müssen auch die Seitenflächen mitbestrahlt werden, da sich auch hier Keime ansammeln können. Formaldehyddämpfe sind wegen der langen Einwirkungszeit und der anschließend notwendigen langen Lüftungszeit nicht empfehlenswert.

Kontaktlinsen können mit den kommerziell angebotenen Reinigungslösungen desinfiziert werden. Für weiche Kontaktlinsen empfiehlt sich das Einlegen in Wasserstoffsuperoxyd 3 %ig für 10 Minuten, anschließend das Neutralisieren nach Herstellerangabe und das Einlegen in Aufbewahrungslösung. Die Kontaktlinse darf bei der Anpassung nicht berührt werden, hierzu sollten Gummihandschuhe bzw. Gummifingerlinge verwendet werden. Der Patient ist eindringlich daraufhinzuweisen, daß er Kontaktlinsen nur mit sauberen Fingern berühren darf.

Andere Maßnahmen. Handschuhe müssen bei jedem Kontakt mit Blut und Serum getragen werden, weiterhin bei Kontakt mit infektiösem Material z. B. bakterieller Conjunctivits, Dacryocystits usw.

Infektiöse Patienten z. B. mit Keratoconjunctivitis epidemica sind über ihre Infektiosität und das dementsprechende Verhalten aufzuklären. Bei bekannt infektiösen Patienten empfehlen sich Untersuchungs- und Behandlungstermine außerhalb der normalen Sprechzeiten. Das Praxispersonal ist daraufhinzuweisen, daß ein Patient, der mit stark geröteten Augen in die Praxis kommt nicht in das Wartezimmer gesetzt werden darf, sondern separat möglichst schnell behandelt werden muß. HIV-serokonvertierte Personen müssen nicht zeitlich und örtlich separat behandelt werden.

Nadeln, Spritzen und andere schneidende Instrumente sollten in stabilen Behältern, nicht zum Beispiel in Müllsäcken entsorgt werden. Es gibt kommerziell angebotene stabile Kanülencontainer, in die Kanülen ohne Verletzungsrisiko eingebracht werden können (Tabelle 2).

Perioperative Infektionsprophylaxe

Um das Risiko einer postoperativen Endophthalmitis zu minimieren, wird ein Bindehautabstrich und das Anlegen einer Kultur 16-24 Stunden präoperativ empfohlen. Bei einer Kultur von potentiell pathogenen Erregern sollte die Operation verschoben werden. Die präoperative lokale Antibiotikagabe ist kontrovers diskutiert. Auf keinen Fall sollte sie über einen längeren Zeitraum durchgeführt werden, weil dadurch hochpathogene resistente Keime wie Staphylokokkus aureus oder Pseudomonas aeruginosa dominierend werden können. Die Wahl des Antibiotikums sollte sich nach dem in der Region typischen Keimspektrum richten. Um eine möglichst breite Wirkung gegen Grampositive und Gramnegative Erreger zu haben, kann heute die gleichzeitige Gabe von Erythromycin und Tobramycin empfohlen werden. Bei Gentamycin werden zunehmend Resistenzen bei Pseudomonas aeruginosa und Staphylokokken beobachtet.

Präoperativ trägt der Patient an dem zu operierenden Auge eine Schutzklappe, um die Berührung durch Finger zu erschweren. Präoperatives

Tabelle 2. Zusammenfassung der Maßnahmen zur Infektionsprophylaxe im ambulanten Bereich

Händedesinfektion
Handschuhe/Mundschutz
"No touch" Untersuchung = Zuhilfenahme von Watteträgern
Örtlich/zeitlich separate Behandlung von bekannt infektiösen Patienten
Aufklärung des Patienten über Infektionsrisiko
Einmaltropfen in Diagnostik und Therapie
Desinfektion von Tonometerköpfen, Kontaktgläsern, Ultraschallköpfen, die mit Patienten-Auge in Berührung kommen
Sterilisation von CL-Anpaßsätzen
AIDS Test bei Honrhautspendern

Schneiden der Wimpern und Abkleben des Op-Bereichs werden empfohlen, so daß die keimtragenden Wimpern, Lidhaut- und Brauenbereich abgedeckt sind. Die präoperative Tränenwegsspülung ist empfohlen, um die Durchgängigkeit der Tränenwege zu prüfen und die abführenden Tränenwege mechanisch zu reinigen.

Intraoperativ hilft eine Reihe von Maßnahmen das Infektionsrisiko zu minimieren: eine möglichst kurze Op-Dauer sollte angestrebt werden, da das Infektionsrisiko mit Dauer der Bulbuseröffnung und mit vermehrten Manipulationen steigt. Spülflüssigkeiten müssen zuverlässig steril sein und sollten möglichst sparsam benutzt werden. Bei extrakapsulärer Kataraktextraktion dient eine intakte hintere Linsenkapsel als Barriere zwischen vorderem und hinterem Augenabschnitt. Die einzusetzende Intraokularlinse darf Wimpern oder Lidhaut auf keinen Fall berühren. Ein dichter Wundverschluß ist abzustreben. Postoperativ ist die lokale Gabe von Antibiotika in Form von Augentropfen und subkonjunktivaler Injektion angezeigt. Hierbei sollten Einzeldosisbehältnisse für die Tropfen benutzt werden, auf der Station ist für jeden Patienten eine separate Tropfflasche zu halten (Abb. 5).

Eine Reihe von Patienten trägt ein besonders hohes bereits präoperativ bekanntes Infektionsrisiko. Hierzu müssen gerechnet werden Patienten mit Conjunctivitis, Blepharitis und Dacryocystitis sowie Patienten mit Sicca-Sydrom und Kontaktlinsenträger, bei denen die Hornhautsensibilität herabgesetzt ist. Eine länger dauernde Antibiotika- oder Steroidtherapie präoperativ muß ebenfalls als erhöhtes Risiko angesehen werden. Diabetes mellitus, Immunsuppression, Alkohol und Drogenabusus stellen begünstigende Faktoren für eine Infektion dar. Liegen eine oder mehrere dieser Risikofaktoren vor, sind besondere Maßnahmen zu ergreifen. Erkrankungen des äußeren Auges wie Conjunctivitis, Blepharitis und Dacyocystitis sind entsprechend zu therapieren. Bei Patienten mit allgemeinen Erkrankungen kann eine systemische Antibiotikagabe indiziert sein (Tabelle 3).

Verhalten bei akzidentellen Verletzungen des Operateurs. Bei Operationen von bekannt HIV-positiven Patienten sind besondere Schutz-

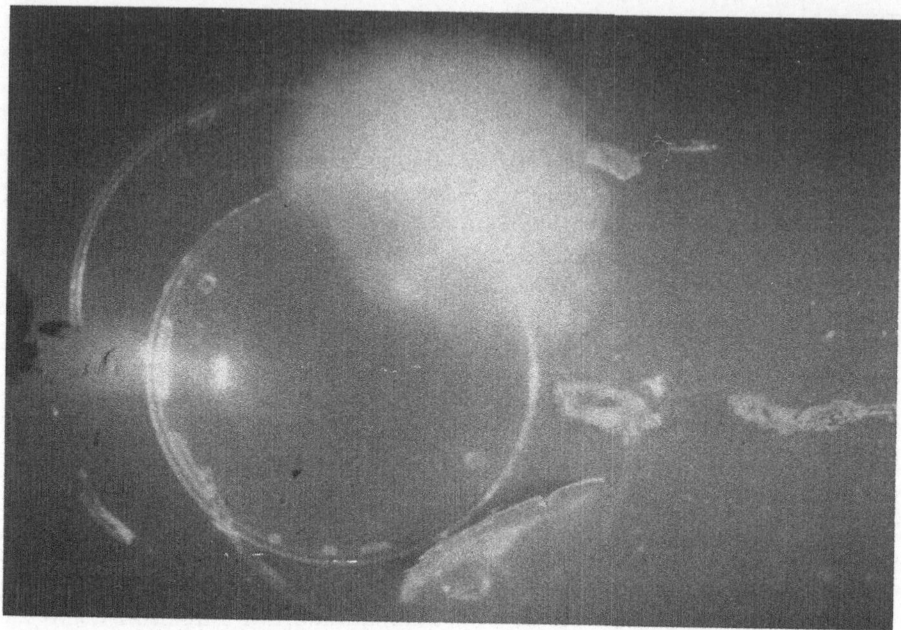

Abb. 5. Explantierte Hinterkammerlinse bei Endophthalmitis durch Mykose: Nachweis von Acremonium roseum sp.

Tabelle 3. Zusammenfassung der infektionsprophylaktischen Maßnahmen im perioperativen Bereich

Präoperativ
   Tränenwegsspülung
   Bindehautabstrich
   Antibiotika lokal
   Schutzklappe
   Schneiden der Wimpern
   Abkleben von Lidhaut, Braue, Wimpern

Intraoperativ
   kurze Op-Dauer
   sterile Spülflüssigkeit (wenig)
   bei EC CE: unverletzte hintere Linsekapsel
   IOL Implantation, ohne Wimpern-/Lidkontakt
   dichter Wundverschluß

Postoperativ
   Antibiotikagabe lokal
   häufige Kontrollen

maßnahmen wie das Tragen einer Brille anzuraten. Vor Keratoplastik ist bei dem Spender ein Test auf HIV-Antikörper durchzuführen. Bei Kontakt von Schleimhäuten mit infektiösem Material bzw. Stichverletzungen ist die sofortige Spülung und Desinfektion angezeigt. Bei Kontakt mit HIVkontaminiertem Material wird die Gabe von AZT für einige Tage angeraten.

Die strikte Einhaltung aller infektionsprophylaktischen Maßnahmen im perioperativen Bereich ist Aufgabe des beratenden Krankenhaushygienikers sowie eines Hygienebeauftragten innerhalb der Klinik, also eines Ophthalmologen, der mit dem Operationsablauf vertraut ist.

Durch Einhaltung aller geschilderten Maßnahmen lassen sich Infektionen im ambulanten und stationären/operativen Bereich fast vollständig ausschließen.

Literatur

Becker CE, Cone JE, Gerberding J (1989) Occupational infection with human immundeficiency virus (HIV). Risks and risk reduction. Ann Int Med 8:653-656

Boltze HJ, Rummelt V, Röllinghoff M, Naumann GOH (1989) Bakterielles Keim- und Resistenzspektrum der reizfreien Conjunctiva. 7845 präoperative Abstriche der Erlanger Universitäts-Augenklinik. Klin Mbl Augenheilk 197:172-175

Burkhardt F, Steuer W (Hrsg) (1989) Infektionsprophylaxe im Krankenhaus. Leitfaden für das Krankenhauspersonal. 2. neubearbeitete und erweiterte Auflage, Thieme, Stuttgart

Duane TD, Jaeger EA (Hrsg) (1987) Clinical ophthalmology. Harper and Row, Cambridge

Klauß V, Lund OE (1988) Augenveränderungen bei AIDS. Fortschr Med 19:27-31

Mueller AJ, Geier S, Klauß V, Gürtler L (Hrsg) (1990) Semiquantitativer Nachweis von HIV in der Tränenflüssigkeit. Deutscher AIDS-Kongreß Hamburg

Opferkuch W, Lehner T (1989) Mikrobiologische Diagnostik und antimikrobielle Chemotherapie. Hippokrates, Stuttgart

Korrespondenzadresse
Professor Dr. med. V. Klauß
Universitätsaugenklinik München, Mathildenstr. 8, D-8000 München 2

Chemotherapy of Bacterial Infections of the Eye

A. A. Bialasiewicz

History

The founder of modern diagnostic bacteriology, *Robert Koch,* laid the grounds for the substantial advances in the knowledge of infectious diseases of the eye that were made by *Theodor Axenfeld* around the turn of the century. The far-reaching insights into the etiology and pathogenesis of infectious diseases of the eye reported by T. Axenfeld in his fundamental textbook "Die Bakteriologie in der Augenheilkunde" (edited by Fischer Verlag, Jena 1907) did not keep pace with research into antiinfective chemotherapeutic agents. Routine modern chemotherapy only began with the clinical application of Salvarsan in 1910, discovered by *Paul Ehrlich* and *S. Hata* and was used for the treatment of Syphilis.

In 1935, five years after Theodor Axenfeld had deceased, sulfanilamides became available after the discovery of antibacterial activity of a synthetic azo dye, Prontosil by *G. Domagk* in 1932.

Many bactericidal and bacteriostatic antiinfective drugs have been discovered or synthesized since. Hallmarks in the development of topical or local antibiotics in Ophthalmology include:

Bacitracin (1945), Cloramphenicol (1947), Polymyxins (1947), Neomycin (1949), Oxatetracycline (1950), Erythromycin (1952), Vancomyin (1956), Kanamycin (1957), Gentamycin (1963) and Tobramycin (1967).

Furthermore, *New Quinolones* like Norfloxacin (1990) and Ciprofloxacin (1990) as well as Ofloxacin have passed clinical trials on their way to routinely benefit patients with external or anterior segment infections (Jacobson et al., 1988). Carbapenemes like *Imipenem* have only recently been studied in patients with ocular infections (Axelrod et al., 1987).

Some systemically administered antibiotics include Cephalosporins (1970), Carbapenems (1974) and New Quinolones (1990) besides the mainstay of therapy, aminoglycosides, and have provided better coverage of potential pathogens for "ad hoc" immediate therapy of severe intraocular infections.

Recently, modern insights into infection pathogenesis have resulted in a multi-faceted approach for the management of severe bacterial anterior segment and intraocular infections using a combination of antibiotics, corticosteroids and surgical intervention.

Gramer/Kampık (Hrsg.) Pharmakotherapıe am Auge
© Sprınger-Verlag Berlın Heıdelberg 1992

Microbiological Prerequisites for the Use of Antibiotics in Ophthalmology

The selection of therapeutic options in infectious bacterial eye diseases must be preceded by adequate microbiologic work-up of probes accurately isolated from the respective sites of infections.

In detail, swabs should be taken from the lid margins in cases of blepharitis, the cul de sac of the conjunctiva in cases of conjunctivitis, from the cornea in cases of keratitis and aspirates from the vitreous in intraocular infection. Probing with a platinum loop is less effective for the isolation of organisms than the use of a cotton- (or alginate-) tipped swab. After an immediate preclassification and cytological evaluation with Gram and Giemsa stains, cultures on solid media should always be performed, even if a monoclonal antibody direct test has resulted in a positive result for a specific pathogen. Culturing for commonly found pathogenic aerobic bacteria on blood, chocolate, Endo and Sabouraud agar plates at 37°C, 5 % CO_2 may be performed in an appropriate setting of an established infection unit inside an eye hospital. In particular situations, different isolation techniques for anaerobes or mycobacteria must be used. Evaluation of cultures should be performed in close cooperation with a microbiologist, and differentiation and antibiotic susceptibility tests should follow in a specialised department of microbiology in order to select the best therapeutic choice. Thus, an immediate clinico-microbiologic correlation secured by mutual cooperation is the prerequisite for successful management of infectious eye diseases.

Immediate therapy of bacterial infections relies primarily on the evaluation of antibiotic susceptibility data of these patients. Thus, antibiotic suscepti-bility testing will not only be valuable for the patient in quest, but primarily for future considerations in similar disease entities as well as epidemiologic monitoring. The monitoring of asymptomatic eyes should be restricted to cultures and antibiotic susceptibility testing for traditionally pathogenic agents.

There is no doubt as to the rationale of an infectious disease unit inside a surgically active eye department, which can interpret microbiological results and represent the missing link between microbiological data and clinical features and the application and monitoring of treatment.

Classic criteria for treatment with antibiotics apply to ophthalmic antibiotics as well. These should include

– spectrum and susceptibility,
– kinetics and bioavailability,
– stability and decay/turn-over-rate,
– toxicity and
– tissue contact time.

Indications for the Use of Antibiotics in Ophthalmology

General Considerations

The bulk of *topical or local antibiotics* prescribed in Ophthalmology comprises the prevention of severe infections. This includes primarily prophylactic antibiotics applied before an elective intraocular intervention as well as perioperatively, and the prevention of bacterial keratitis after the superficial impact on the cornea of a contaminated foreign body.

The sole use of topical antibiotics in the treatment of *blepharitis* has not been proven nor has the use of topical antibiotics for infections of the ocular adnexae or *canaliculitis*. Practically, the cure of blepharitis and canaliculitis relies on additional measures such as lid hygiene, routinely squeezing Meibomian glands or dermatologic medications (blepharitis) and surgical excision of dacryoliths (canaliculitis).

Although topical antibiotics may be helpful as an adjunct in the treatment of *conjunctivitis,* their primary role is restricted to the prevention of keratitis in this disease category. Work by Leibowitz and others has not been able to demonstrate a significant reduction of morbidity when antibiotics were used for the treatment of conjunctivitis (Leibowitz et al., 1976).

The use of topical antibiotics remains most beneficial and most reasonable theoretically as well as practically for the treatment of bacterial *keratitis*. The outstanding role of appropriate formulae of topical antibiotics for bacterial keratitis relies on their sufficient penetration into the epithelial layer and enrichment in the corneal stroma with the stroma serving as a slow-release drug depot. Most substances cannot penetrate significantly further into the anterior chamber. If, however, the blood-aqueous barrier is compromised notably (accompanied by inflammatory cells in the anterior chamber or a hypopyon), the use of topical antibiotics is only adjunctive with respect to the application of subconjunctival and systemic antibiotics (see later).

Subconjunctival antibiotics have been used routinely to lessen the risk of postoperative endophthalmitis and systemic antibiotics have been applied prophylactically during the *perioperative period* in high-risk patients with intraocular elective surgery. This approach has been recommended for patients suffering from diabetes mellitus and immunocompromising diseases (malignancies, immunodeficiencies, medical immunosuppression).

Otherwise, medication with systemic antibiotics seems only indicated for *intraocular infections* that suffer from compromised blood-retinal and blood-aqueous barriers (Bardenoch et al., 1986; Kanski et al., 1982). The rationale to use systemic antibiotics in such compromised eyes relies on data showing that systemically administered antibiotics may result in very high drug levels intraocularly thereby rendering this mode of therapy effective (Kanski et al., 1982; Axelrod et al., 1987). Treatment indications for systemic antibiotics include perforating injuries, since every foreign body must be suspected contaminated necessitating broad-spectrum antibiotic immediate therapy.

The use of systemic antibiotics like tetracylines may be necessary for *selected external eye diseases* (blepharitis), since their lipophilic features may enhance therapeutic effects inside glandular tissues like Meibomian glands. Some workers believe in the stimulation of interleukin 2 secretion by specific tetracyclines (minocycline) adding to the antiinfective (MIC-dependent) effects.

Choice of Topical Antibiotics - Pros and Cons

Five criteria must be fulfilled to render any given antibiotic solution useful for topical ophthalmic application: tonicity (225-482 mOsm/kg), pH (3.5-10.5), maintenance of stability during treatment. viscosity and sterility (Riegelman et al., 1958).

Therefore, the use of topical antibiotics for external eye diseases has up to now been limited to

bacteriostatic medications like
– Sulfanilamides,
– Cloramphenicol,
– Erythromycin,
– Tetracylines and
bactericidal drugs like
– Bacitracin,
– Polymyxins B and E,
– Neomycin,
– Kanamycin,
– Vancomycin,
– Gentamycin and
– Tobramycin.

Additional antibiotics like the New Quinolones (Ciprofloxacin, Norfloxacin, Ofloxacin) and Carbapenems (Imipenem) have been developed for topical and local use and will be commercially available soon.

Cephalosporins like Cefazolin have been prepared in "fortified" aqueous solutions and are widely used in the USA. Trimethoprim has also been considered a valuable topical antibiotic in the USA (Lambertz et al., 1984).

Infectiological common sense demands that topical antibiotics should be selected having in mind their potential use in systemic disease. This means to prefer topical treatment with drugs that will never be applied systemically for life-threatening infections (Sack, 1979). With respect to the primary goal of preventing serious corneal complications in external bacterial eye disease, foremost the prevention of Pseudomonas keratitis, and the availability of few antibiotic combination ointments including such substances as *Gramicidin,*

Polymixin B or *Polymixin E* (=Colistin), this theroretical consideration is not very helpful for everyday routine and must be individualised for each case.

Topical (as well as systemic) *Sulfanilamides* bear the specifically ocular complication of calcific band-shaped keratopathy (sulfamethoxazole) (Stern et al., 1989) and potentially fatal side-effects of Stevens-Johnson syndrome (sulfacetamide) (Genvert et al., 1985) besides their very limited effectiveness against common bacterial pathogens including Pseudomonas. Only sulfacetamide has been approved as a third-line topical antibiotic for the treatment of chlamydial infections (in Third-World countries) when other antibiotics are not available.

Tetracyclines may not be helpful any more in the prevention or treatment of external eye infections except for endemic trachoma. Effectiveness against most gram-positive and gram-negative bacteria is limited. Evolvement of R-plasmids in Neisseria gonorrhoeae for tetracyclines has made this ointment a contraindication for the general routine substitute of Credé's prophylaxis (Jahn et al., 1982).

Chloramphenicol should not be prescribed as a first-line topical antibiotic, since doubts of sensitisation or immediate-type allergic agranulocytosis have not been eliminated and better antibiotics with activity against Pseudomonas are on the market. Topical Chloramphenicol may have fatal consequences when given to neonates (Abrams et al., 1986; Stern et al., 1989). The defenders of Chloramphenicol (Besamuca et al., 1986) like the substance, because it is well tolerated, tissue penetration is good and its epithelial toxicity is low, although some delay in corneal wound healing has been reported. Chloramphenicol accumulates in macrophages and may be successfully used in cases of porin-associated bacterial resistance, particularly due to New Quinolones.

Erythromycin has a limited spectrum of activity in general, but its effectiveness on gram-positive bacteria may be considerable. In a study of 163 corneal ulcers, overall antibiotic susceptibility was greater than 80 % ranging second only to Ciprofloxacin. However, a one step-mutation ("Streptomycin-type") mode of resistance has been confirmed for Erythromycin in staphylococcal infections, which limits its use for prolonged therapy.

Bacitracin and *Gantrisin* are antibiotics often included in combined preparations for coverage of gram positive organisms. They should never be used as a sole medication, since both substances are not effective against Pseudomonas aeruginosa. In preparations with Gantrisin, Polymyxin B or Polymyxin E (=Colistin) is added for coverage of P.aeruginosa. In preparations with Bacitracin, Polymyxins are added to cover Hemophilus, P.aeruginosa, Acinetobacter, and Enterobacter; Proteus and Serratia are not included in the antibacterial spectrum of such a combination.

Neomycin bears the risk of about 14 % sensitisation (42). Therefore, besides its inefficacy against Streptococci, Pneumococci, Hemophilus and Pseudomonas, "red" eyes that have been cured from bacterial infections may become even "redder" after treatment and clinical distinction between a persisting or worsening infection and cure is often not possible. Neomycin is an unsafe substance for the prevention of gonococcal neonatal blennorrhea and no valid substitute for Credé's prophylaxis. However, its activity against Staphylococci, Proteus and other gram negative organisms has made it a popular ointment, particulary in preparations with steroids (!).

Kanamycin exerts activity against many staphylococcal isolates from conjunctivitis patients as well as most commonly found gram negative agents. However, the lack of activity against Pseudomonas is unfavorable for its use in bacterial (kerato) conjunctivitis and a one–step mutation mode of resistance limits its use for prolonged therapy. Kanamycin has also been reported a useful topical drug for gonococcal neonatal, mycobacterial and acanthamebic keratitis.

Vancomycin is an extremely valuable glycopeptide antibiotic for multi-resistant staphylococci, which play a significant role in some patients suffering from blepharoconjunctivitis (Fleischer et al., 1986). Although there have been reports of Vancomycin resistant Staphylococci, susceptibility is still better than 90 % (Schwalbe et al., 1987). Vancomycin has been limited in its topical use because of irritation due to low osmolality and pH. Made-up solutions in phosphate-buffered saline, however, have shown this topical antibiotic to be a useful second choice for Methicillin-resistant staphylococci (Smith et al., 1986).

The best choice of traditional topical antibiotics to prevent Pseudomonas keratitis remains to be *Tobramycin,* since *Gentamicin* is said to be a little less active against Pseudomonas (Wilhelmus et al., 1987; Wilson et al., 1982). (When Gentamycin and Tobramycin resistant organisms occur, Amikacin may sometimes be superior to these substances. Amikacin has only been used systemically and shows strong binding to pigmented tissue, and free substrate is only available after multiple applications.) Gentamycin and Tobramycin are not effective against streptococci and pneumococci at all, and S. aureus and coagulase negative Staphylococci may be resistant in up to 15-25 %. Gentamycin and Tobramycin have a multistep mode of resistance, which is favorable for a prolonged therapy. Marginal punctate keratitis and delayed healing rates have been reported for Gentamycin (Alfonso et al., 1988) and Tobramycin (Wilhelmus et al., 1987). Gentamycin has been shown to inactivate Lysozyme, a fact, which is of no practical importance.

The new Quinolones, *Ofloxacin, Norfloxacin* and *Ciprofloxacin* have been tested against pathogens of external ocular infections (Jacobson et al., 1988). From in vitro data, their activity vs. Pseudomonas aeruginosa is better compared to traditional aminoglycosides (Chi et al., 1984); O'Brien et al., 1988). Topical Ciprofloxacin may be best to cover the whole spectrum of pathogenic isolates of external ocular infections from the standpoint of in vitro susceptibility testing, however, double-masked clinical evaluations have to further substantiate its role for severe external infections. Considering the emergence of Propionibacterium acnes postoperative endophthalmitis, the New Quinolones may not be a useful tool for preoperative conjunctival antisepsis as they lack activity against anaerobes. Mycobacterial infections may be susceptible to the New Quinolones, although ophthalmic use has not yet been reported (Gay et al., 1984). – Another problem concerning the use of all of the new Quinolones for ocular infections is threefold in that they

– are not effective against P.maltophila causing selection of this organism,
– are not effective for infections with streptococci or pneumococci, which may occur frequently in ocular infections and
– may induce porin-associated resistance that can often only be overcome by smaller molecular agents like Chloramphenicol (which is hazardous in itself (see Chloramphenicol) (Kotilainen et al., 1990).

The newer β-Lactam antibiotics like *Imipenem* may prove even better than Ciprofloxacin for broad-spectrum coverage of Gram positive and Gram negative organisms (Kropp et al., 1985). P.aeruginosa has been reported up to 8 times more susceptible to Imipenem than to Tobramycin and experimental models of endophthalmitis have proven this finding in vivo (Sawusch et al., 1988). Imipenem effectiveness is not compromised in the gram positive spectrum and may therefore be a good antibiotic for ophthalmic use, however, clinical trials have to further establish its role in this regard.

Choice of Local Antibiotics

Local applications (subconjunctival, sub-Tenon's and intraocular/intravitreal) have been advocated for any setting requiring high amounts of antibiotics in the anterior segment of the eye (Baum et al., 1983).

Subconjunctival/Sub-Tenon's. Most data concerning intraocular concentrations of subconjunctivally given antibiotics, have been reported from uninflamed eyes with an intact blood-aqueous humor barrier and intact posterior capsule. These data indicate sufficient (above MIC amounts of most antibiotics up to 2-5 hours after injection in the anterior chamber (Axelrod et al., 1980; Baum et al., 1983; Rubinstein et al., 1985; Utermann et al., 1977) and in the vitreous if the posterior capsule is nonexistent (Duncker et al., 1988). Some substances can also be determined at above-MIC levels in serum. However, these data seem controversial with respect to a study of Driebe and coworkers stating a high incidence of postoperative bacterial infections in patients harboring Gentamycin-sensitive organisms who had been given subconjunctival Gentamycin at the end of surgery (Driebe et al., 1986). Neuromuscular blockade including mydriasis and conjunctival paresthesia has been reported after subconjunctival injection of 20 mg/ml Gentamycin (Awan 1985) and may theoretically occur with any aminoglycoside, although this is a rare event.

Nowadays, most antibiotics given subconjunctivally are applied at the end of intraocular surgery in order to prevent postoperative endophthalmitis. Agents inculde broad-spectrum Aminoglycosides (*Gentamycin* and *Tobramycin*) or Cephalosporins (e.g. *Cefazolin, Cefmenoxim*). Other antibiotics tested for intraocular penetration after subconjunctival application in man are Azlocillin (Behrens-Baumann et al., 1983), Mezlocillin (Behrens-Baumann et al., 1985) and Cefsulodin (Rubinstein et al., 1985).

Second in frequency comes the use of antibiotics for the treatment of keratitis/corneal ulcers. This mode of application is advantageous in that it may allow the use of otherwise extremely toxic substances like *Vancomycin*.

Intravitreal. Intraocular application of antibiotics has been suggested in the nineteen-seventies and has since then become the preferred route for the management of bacterial endophthalmitis (Baum et al., 1982). Reports on the toxicity of certain agents (e.g. Gentamycin, Tobramycin) may partly be ascribed to phenolic preservatives, partly to the substances themselves and will be further disussed in the chapter on endophthalmitis by Heidenkummer and Kampik.

Preferred antibiotics instilled intraocularly are *Gentamycin, Netilmicin, Tobramycin, Amikacin, Vancomycin* (D'Amico et al., 1985; Smith et al., 1986); Amikacin is known to exert the least retinal toxicity compared to the other aminoglycosides mentioned. Recommended drug concentrations vary for each substance, and the author of this article wishes not to take any responsibility for the validity of data (recommended concentrations from the literature are: Gentamycin: 0.1-1.0 mg, Tobramycin 0.2 mg, Amikacin 0.4 mg, Vancomycin 0.1-1.0 mg).

Choice of Systemic Antibiotics

When the application of systemic antibiotics is considered, pharmacokinetics and -dynamics may limit the potential benefits expected from in vitro antibacterial activity (MIC) data (Baum et al., 1983). Most data reported from intraocular concentrations of systemic antibiotics have been recruited from uninflamed eyes with intact blood-ocular barriers. Only few experimental and patient observations have been reported up to now indicating that triple (Kanski et al., 1982) and higher (up to six times (Axelrod et al., 1987)) the serum concentration may be found intraocularly in case of inflamed compared to uninflamed human eyes. Therefore, studies measuring levels of systemic antibiotics in the uninflamed human eye are essentially of no practical value but may only give a hint at the ease of penetration.

Intravenous Antibiotics. Nowadays, the most widely applied standard combination of intravenous antibiotics with acceptable pharmakokinetic data even in the uninflamed eye consists of aminoglycosides (Amikacin, Tobramycin) in combination with the newer second or third generation Cephalosporins (Cefazolin (Axelrod et al., 1985), Cefotaim or Cefotaxim etc.). Most organisms responsible for infectious endophthalmitis may be covered by these agents, including anaerobes (e.g. P.acnes). This combination, however, bears the risk of a selection of enterococci, since neither

Cephalosporins nor Aminoglycosides are effective against enterococci. Enterococcal ocular infections infrequent, but in tertiary referral centers treating non-ophthalmic patient populations, hospitalised patients in Ophthalmology departments may acquire these organisms. In future, combination strategies including Carbapenems and New Quinolones may evolve as a superior choice, if the pharmacokinetic data and in vivo tests will support these findings.

Oral Antibiotics. Great caution with respect to uptake and intraocular penetration must be taken when oral antibiotics are prescribed.

Pharmakokinetic data of most oral *Cephalosporins* are unreliable, however, as newer oral Cephalosporins become available soon, they may be prescribed on an out-patient basis for selected intraocular bacterial infections. In my experience, selected patients with a "toxic lens" syndrome caused by slowly replicating bacteria may be treated successfully with oral Cephalosporins currently available.

Most oral antibiotics are indicated for multi-site mucosal infections (chlamydial, gonococal etc.). The classical choice for the management of these infections has included *Tetracyclines* and *Erythromycin,* however, *Ciprofloxacin* and other *New Quinolones* have been reported effective as well.

Oral *Tetracyclines* may be used for the successful adjunctive treatment of meibomianitis with or without rosacea on a long-term basis.

Indications for the Use of Antibiotics in Ophthalmology Specific Considerations

Antibiotics for External Eye Infections

Conjunctiva – Interpretation of Conjunctival Smears. The significance of conjunctival smears of asymptomatic and symptomatic patients should be clarified before the role of antibiotics in external eye diseases may be dicussed.

Conjunctival tissue is, of course, very exposed towards external inoculation. In contrast to the intraocular germ-free situation in asymptomatic healthy persons, 15-20 % of asymptomatic conjunctivae grow aerobic bacteria in a 24 hour culture. It is known that after 48 hours of incubation, approximately 40 % of probes and after 72 hours, 60 % or more cultures grow organisms from the normal asymptomatic "healthy" conjunctiva.

Thus, etiologic therapy of conjunctivitis is hampered by the daily change of the "naturally" occurring flora and mainly consists in the prevention of corneal complications, primarily Pseudomonas infections.

Spectrum of Isolated Organisms. In the USA, aerobic isolates feature coagulase negative Staphylococci (CNS), S. aureus, Proteus, Diphtheroids and gram negative organisms in dcesending order. In Germany, CNS are followed by Diphtheroids, Staph aureus, streptococci, Hemophilus and gram negative organisms (Perkins et al., 1975). The spectrum of isolated bacteria varies with respect to geography (tropical/northern climates, rural/urban neighborhood), social environment and the age of the population studied. Anaerobic bacteria have been reported in up to 50 % of asymptomatic conjunctivae in longterm cultures (7-40 days) with Propionibacterium acnes dominating in 80 % followed by Peptostreptococci (5 %), Proionibeaacterium granulosum (1 %), Propionibacterium avium (1 %) and some Lactobacilli, Veilonella and Fusobacteria.

Transient and Resident Flora. Considering the results of a multicenter study conducted in Germany involving the evaluation of conjunctival smears of more than 300 hospitalised asymptomatic patients, and results from the other workers, a newly acquired flora in previously culture-negative patients can be found in 5-15 % after a 24 hour incubation time. The newly acquired flora in culture-postive patients can be estimated at 10-20 % after a 24 hour incubation time. These data, however, must be interpreted with respect to a "normal" not overly pathogenic environment of the Western Hemisphere. Rates may differ according to increased pathogen loads (cf. monsoon in tropical countries) (Bialasiewicz et al., 1990).

Transient and Resident Flora under Topical Aminoglycosides. Interestingly, evaluation of cultures after the application of Tobramycin (3.Omg/ml five times daily) has resulted in a newly acquired flora in previously culture-negative patients of 5.2 % and 11 % of previously culture-positive patients in a multi-center study conducted in Germany recently. Whereas gram negative bacteria could be eliminated after one day of topical prophylaxis with Tobramycin in this study, coagulase-negative Tobramycin-sensitive Staphylococci persisted in 37 % of isolates and coagulase-positive Tobramycin-sensitive in 13 %. This must be compared to a persisting flora in untreated eyes of about 50% of smears. The elimination rate for Tobramycin in the aforementioned study was 84.4 % with a confidence interval of 77.5-89.8 %. Antibiotic susceptibility data revealed resistance patterns of 11 % for gram positive and 8.6 % of gram negative agents.- In 1972, elimination rates of the flora of the asymptomatic conjunctiva have been estimated at 41 % for Gentamycin vs. none for Chloramphenicol by Burns and Oden. The daily changes of bacterial flora casts a doubt on the interpretation of any single conjunctival swab result in patients suffering from conjunctivitis.

Spectrum of Organisms in Infectious Symptomatic Conjunctivitis. Bacteria isolated from infectious follicular conjunctivitis in adults of countries of the Western Hemisphere include Staph aureus (35-50 %), CNS (30-60 %), streptococci and pneumococci (5-15 %), Hemophilus (5-10 %) and gram negative rods (5-15 %) ‹C.trachomatis (5-8 %, fungi (5 % or less)› in 24 or 48 hour cultures. The main infectious agents in patients suffering from conjunctivitis of suspected bacterial etiology are gram positive organisms, particularly Staphylococci. Elimination rates with Chloramphenicol have been reported at 40 %, Gentamycin at 84 % and Tobramycin at 91 %.

Cornea – Spectrum of Keratitis Organisms. From the epidemiologist's point of view, virus infections represent the most frequent cause of keratitis (Adenovirus 92 %, Enterovirus 4 %, Herpes simplex Virus 4 %) and bacterial infections range second in developed countries.

While there is an appreciable amount of transient pathogenic organisms in conjunctivitis patients, resident bacteria dominate the spectrum of keratitis patients. Organisms most frequently encountered in bacterial keratitis of adult patients include Staphylococci (CNS 10-40 %, S. aureus 10-15 %) other gram positive agents (5-10 %), gram negatives (15-30 %, in some studies up to 44 %). In children, Pseudomonas has been reported by far the most frequently isolated agent. Mycobacterial, parasitic, fungal and other infectious lesions account for less than 1 % of infectious keratitis in adults and children of the industrialised countries.

Keratitic lesions present the primary indication for the use of topical antibiotics. If there are signs of a severe break-down of the blood-aqueous barrier (inflammatory cells in the anterior chamber) or of a hypopyon, the use of systemic antibiotics in combination with topical/local antibiotics is indicated.

Antibiotics for Intraocular Infections

Diagnosis. Intraocular infections may generally be subdivided into a group with or without loss of integrity of the globe. For the establishment of the diagnosis, aspiration of the vitreous seems rewarding in postoperative or posttraumatic endophthalmitis, whereas blood cultures remain the mainstay of bacterial "metastatic" endophthalmitits. Culturing and testing for antibiotic susceptibility will always take a least 2 days; thus, the probable spectrum of pathogens must be known when an immediate therapeutic regimen is installed.

Management/Special Antibiotics. Posttraumatic and postoperative endophthalmitis may require different therapeutic strategies than those intraocular infections, which result from intraocular hematogenous embolisation from distant sites. Starters for the management of posttraumatic endophthalmitis should include an agent against Bacillus, e.g. Clindamycin, whereas immediate therapy of postoperative endophthalmitis should include a potent anti-Staphylococcal regimen, e.g. Vancomycin (Davis et al., 1988). Metastatic bacterial endophthalmitis leaves us with Bacillus cereus as the most frequently encountered organism, which must be included in devising immediate therapy (e.g. Clindamycin).

Management Strategies for Endophthalmitis. Indications for the therapy of intraocular infections in the surgically or traumatically opened eye must include systemic and local/topical or intravitreal antibiotics and vitrectomy as an adjunct therapy. Vitrectomy has not been proven effective for metastatic infectious eye disease and antibiotics are the mainstay of therapy.

Management of Systemic Bacterial Disease and Ocular Involvement. Intraocular inflammation may also occur as a predominant or even sole feature of *systemic disease*. Particularly in spirochetal infections (Syphilis, Bejel, Leptospirosis, and Borreliosis), clinical features and history should call attention to detailed serology and extensive discussion with a microbiologist in case of negative laboratory results and a positive clinical history. Monitoring of clinical features through the "ocular window" is a helpful adjunctive tool for the successful management of disseminated infections using an effective treatment with systemic antibiotics. Recently, preferred treatment for spirochetal infections has evolved to be Ceftriaxon.

Intraocular inflammations may also be part of aberrant immune responses following genital or gastrointestinal infections with gram negative organisms, chlamydiae or mycoplasmas/ureaplasmas in HLA B27 positive patients. Ocular manifestations of this so-called "Reiter's" syndrome may be linked to persistence of pathogenic agents. Isolation of etiologically conclusive organisms is difficult, and serological tests (antibody titer dynamics) must be relied on. Under these circumstances, systemic antibiotic therapy (preferrably oral doxycycline) combined with topical ocular corticosteroids is warranted.

Controversial Modes of Action of Antibiotics in Ophthalmology

Topical Antibiotics – Arguments for Efficacy

Many different factors are known to influence the efficacy of topical antibiotics in external eye disease. Efficacy depends mainly on tissue contact time. Therefore, the application formula or the strength may be altered.

Application Formulae – Hypothesis. Most applications consist in *drops* or *ointment*, which must be in a partly lipophilic condition to pass through the epithelium and in a partly aqueous solution to get into the stroma (Shell 1982). Corneal epithelial permeability, however, is commonly compromised already due to local anesthetics (such as Oxybuprocaine or Tetracaine) or preservatives (Chlorhexidine, Benzalkonium Chloride) added to the antiinfective medication (Raselaar et al., 1988). It is commonly accepted that gels or ointment as well as inserts or soaked therapeutic contact lenses (Waltman et al., 1970) will maintain higher drug concentrations for an extended period of time than drops. It has been estimated that the physiological turn-over rate of tears and aqueous solutions is 16 %, whereas this rate for ointments in the cul de sac is 0.5 %. Controlled studies, however, have never been performed and are difficult to conceive. *Iontophoresis* (Rootman et al., 1988), *liposome-encapsulation* (Barza et al., 1984) and *ocular inserts* have been tried for increasing and maintaining the amount of effective substance in the cornea and the aqueous humor. These modes of application, however, have mostly been experimental.

Application Strength – MIC Hypothesis. Topically instilled antibiotics may achieve highly effective drug concentrations far *above the minimal inhibitory concentrations (MIC)* of the respective pathogen particularly in the cornea, which acts as a depot in that respect.

Sidikaro and Jones have found in 1981 that initial levels of 18 µg/ml after 15 minutes decreased to as low as 2.2 µg/ml after 60 minutes when a 0.3 % Gentamycin solution was used (Sidikaro et al., 1981). "Fortified" solutions have been recommended by several authors because of higher drug concentrations measured after routine hourly administrations with Tobramycin 14 mg/ml, Cefazolin 33-50 mg/ml, Erythromycin 10 mg/ml, Neomycin 33 mg/ml, Polymixin B 33 000 U/ml and Bacitracin 10 000 U/ml applied hourly, half-hourly or less. Thus, clinical rationale may be delineated as: the more a drug is concentrated and the higher the frequency of instillation, the higher will be effective concentrations and the greater will be a therapeutic success. However, data from experimental work do not lend evidence for increased effects of "fortified" solutions compared to commercially available formulae. Excessively high topical drug concentrations will result in potentially toxic serum concentrations particularly in children, increase cytopathic effects for the whole of the cornea and may also result in unforeseen cytotoxic effects at the site of a corneal ulcer resulting in increased morbidity. Therefore, work has been carried out to show that Gentamycin "loading doses" of drops applied every minute for 5 min. followed by hourly applications to maintain the drug concentration in the cornea may be superior to the fortified approach (Glasser et al., 1985).

From the studies mentioned, one may deduce that topical aminoglycosides for external infections without structural defects must be applied more than hourly in order to achieve above MIC concentrations, a fact, that has been advocated by most researchers and clinicians. When a corneal ulcer is present, however, frequency of applications should be individualised according to progress in infection management and the state of the cornea and other ways of drug application should be sought.

Adherence Hypothesis. Another mechanism considered for the effectiveness of topical antibiotics may be the *interference with bacterial adherence*. This idea, however, remains mostly speculative for routinely used antibiotics in Ophthalmology.

Flushing Hypthesis. A third mechanism has been proposed with the *flushing action* of applied solutions. Since flushing of the eye with physiologic NaCl in perioperative antisepsis studies has been demonstrated not to reduce the resident flora, this effect may be not be critical.

Topical Antibiotics – Cautionary Tale

Aqueous suspensions have been found to crystallise or precipitate when exceedingly strong "fortified" formulations are used. If shaking a vial for a considerable time is omitted, differences in drug concentrations of up to factor 20x can occur (Shell et al., 1982). Furthermore, "fortified" and other highly concentrated aqueous drug solutions have not been shown to increase cure. Possibly, ointments are superior to drops, since bioavailability is increased including higher effective concentrations, increased tissue contact time, inhibition of dilutions by tears and resistance to nasolacrimal drainage.

Ocular factors like blinking, rubbing, epithelial desquamation, compromised structural integrity of the globe, flushing action of the tears and modifications of the precorneal tear film as well as the localization of applications (nasally vs.laterally) and lacrimal drainage are decisive to reach adequate concentrations of medications at the sites of lesions and will render reproducible study results almost impossible. Particularly neonates and patients with predictably low compliance must be considered candidates for additional local systemic therapy and possibly inpatient therapy. In neonates, perilous overdosing of topical aminoglycosides or Chloramphenicol (which may be rapidly absorbed by mucosal sites nasally and through the laryngeal regions) should be considered (Stern 1989).

Concentrations achieved at the sites of infection are totally unpredictable.

Local Antibiotics (Subconjunctival Antibiotics) – Arguments for Efficacy

Subconjunctival antibiotics are the best way to achieve effective concentrations in the cornea, anterior segment and aqueous humor. Ten percent of subconjunctivally administered medication is lost to the tears, a minor part to reflux or systemic circulation, and the rest diffuses into ocular tissues. This has been shown experimentally as well as in man. A certain amount of drug reaches the cornea via the conjunctival vessels and epibulbar plexus, whereas the aqueous is reached by the anterior ciliary vessels. For these anatomic reasons, subconjunctival injections achieve higher intraocular drug levels than periocular/retrobulbar. Highest concentrations are found at the site of injection. The diffusion rate is not increased in inflamed eyes, which may be due to increased blood flow flooding the tissues and carrying the drug away simultaneously at an increased speed. The precorneal tear film is not significantly involved as a drug carrier (Baum 1983, Johnson et al., 1985).

Significant drug levels 10 times as high as in the aqueous humor of comparable individuals have been observed in the vitreous of patients with a compromised posterior lens capsule (Duncker et al., 1988).

Local Antibiotics (Subconjunctival Antibiotics) – Cautionary Tale

Most data for the efficacy of subconjunctival antibiotics have been accumulated from rat or rabbit models, fewer from guinea pig models and only rare data exist on human non-compromised eyes. Accepting a theory of diffusion of subconjunctival antibiotics, the rabbit may be the wrong model to study pharmakokinetics compared to man, since corneal permeability of the rabbit is known to be 10^{-3} cm/h (man 10^{-5} cm/h, rat 6.4×10^{-4} cm/h) and the elimination rate of Gentamicin from the aqueous humor is 10^{-2}/h (man 0.15/h, rat 0.67/h).- Additionally, it has been shown that subconjunctival antibiotics result in very different regional concentrations (Oakley et al., 1976).

Subconjunctival injection of agents in man has been shown to result in MIC-effective levels in the aqueous humor averaging 2 hours (5 hours at most with selected antibiotics). Studies for the determination of turn-over and clearance of intravitreal antibiotics in inflamed human eyes have not been performed sufficiently. From those data one might deduce that subconjunctival antibiotics be given every two hours, which is not practical and would probably not be tolerated by patients. Therefore, frequent topical treatment with "normal strength" – antibiotics and systemic antibiotics (see later) may be recommended to accompany subconjunctival injections for maintaining sufficient drug concentrations in the cornea and aqueous humor for external or anterior segment infections. In this context it must be considered that prophylactic antibiotics applied at the end of surgery will not be a guarantee against endophthalmitis. It has been shown that 90 % of organisms isolated from postoperative endophthalmitits were susceptible to the antibiotic given subconjunctivally at the end of pseudophakic cataract extraction.

A slight risk of perforation of the globe must be mentioned, which cannot occur with topical and systemic therapy.

Subconjunctival injections of antibiotics may also result in measurable serum concentrations and may therefore bear a substantial risk of sensitisation.

Local Antibiotics (Intravitreal Antibiotics) – Arguments for Efficay

The reason for an effectiveness of intravitreal antibiotics needs not to be discussed, since the direct application of antibiotics to the site of infection may always be considered the best way of treatment, if the infecting organism is susceptible to the antibiotic (Baumet et al., 1982; Baum 1983, Stern et al., 1989).

The effects are directly related to the MIC-values in vitro. Pharmakokinetics have shown very high starting levels and clearance rates of 48h and therapeutic levels still demonstrable after 6 days in experimental endophthalmitis models.

The same applies to vitrectomy infusion fluids used during surgery for endophthalmitis. Very high and constant levels of antibiotics may be maintained to literally "soak" the eye with antibiotic.

Local Antibiotics (Intravitreal Antibiotics) – Cautionary Tale

Recommendations concerning the dosages and the time periods regarding repeat (and, therefore, toxicity)of antibiotics in the infected human vitreous have mostly been derived from experimental models. Possible toxicity of drugs (and their phenolic preservatives)is still a reason for major concern (D'Amico et al 1985, McDonald et al 1986); even more so are highly concentrated antibiotics in infusion fluids, although some data have been recommended to stay below toxicity (Morgan et al 1979).

Systemic antibiotics (only safe with appropriate drug monitoring in case of aminoglycosides!)in combination with local/topical solutions can circumvent this peril.

Perspectives

The distinctive requirements for antibiotics in Ophthalmology and future avenues of research are twofold:

1) everyday prescription of mostly prophylactic antibiotics in the office or prophylactic antibiotics before elective intraocular surgery and
2) therapy of severe external or intraocular infections

Therefore, two ways of antibiotic development should be pursued: one way is to develop medications effective against Pseudomonas, which are least toxic and least sensitising, the other way should pursue research into the most effective broad-spectrum antibiotics. However unpractical this may seem, the clinicians's point of view for the prevention and treatment of infections in Ophthalmology must be born in mind.

References

Abrams SM, Degnan TJ, Vinciguerra V (1986) Marrow aplasia following topical application of chloramphenicol eye-drops. Arch Intern Med 140:576-577
Alfonso E, Kenyon KR, D'Amico DJ, Saulenas AM, Albert DM (1988) Effects of

gentamycin on healing of transdifferentiating conjunctival epithelium in rabbit eyes. Am J Ophthalmol 105:198-202

Awan KJ (1985) Mydriasis and conjunctival paresthesia from local gentamycin. Am J Ophthalmol 100:723-724

Axelrod JL, Kochman RS (1980), Cefoxitin levels in human aqueous humor. Am J Ophthalmol 90:388-341

Axelrod JL, Klein RM, Bergen RL, Sheikh MZ (1985) Human vitreous levels of selected antistaphylococcal antibiotics. Am J Ophthalmol 100:570-575

Axelrod JL, Newton JC, Klein RM, Bergen RL, Sheikh, MZ (1987) Penetration of imipenem into human aqueous and vitreous humor. Am J Ophthalmol 104:649-653

Badenoch PR, McDonald PJ, Coster DJ (1986) Effect of inflammation on antibiotics penetration into the anterior segment of the rat eye. Invest Ophthalmol Vis Sci 27:958-965

Barza M, Baum J, Szoka F (1984) Pharmakokinetics of subconjunctival liposome-encapsulated gentamycin in normal rabbit eyes. Invest Ophthalmol Vis Sci 25:486-489

Baum JL (1983) Antibiotic mechanisms in: The cornea-scientific foundations and clinical practice. Smolin G, Thoft RA (eds.) Little Brown & Co, Boston pp. 134-143

Baum JL, Peyman GA, Barza M (1982) Intravitreal Administration of antibiotics in the treatment of bacterial endophthalmitis III Consensus. Surv Ophthalmol 26:204-206

Behrens-Baumann W, Ansorg R (1983) Azlocillin concentrations in human aqueous humor after intravenous and subconjunctival administration. Graefes Arch Clin Exp Ophthalmol 220:292-293

Behrens-Baumann W, Ansorg R (1985) Mezlocillin concentrations in human aqueous humor after intravenous and subconjunctival administration. Chemother 31:169-172

Besamuca FW, Bastiaensen LA (1986) Blood dyscrasias and topically applied chloramphenicol in ophthalmology Doc Ophthalmol 64:87-95

Bialasiewicz AA, Welt R, Werry H (1990) Prophylactic topical antibiotics for elective intraocular surgery: results of an open multicenter study with tobramycin. Zbl Bakteriol II 273:72-73

Chi NX, Neu HC (1984) Ciprofloxacin, a quinolone carboxylic acid compound active against aerobic and anaerobic bacteria. Antimicrob Ag Chemother 25:319-326

Davis JL, Koidou-Tsiligianni A, Pflugfelder CS, Miller D, Flynn HW, Forster RK (1988) Coagulase negative staphylococcal endophthalmitis. Ophthalmology 95:1404-1410

Driebe WT, Mandelbaum S, Forster RK, Schwartz LK, Culbertson WW (1986) Pseudophakic endophthalmitis: diagnosis and management. Ophthalmology 93:442-448

Duncker G, Eckardt C, Ullmann U (1988) Cefmenoxin-Penetration in den Glaskörpern des menschlichen Auges nach subkonjunktivalter Injektion. Fort Ophthalmol 85:210-212

D'Amico DJ, Kenyon KR, Albert DM et al., (1985) Comparative toxicity of intravitreal aminoglycoside antibiotics. Am J Ophthalmol 100:264-275

Fleischer AB, Hoover DL, Khan JA, Parisi JT, Burns RP (1986) Topical vancomycin formulation for methicillin-resistant staphylococcus epidermidis blepharoconjunctivitis. Am J Ophthalmol 101:283-287

Gay JD, DeYoung DR, Roberts GD (1984) In vitro activities of norfloxacin and ciprofloxacin against M.tuberculoisis, M.avium complex, M.chelonei, M.fortuitum and M.kansasii. Antimicrob Ag Chemother 26:94-96

Genvert GI, Cohen EJ, Donnenfeld ED, Blecher MH (1985) Erythema multiforme after use of topical sufacetamide. Am J Ophthalmol 99:465-468

Glasser DA, Gardner S, Ellis JG, Pettit TH (1985) Loading doses and extended dosing intervals in topical gentamycin therapy. Am J Ophthalmol 99:329-332

Jacobson JA, Call NB, Kasworm AM, Dirks MS, Turner RB (1988) Safety aand efficacy of topical norfloxacin versus tobramycin in the treatment of external ocular infections. Antimicrob Ag Chemother 32:1820-1824

Jahn GJ, Bialasiewicz AA, Blenk H (1985) Evaluation of plasmids in tetracycline resistant strains of N.gonorrhoeae and U.urealyticum in a case of severe urethritis. Eur J Epidemiol 1:294-300

Johnson AP, Scoper SV, Woo FL, Caldwell DR, George WJ (1985) Azlocillin levels in human tears and aqueous. Am J Ophthalmol 99:469-472

Kanski JJ, Young JH, Vogel R (1982) Penetration of intravenously administered cefoxitin into the aqueous humor of inflamed human eyes. Am J Ophthalmol 94:516-519

Kotilainen P, Nikoselainen J, Huovinen P (1990) Emergence of ciprofloxacin-resistant coagulase-negative staphylococcal skin flora in immunocompromised patients receiving ciprofloxacin. J Inf Dis 161:41-44

Kropp H, Gerckens L, Sundelof JG, Kahan FM (1985) Antibacterial activity of imipenem. The first thienamycin antibiotic. Rev Infect Dis 75:389-397

Lamberts Dl, Buka T, Knowlton GM (1984) Clinical evaluation of trimethoprim-containing ophthalmic solutions in humans. Am J Ophthalmol 98:11-16

Leibowitz HM, Pratt MV, Flagstad IF (1976) Human conjunctivitis: treatment. Arch Ophthalmol 94:1752-1756

McDonald HR, Schatz H, Allen AW et al., (1986) Retinal toxicity secondary to intraocular gentamicin injection. Ophthalmolgy 93:871-877

Morgan BS, Larson B, Peyman GA, West CS (1979) Toxicity and antibiotic combinations for vitrectomy infusion fluid. Ophthalmic Surg 10(10):74-77

Oakley DE, Weeks RD, Ellis PP (1976) Corneal distribution of subconjunctival antibiotics. Am J Ophthalmol 81:307-311

O'Brien TP, Sawusch MR, Dick JD, Gottsch JD (1988) Topical ciprofloxacin treatment of pseudomonas keratitis in rabbits. Arch Ophthalmol 106:1444-1446

Perkins RE, Kundsin RB, Pratt MV (1975) Bacteriology of normal and infected conjunctiva. J Clin Microbiol 1:147-152

Ramselaar JAM, Boot JP, von Haeringen NJ, van Best JA, Oosterhuis JA (1988) Corneal epithelial permeability after instillation of ophthalmic solutions containing local anesthetics and preservatives. Curr Eye Res 7:947-950

Riegelmann S, Vaughan DG (1958) A rational basis for the preparation or ophthalmic solutions. Surv Ophthalmol 3:471-478

Rootman DS, Jantzen JA, Gonzales JR, Fischer MJ, Beuermann R, Hill JM (1988) Pharmakokinetics and safety of transcorneal iontophoresis of tobramycin in the rabbit. Invest Ophthalmol Vis Sci 29:1397-1401

Rubinstein E, Avni I, Tuizer H, Treister G, Blumenthal M, Cefuslodin levels in the human aqueous humor. Arch Ophthalmol 103:426-427

Sack RB (1979) Prophylactic antibiotics? the individual vs. the community. N Engl J Med 300:1107-1108

Sawusch MR, O'Brien TP, Valentine J, Dick JD, Gottsch JD (1988) Topical imipenem therapy of aminoglycoside-resistant pseudomonas kreatitis in rabbits. Am J Ophthalmol 106:77-81

Schwalbe RS, Stapleton JT, Gilligan PH (1987) Emergence of vancomycin resistance in CNS. New Engl J Med 316:927-931

Shell JW (1982) Pharmakokinetics of topically applied ophthalmic drugs. Surv Ophthalmol 26:207-218

Sidikaro J, Jones DB (1981) Concentration of gentamycin in Preocular tear flow following topical application. Invest Ophthalmol Vis Sci 20(S):109

Smith MA, Sorenson JA, Lowy FD, Shakin JL, Harrison W, Jakobiec FA (1986) Treatment of experimental methicillin-resistant staphylococcus epidermidis endophthalmitis with intravitreal vancomycin. Ophthalmology 93:1328-1335

Stern GA, Killingsworth DW (1989) Complications of topical antimicrobial agents. Int Ophthalomol Clin 29:137-142

Stern GA, Engel HM, Driebe WT (1989) The treatment of postoperative endophthalmitis. Ophthalmology 96:62-67

Utermann D, Math K, Meyer K (1977) Gentamycinspiegel im Kammerwasser des Menschen nach parenteraler, subkonjunktivaler und lokaler Applikation. Klin Mbl Augenhlk 171:579-583

Waltman SR, Kaufman HE (1970) Use of hydrophilic contact lenses to increase ocular penetration of topical drugs. Invest Ophthalmol Vis Sci 9:250-253

Wilhelmus KR, Gilbert ML, Osato MS (1987) Tobramycin. Surv Ophthalmol 32:111-123

Wilson LA, Weinstein AJ, Wood TO et al., (1982) Treatment of external eye infections: a double-masked trial of tobramycin and gentamycin. J Ocular Ther Surg I:364-367

Corresponding Address

Priv.-Doz. Dr. med. A. A. Bialasiewicz

Universitätsaugenklinik Münster, Domagkstraße 15, D-4400 Münster

Sachverzeichnis

Glaukom ohne Hochdruck   29, 52, 65,
  158, 163
- Pathogenese   62
glaukomspezifisches Prüfpunktraster
  160, 171
Glaukomtherapie   12, 19, 72, 80, 92,
  100, 111, 112, 121, 125, 134
Gliazellen   244
Gramfärbung   226
Gramicidin   269
Guanethidin   136, 150

halbsynthetische Zellulosederivate   205
hämatogene Endophthalmitis   221
Heidelberger Retina Tomograph
  (HRT)   30
Heparin   249
Herpes simplex type 1 and 2   232
Herpes-Virus   255
Herpes Zoster   232
high-tension glaucoma   8
histopathological studies, low-tension
  glaucoma   12
HIV-Infektion   256
Hornhautepithel   223
Hornhautpenetration   147
Hornhautstroma   223
5-HT-1A
- agonist   130, 131
- antagonist   131
- receptor   130
5-HT-1C receptor   128
5-HT-receptors   131
Humphrey Perimeter   178, 180
Hyaluronsäure   205, 206
Hypotonie   64

IC_{50} 127
ICI   118.551 130
Indomethazin   97
infectious retinitis   231
Infektionsprophylaxe   253
Infektionsprophylaxe in der Praxis/Am-
  bulanz   260
Inserte   205
intraocular infections   276
- diagnosis   276
- management   276
intraocular microendoscopy   100
intraocular Pressure (IOP)   72, 111
- asymmetry   24
- lowering beta-blockers   132
- normative   8
- treatment   19
intraokuläre Halbwertszeit   225
intravenous antibiotics   273

intravitreal   273
intravitreal ganciclovir   234
intravitreal injection   234
intravitreale Medikamentenapplikation
  227
intravitrealer Wirkspiegel   224
IOP (see intraocular pressure)
ipsapirone   130
isoprenaline   126
Isopto-Pilomin   138

Kammerwasser   92
Kammerwasserproduktion, Verminde-
  rung   140, 143
Kammerwassersekretion   95
Kanamycin   271
K_d 126, 127
Keratoconjunctivitis epidemica   255
keratoconjunctivitis sicca   187, 192, 194
K_i 127, 128, 129
Kölner Schema   250
Kombination   250
Kombinationspräparate   134, 137
Kombinationstherapie   121
konfokale Blende   34
konfokales Untersuchungsprinzip   29
Konservierungsmittel   152, 153, 154
- in Augenmedikamenten   200
- in der Glaukomtherapie   152
Kontaktlinsen   207
kontrolliertes Blinken   201
Kosmetika   200

lactoferrin tear fluid concentration   190
Lage   159
Laser Tomographic Scanner (LTS)   29,
  30, 34
lasers   111
Levobunolol   148
Lidschlag, unvollständig/selten   201
liposome   231, 238, 240
Liposome   249
Littmann-Formel   38
local antibiotics   272, 279, 280
low-tension glaucoma (LTG)   3, 12, 19
- asymmetry in IOP   19
- asymmetry in outflow facility   19
- asymmetry in visual field loss   19
- diurnal tension variation   19
- epidemiology   3
- intraocular pressure treatment   3, 12,
  19, 80, 92, 100, 111, 116, 121, 125,
  134
- IOP-related damaging factors   19
- pathogenesis   19
- systemic risk factors   19